SELF-CARE
NURSING

Promotion of Health

second edition

Lyda Hill, RN, CS, PhD
Associate Professor
Department of Nursing
California State University—Long Beach
Long Beach, California

Nancy Smith, MS, RNC
Adult Nurse Practitioner/Senior Instructor
Primary Health Care of Adults
School of Nursing
University of Colorado Health Sciences Center
Denver, Colorado

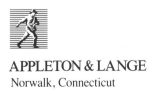

APPLETON & LANGE
Norwalk, Connecticut

0-8385-8528-0

Notice: Our knowledge in clinical sciences is constantly changing. As new
information becomes available, changes in treatment and in the use of drugs
become necessary. The authors and the publisher of this volume have taken
care to make certain that the doses of drugs and schedules of treatment are
correct and compatible with the standards generally accepted at the time of
publication. The reader is advised to consult carefully the instruction
and information material included in the package insert of each drug or
therapeutic agent before administration. This advice is especially
important when using new or infrequently used drugs.

Prentice Hall International (UK) Limited, *London*
Prentice Hall of Australia Pty. Limited, *Sydney*
Prentice Hall Canada, Inc., *Toronto*
Prentice Hall Hispanoamericana, S.A., *Mexico*
Prentice Hall of India Private Limited, *New Delhi*
Prentice Hall of Japan, Inc., *Tokyo*
Simon & Schuster Asia Pte. Ltd., *Singapore*
Editora Prentice Hall do Brasil Ltda., *Rio de Janeiro*
Prentice Hall, *Englewood Cliffs, New Jersey*

Library of Congress Cataloging-in-Publication Data
Hill, Lyda, 1947-
    Self-care nursing : promotion of health / Lyda Hill, Nancy Smith :
foreword by Jean Watson.—2nd ed.
        p. cm.
    Includes bibliographical references.
    ISBN 0-8385-8528-0
    1. Patient education—Study and teaching. 2. Self-care, Health—
Study and teaching. 3. Nurse and patient. 4. Health education.
I. Smith, Nancy, 1947- . II. Title.
    [DNLM: 1. Health Promotion/nurses' instruction. 2. Self
Care/nurses' instruction.   WA 590 H646s]
    RT90.H55   1989
    613'.07—dc20
    DNLM/DLC
    for Library of Congress   89-17925
                                                                             CIP

Acquisitions Editor: Marion K. Welch
Production Editor: Susan Meiman
Designer: Steven Byrum

PRINTED IN THE UNITED STATES OF AMERICA

To my Grandmother, Lyda Murray Ryan;
now in her 93rd year of self-care.

LH

To Jim Smith, our #1 model of self-care;
with appreciation for all he has taught
us by living his beliefs.

NS

Contributors

Susan C. Baldi, RN, MS
Assistant Dean of Instruction
Santa Rosa Junior College
Santa Rosa, California

Beverly Bauer Hatch, RNC, MS
Certified Psychiatric and Mental Health Nurse
Saint Joseph's Hospital
Orange, California

Lyda Hill, RN, CS, PhD
Associate Professor
Department of Nursing
California State University—Long Beach
Long Beach, California

Mary Paquette, RN, MN
Nurse Psychotherapist in Private Practice
Van Nuys, California

Sylvia A. Puglisi, RN, MS
Nurse Psychotherapist in Private Practice
Desanzano, Italy

Brenda Smith, RNC, MSN
OB/GYN Nurse Practitioner
Private Practice
Educational Consultant
Long Beach, California

Nancy Smith, MS, RNC
Adult Nurse Practitioner/Senior Instructor
Primary Health Care of Adults
School of Nursing
University of Colorado Health Science Center
Denver, Colorado

Gale J. Taucher, RN, CS, PhD
Clinical Psychologist
Director of Psychiatric Assessment Team
Santa Ana Psychiatric Hospital
Santa Ana, California

Patricia A. Ticken, RN, MSN
Lecturer
University of California, Los Angeles
Los Angeles, California

Carol G. Wells, RN, MS, CST
Director of Psychological Services
Center of Allied Sexual Treatment
Los Alamitos, California

Contents

Foreword

The fate and the future of nursing, and indeed, the entire health care system are now more than ever dependent upon self-care, health promotion, and self-generated coping and healing modalities. While the traditional system is still perpetuating technocure and high cost medical care, the minds and actions of an increasingly well-informed, health-oriented, cost-conscious society are no longer patient with such a one-sided system of care.

American society is no longer willing to accept the rising costs, decreased quality, and limited access contained within an outdated medical system. Caring, healing, and health needs have changed, as the United States population is required to cope with more members who are aging, poor, chronically ill, and uninsured.

Nursing is the health profession of unmet expectation in the field of primary health and self-care knowledge and practices. Nurses have generally been the care providers who help people learn how to stay healthy, reduce their dependency on high cost technocure procedures and hospitalization. While nurses provide numerous health care services of the highest quality, nursing is highly underused and therefore incomplete in its mission to society.

As nursing makes its transition into the twenty-first century, it will be increasingly necessary for the nursing profession to come of age, and more fully realize its health, caring, and healing role in society. Such a changing role is dependent upon advanced knowledge and practices associated with self-care and health promotion. Hill and Smith's second edition of *Self-Care Nursing* is a major resource for curricular and practice changes that are necessary as nursing assumes a more prominent role in primary health care, including prevention of disease.

As nursing matures in its self-care knowledge, it can become more capable of actualizing its human caring, healing, and health care mission to society. Hill and Smith offer a definitive work on self-care in nursing that will continue to assist students and practitioners in obtaining the essential self-care theory and practice so critical to nursing's evolution.

This book is a comprehensive, self-guiding, theory and research-based work. It is based upon extensive educational and practice experiences of the authors. Self-care nursing practice lights the way for a prominent future for nursing. Nursing must establish a rightful place for itself in a system that is in dramatic flux. Hill and Smith provide a long overdue, different order of priorities, that can create a new social and professional order in nursing and society, a set of self-care priorities and practices that will carry us into the next century.

Jean Watson, RN, PhD, FAAN
Dean and Professor of Nursing
Director of Center for Human Caring
University of Colorado, Health Sciences Center
Denver, Colorado

Preface

Since the first edition of *Self-Care Nursing* came out in 1985, changes in the American health care system have continued at an ever-increasing rate. Thirty-seven million Americans currently have no health insurance coverage and enrollment in health-maintenance organizations and managed-care systems are rapidly rising. Along with these changes, both the deductibles and co-payments for clients continue to rise while the covered services continue to decline. In this new environment, it has become even more imperative for nurses to provide leadership efforts to promote wellness and prevent illness. How can this type of leadership be integrated into nursing curricula? How can nurses help clients learn to develop healthy lifestyles? What role do nurses have in promoting this approach in conjunction with traditional health systems?

This new edition represents our continued efforts to answer these questions. *Self-Care Nursing: Promotion of Health* is designed for the health care professional interested in learning about self-care theory, process, and application. The primary focus is on *application* of the self-care process. The text centers primarily on normalcy and health maintenance. However, attention is also given to integration of self-care within hospital settings. A secondary focus of the book is on *modeling* and the specific role of the nurse as a model of self-care.

This text can be used by nursing students in both undergraduate and graduate programs. It will be particularly useful in schools that have adopted self-care as a conceptual framework. For schools with other frameworks, the text can be used wherever wellness, holistic health, stress management, and self-care nursing are discussed. This might be in a beginning level nursing trends course, a nursing process course, a baccalaureate program for returning registered nurses in which new roles and health care concepts are presented, or in a graduate seminar for nurse practitioners interested in assisting clients to change health care behaviors. In addition, clinicians in a variety of areas can use this book to expand their skills in teaching self-care.

The text is divided into three sections. The first section includes the theoretical basis for the self-care process and its application to clinical practice. This section begins with perspectives on self-care from both an historical focus and from a variety of experts in the field. In addition, current socioeconomic issues affecting self-care are reviewed. Self-care is then explored from a nursing perspective. The commonalities between the self-care process and nursing process are presented. Orem is the primary nursing theorist discussed. In addition, the models of Hall, Blattner, Watson and Roy are briefly presented. Related theories of teaching/learning, psychoanalysis, communication, systems, development, stress/adaptation, and biology are discussed in reference to their applications to self-care.

Another focus of the first section is on the nurse as a model of self-care. A chapter on the self-contracting process, based upon behavioral reinforcement theory, is presented as a primary mechanism for behavior change and is used in each clinical application in the second and third sections.

The second and third sections focus on eleven different areas of self-care. We believe that the mind, body, and spirit are clearly interrelated. However, for organizational purposes, these sections are divided in the following manner. The second section contains topics that deal primarily with *self-care of the mind*. These include relationships, psychological self-care, relaxation, spirituality, and humor and play. Section three is comprised of self-care areas that focus primarily on *self-care of the body*. These areas include movement and exercise, sleep and dreams, nutrition, sexuality, environmental self-care, and physical self-care.

Within these chapters, the current trends, characteristics, developmental considerations, and self-care activities related to each topic are explored. The nurse as a model of self-care in each particular area is presented. A nursing process approach is applied to each of these components with the use of a clinical case presentation. These cases illustrate how nursing process can be effectively integrated with the self-care process in clinical settings. Each case presentation includes sample assessment tools, nursing care plans, and self-contracts.

Each chapter has objectives, definitions, summary, and study questions. Figures, tables, and photographs are used to emphasize important points. Many specific tools are presented that can be used directly with clients. The format of this text facilitates use by both students and faculty. An appendix provides supplementary materials for the reader.

Lyda Hill, RN, CS, PhD
Nancy Smith, MS, RNC

Acknowledgments

The preparation of the second edition of *Self-Care Nursing* has provided us with sometimes joyous and sometimes painful opportunities to reexamine our values and beliefs about wellness and self-care. Through our continuous contacts with friends, families, colleagues, and clients, the benefits of these self-care skills have become increasingly apparent. We have had two dramatic examples of this recently in our own lives.

After years of increasing compromise to renal function, Nancy's husband Jim went into end-stage renal disease in spite of conservative treatment. Working with his nephrologist Joseph Shapiro, MD, as a professional resource and collaborator, he made decisions about controversial surgery done at an academic medical center on the west coast and therapeutic diets from Europe to improve and maintain renal function for as long as possible. Compliance was nearly perfect in spite of the major lifestyle changes required.

When it became apparent that these interventions were insufficient, home dialysis training for continuous ambulatory peritoneal dialysis was initiated. Almost simultaneously he began screening transplant surgeons and programs. After twenty-three days on the transplant list and five weeks on CAPD, a successful renal transplant was completed. He continues to work with his surgeon, Warren Kortz, MD, and his nephrologist Chakko Kuruvila, MD, making joint decisions regarding his care. His compliance is high. He is able to fit appointments, rest, exercise, relaxation, work, play, nutrition, and psychological self-care into his busy day. His modeling of self-care for his two children and all of us has been inspiring.

Lyda's grandmother, Lyda Murray Ryan, underwent a major colon resection at ninety-one. During the pre-operative visit, she surprised her surgeon by interrupting discussion of the impending surgical procedure with a request that family members secure an absentee ballot for her to vote in the upcoming Presidential election. She was clearly still actively involved in her community and environment.

Lyda Ryan not only survived the major surgical procedure, she began ambulating on the second post-operative day and soon returned to her own home and independent living situation. During her recuperation, she performed all of her activities of daily living independently and even changed her own dressings. Her active interest in her environment continues; maintaining telephone contact with each of her 23 grandchildren regularly—dialing each of the telephone numbers from memory.

These crucial events had major impact on both of our families. We have learned more about how to realign priorities and develop new ways to find time and energy for our own self-care. Our students have continued to listen to our ideas, developing their own self-care programs and struggling with the integration of behavior changes into their own lives. They have also developed an incredible ability to promote self-care skills with clients in a variety of health care settings, teaching clients new ways in which to care for themselves. We are continually grateful to our own clients for reminding us of what self-care is all about, and the many ways in which we are not needed.

Lyda Hill, RN, CS, PhD
Nancy Smith, MS, RNC

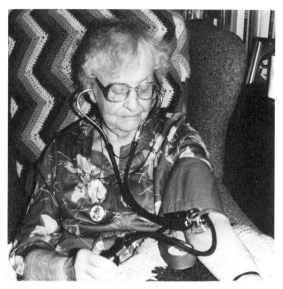

"Self-care asks: What can I do for myself? What can I do for you? To what purpose? At what cost?"

Yetta Bernhard, Self-Care (Millbrae, CA: Celestial Arts, 1975), pp. 26–29.

1   Self-Care in Perspective

LEARNING OBJECTIVES

Upon completion of this chapter, readers will be able to:

1. Define and discuss the concept of self-care.
2. Give a brief historical background of the self-care movement.
3. Compare and contrast self-care with activities of daily living, stress management, patient education, alternative medicine, holistic health and wellness, and self-help.
4. Differentiate between the terms *patient* and *client*.
5. Identify four roles for self-care and give clinical examples of each.
6. Identify factors influencing current transitions to self-care.
7. List and discuss two studies that support the cost effectiveness of self-care.

8. List seven self-care activities that have been linked to a marked increase in life span.

DEFINITIONS

Health/Wellness   Two terms that are used interchangeably and involve a continuum in which the mind, body, and spirit are in balance, providing a sense of well-being. In a state of health, the individual's developmental and behavioral potential is realized to the fullest possible extent.[1]

Self-Care   "The production of actions directed to self or to the environment in order to regulate one's functioning in the interests of one's life, integrated functioning, and well-being."[2]

Client   A person who has a collaborative relationship with a health care provider for the purpose of receiving health care services or consultation. This person may be well.

Patient   A person who has a dependent relationship with a health care provider for the purpose of receiving health care services. This person is typically ill.

Consumer   A person who uses health care services. May be a client or a patient.

Health Care Provider   A person who provides health care services, including consultation and collaboration. Includes nurses, physicians, nutritionists, and so on.

INTRODUCTION: CONCEPT OF SELF-CARE

Susan is a 26-year-old school teacher. She is married with two children, aged 2 and 4. When she awoke this morning, she had a sore throat. She went to her kitchen and sat down at her multiple-services computer terminal and entered the following information:

```
Ready? ==>MY NAME IS SUSAN ANDERSON.
What is your address? ==> 42 BEECH TREE LANE
Good morning Susan. How are you today?
==>I HAVE A SORE THROAT AND WOULD LIKE TO USE THE SELF-CARE
    PROGRAM.
```

The exchange went back and forth for several minutes. The computer asked Susan many historical questions about how she had been caring for herself and about changes in her life over the previous two or three weeks.

She was asked to take Test Kit 4 from her Self-Care Pack and follow the instructions. Susan swabbed the inside of her mouth with a specially treated swab and then compared it with the color chart on the instruction sheet.

She entered the coded results into her terminal and received the following information:

```
Get two hours more sleep tonight and for the next three nights.
Drink at least eight glasses of water today and for the next ten
 days.

Limit direct contact with other people, particularly children
     until your test results are returned.

Return to Self-Care Program if temperature is above 100°
  or other symptoms develop.
```

This interaction may seem futuristic to some people. The concept of self-care, however, is as old as humankind. It has recently undergone a revival, with many people becoming interested in learning how to prevent the onset of illness, decrease the severity of disease, and generally increase their sense of well-being.

The term *self-care* has many definitions in both lay and professional literature. Commonly associated descriptions include: self-responsibility, independence, interdependence, attendance to the mind, body, and spirit, health maintenance, preventive care, and health promotion. To many nurses, self-care is synonymous with *activities of daily living* (ADL): the clients' ability to brush their own teeth or wash their own faces. Others associate the term with patient education.

These terms have their roots in a health care system based on an illness model. A new paradigm of medicine that integrates ideas and practices from holistic health has provided a different focus (Table 1–1). For economic and other reasons, people are becoming more interested in improving their health, not merely in curing their illnesses.

It is becoming widely known that people have the ability to make decisions or choices that can influence the state of their health. Popular magazines such as *Newsweek, Time, Redbook,* and *Ladies' Home Journal* feature self-care concepts, giving attention to physical and emotional fitness. Many national television networks have health programs that feature self-care approaches.

Nurses are also involved in helping people make choices that keep them well. They are teaching clients to examine their life-styles with regard to health maintenance and health care. Self-care holds many implications for nursing practice. In order for the nurse to integrate these concepts into clinical practice, relevant terms, issues, and trends must be understood.

HISTORY OF SELF-CARE

Historically, the popularity of self-care practices has risen and fallen like tides in the ocean. Before medical specialization and the easy accessibility of medical services, the "self-care tide" was high.

TABLE 1–1. THE EMERGENT PARADIGM OF HEALTH

Assumptions of the Old Paradigm of Medicine	Assumptions of the New Paradigm of Health
Treatment of symptoms.	Search for patterns and causes, plus treatment of symptoms.
Specialized.	Integrated, concerned with the whole patient.
Emphasis on efficiency.	Emphasis on human values.
Professional should be emotionally neutral.	Professional's caring is a component of healing.
Pain and disease are wholly negative.	Pain and disease are information about conflict, disharmony.
Primary intervention with drugs, surgery.	Minimal intervention with "appropriate technology," complemented with full armamentarium of non-invasive techniques (psychotherapies, diet, exercise).
Body seen as machine in good or bad repair.	Body seen as dynamic system, context, field within other fields.
Disease or disability seen as thing, entity.	Disease or disability seen as process.
Emphasis on eliminating symptoms, disease.	Emphasis on achieving maximum wellness, "meta-health."
Patient is dependent.	Patient is (or should be) autonomous.
Professional is authority.	Professional is therapeutic partner.
Body and mind are separate; psychosomatic illness is mental, may be referred to psychiatrist.	Body-mind perpsective; psychosomatic illness is province of all health-care professionals.
Mind is secondary factor in organic illness.	Mind is primary or coequal factor in all illness.
Placebo effect shows the power of suggestion.	Placebo effect shows the mind's role in disease and healing.
Primary reliance on quantitative information (charts, tests, dates).	Primary reliance on qualitative information, including patient's subjective reports and professional's intuition; quantitative data an adjunct.
"Prevention" largely environmental: vitamins, rest, exercise, immunization, not smoking.	"Prevention" synonymous with wholeness: work, relationships, goals, body-mind-spirit.

With many early health care systems, people used self-assessment, self-diagnosis, and self-treatment both to prevent and to solve health care problems. Before the early eighteenth century, women rarely saw a health care provider for perinatal care. When it came time to deliver, women relied on their mothers, friends, other women who had had children, or perhaps delivered the child alone.[3]

Many primitive people believed that disease and illness were directly related to supernatural causes. Magical cures were used to drive evil spirits from the bodies of the sick. Although these curing tasks were the responsibility of the medicine man or his equivalent, a majority of health care was the responsibility of individuals or their families. Rest, music, and relaxation were all structured and supervised by family members to treat fatigue, "fevers," and so on.[4]

Early health writings are heavily laden with descriptions of faith healers, folk medicine, mystification, and shamans. People seeking help from early healers were taught to use beads, herbs, oils, relationships, mineral baths, sleep and dreams, music, and statuary to care for themselves.

Self-Care Tide Ebbs: Medical Specialization

It was only after medical and nursing schools became prevalent that the tide ebbed for self-care practices. Health care developed a "scientific basis" for practice. Increased specialization and technical developments placed a high level of responsibility on the health care provider to maintain people's health. "Whatever the doctor says," "Get a shot and fix it," "When my body gets sick I'll just go to the doctor and get it fixed," became common phrases heard about health care.

At the beginning of the twentieth century, communicable disease accounted for most illness in the United States. People relied on self-care measures to help fight those illnesses. For example, clients with tuberculosis were sent to sanitariums to rest and get plenty of sunshine. As medical specialization increased, the development of antibiotics and vaccines decreased the incidence of communicable disease and self-care practices became less crucial. When the incidence of communicable disease decreased, diseases that were linked to lifestyle, such as hypertension, cardiovascular disease, and ulcers, became larger problems.

The Self-Care Tide Rises Again

The self-care tide began to rise in the late 1960s. Various economic, political, and social issues precipitated this renewed interest in self-care. People again began to pay more attention to learning and practicing basic self-care skills. The continued escalation of costs for the treatment of illness has played a major role in this new focus.

In the last decade, the federal government has become actively involved in defining the health needs of the people in the United States. Many of the identified needs are pertinent to self-care practice. In 1975, the Department of

Health, Education and Welfare published a *Forward Plan for Health: 1975–1981*. The report identified life-style and psychosocial factors as having the *largest influence* on mortality and morbidity. Specific topics that were addressed included diet, obesity, lack of exercise, alcohol abuse, smoking, and environmental hazards.[5]

In a 1979 report, *Healthy People: The Surgeon General's Report on Health Promotion and Disease Prevention*, the government recognized that improved health has come from *prevention* instead of treatment of illness. *Healthy People* predicted a reduction of 20 to 35 percent in mortality and morbidity through utilization of self-care practices.[6]

The renamed Department of Health and and Human Services issued a follow-up report, *Promoting Health, Preventing Disease: Objectives for the Nation*, in 1980. The objectives, along with strategies for each, focused on health promotion and protection and disease prevention.[7]

In 1981, the government targeted health promotion toward specific ethnic groups within the country: black, Hispanic, Southeast Asian, and American Indian.[8]

The preamble of the World Health Organization identifies health as a fundamental right of every human being. In 1978, the member countries reiterated this by pledging, "Health for all by the year 2000."[9,10] The Canadian government issued a similar document, *A New Perspective on the Health of Canadians*, the purpose of which was to identify funding priorities for its prepaid national health insurance program. The focus was on prevention rather than treatment of illness. Priorities addressed included the areas of weight control; excessive use of medication, alcohol, mood-modifying drugs; smoking; exercise; fitness; stress; and air and water pollution.[11]

At long last, preventive care issues are being acknowledged at the federal level. Ideally this response could be more extensive, but it is an improvement over earlier years, when the development of technology to combat specific diseases was the primary focus. Hopefully, this formal recognition by national governments will add impetus to current transitions in the health care system.

Naisbitt refers to this "megatrend" as a move from institutional help (the medical establishment) to self-help (personal responsibility for health). U.S. society has come full circle in these time-tested practices. Naisbitt identifies three trends:

1. New self-care habits that actualize our new-found responsibility for health.
2. Self-care that illustrates our self-reliance in areas not genuinely requiring professional help.
3. The triumph of the new paradigm of wellness, preventive medicine, and holistic care over the old model of illness, drugs, surgery, and treating symptoms rather than the whole person.[12]

PERSPECTIVES ON SELF-CARE

Nurses, physicians, and other health care providers apply the concepts of self-care to clinical practice in various ways. Some practice within acute care settings, others in ambulatory care, and still others work only with "well" clients. The following are brief sketches of the views of five self-care experts. Each has a different way of utilizing self-care concepts in clinical practice.

Dorothea Orem, R.N., M.S.N.Ed.

Orem defines self-care as "the production of actions directed to self or to the environment in order to regulate one's functioning in the interests of one's life, integrated functioning, and well-being."[2] As a nursing educator and health consultant, Orem has continued to explore self-care concepts, which she first wrote about as early as 1959.

Her model was initially designed for working with ill people in traditional health care settings, helping people regain the ability to care for themselves. Other nurse clinicians have applied her work in a variety of clinical settings and with well people.

She views self-care as a *deliberate* action that is goal oriented. Her model includes three types of self-care: universal (maintenance of air, water, food, etc.), developmental (related to life events such as birth and death), and health deviation (seeking medical assistance, carrying out medical treatment, learning to live with certain conditions).[13] Specific information about her approach and the ways in which it is clinically applied are presented in Chapter 2.

Orem's work has continued to enjoy popularity throughout the nursing profession, in both education and practice.

Tom Ferguson, M.D.

Ferguson's interest in self-care began when he was in medical school. He noticed several related issues in his practice: (1) Clients had physical symptoms that he felt were related to problems with jobs, relationships, and money; (2) clients had difficulty getting information about their illnesses; (3) he and his colleagues were getting little education or support in caring for themselves; (4) neither the doctor nor the clients were taking responsibility for health maintenance, prevention, or illness self-care; and (5) there was poor modeling and teaching of good health practices by health care professionals.[14]

His publication of *Medical Self-Care* is one effort to address these multiple problems. Through that forum both health care providers and clients learn important self-care skills. He continually emphasizes the fact that people have been too dependent on traditional care providers and encourages people to take a more active role in their health care.

Lowell Levin, M.P.H., Ed.D.

Levin sees self-care as a process whereby laypeople function on their own behalf in health promotion, disease detection, and treatment at the level of the *primary health resource* in the health care system.[15] Many of Levin's concerns center on self-care education, particularly for school-age children. He is interested in developing school health classes that promote self-care, self-discovery, and opportunities for increased control over one's life.[16]

Levin sees an expansion of nonprofessional health care resources to include "nuclear and extended families, friendship networks, affinity groups, churches, mutual aid groups, libraries, groups of fellow-workers, and political groups."[16] He sees another impact for the self-care movement as improving the environment and communities through building on the base of individual initiative.[17]

Keith Sehnert, M.D.

Sehnert views self-care as "directed toward a new kind of consumer, what [he] calls the activated patient."[18] In 1970, he developed the concept of self-care classes, in which people are taught specific skills, such as taking blood pressures, giving injections, and using otoscopes. He values alternatives to traditional Western medicine, such as *t'ai chi* and yoga, and includes them in his classes.

He is convinced that a self-care model is a feasible and vital health care approach. This conviction comes from his reasoning that people want to:

1. Save money on their health care expenses.
2. Be able to take better care of their families' health.
3. Feel more comfortable dealing with family members who are ill.
4. Learn how to "hook into" the medical system.
5. Learn more about their bodies and how they work.
6. Take increased responsibility for their own illness care.
7. Know more about healthier life-styles.[19]

His two publications, *How to Be Your Own Doctor (Sometimes)*[20] and *Selfcare-Wellcare*[21] meet some of these consumer needs.

John Travis, M.D.

Travis uses a self-care model at his Wellness Resource Center in California. When clients are sick, they are referred to another physician for diagnosis and treatment and encouraged to come back when they are "well." His goal is to "evaluate and enhance his clients' levels of wellness."[22]

Through consultations with his clients, Travis gives them the information and skills *they* need. He makes clear the professional's limits of responsibility in terms of only *assisting* clients to do things for themselves. Self-assessment tools, risk assessment, and life-span prediction are all integrated to help clients learn self-assessment and self-care.

Although Travis recognizes the importance of self-care skills such as diet and exercise, he places most emphasis on clients getting to know themselves: experiencing themselves directly rather than intellectually, removing self-imposed barriers, communicating feelings, enhancing creativity, visualizing positive outcomes, taking responsibility, and loving themselves.[22]

Each of these experts has a slightly different view of the concept of self-care and its clinical application. Many other health care providers have views that differ from these, but all have overlapping components. A review of the assumptions on which this text is written will assist the reader in understanding the perspective of this particular text.

PHILOSOPHICAL AND THEORETICAL ASSUMPTIONS

The focus of this text is on *promotion of normalcy*. This involves developing a realistic self-concept; fostering growth and development; maintaining and promoting physical health; and identifying and intervening with deviations from the norm.[23] Several assumptions are central to this focus and its integration. These are premises used in the development of this text and clarify its philosophical stance.

Human Care
Human caring is based upon a value system that respects spirituality and the ability of the individual to grow and change. The nurse is a co-participant in the human care process. The way in which the patient and the nurse perceive and experience health and illness conditions are an integral part of nursing assessment.[24]

Health Is a Good Investment
Health behaviors that prevent disease or reduce the severity of an illness are economically valuable to both the individual and to society.

Self-Care Process
Self-care is an ongoing, learned, practical process that is applicable in all settings with all individuals. It parallels the nursing process and may be practiced by the nurse for personal needs. Self-care can be effectively used by people with or without a health care provider.

Self-Care Skills/Health Behaviors
Health behaviors are deliberate actions that people take to influence their health states or to prevent, limit, or cure disease. All human beings have the

potential to learn and develop self-care skills, which may be either internally or externally oriented.

Components of Self-Care

The self-care components that are detailed in this text include behaviors first related primarily to the mind: relationships, psychological health, relaxation, spirituality and play; and then behaviors related primarily to the body: exercise, sleep and dreams, nutrition, sexuality, environmental health, and physical health. They are not intended as a comprehensive list of all possible self-care areas (see Fig. 1–1). This text does not include specific discussion of stress management. It is believed that effective stress management occurs when individuals are working toward their optimum levels of health in all self-care areas.

Conditions Essential to Meeting Self-Care Needs

The essential condition to meet self-care needs is the ability to initiate and persevere in the self-care process. To succeed, the person must have:

1. Essential *knowledge, skills* and *responsibility* for health care needs.
2. Sufficient *motivation* and energy to begin and continue until the desired results are achieved.
3. Placed a high *value* on health; cultural values influence health behavior.
4. A perception that new health behavior will reduce vulnerability to illness.[25,26]

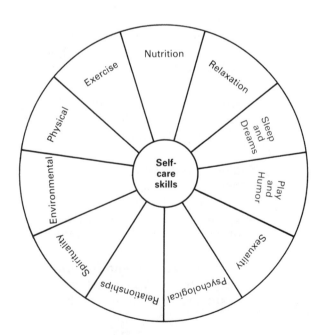

Figure 1–1. Self-care skills used in health maintenance.

New Paradigm of Medicine

The *new paradigm of medicine* (Table 1–1) offers great potential benefit for clients. *Self-care models do not exclude incorporation of traditional medical approaches.* Self-care is not inconsistent with good medical care; it utilizes the medical health care system without being solely dependent on it. In working with a newly diagnosed hypertensive client, for example, diet, exercise, relaxation, and sleep self-care skills may be initially utilized. If practicing these skills does not bring the hypertension under adequate control, antihypertensive medication might be introduced and used in conjunction with the foregoing self-care skills. Ethical nursing care includes a recognition of those instances when individuals need assistance in identifying their self-care limitations and needs for professional assistance.

Health Care Providers Are Models of Health

Health care providers have positive and negative health behaviors that they personally practice on a day-to-day basis. These behaviors are open to inspection, criticism, and adoption by their clients, families, friends, and peers. In addition to being an educator and consultant, the nurse is also a health model. Clients are more apt to value and practice self-care if they perceive that nurses value these skills and have actively integrated them into their own life-styles.

Self-Care Nursing

Self-care nursing is a specific approach to clinical practice that places primary emphasis on the client's ability to attain and maintain health. A primary outcome of effective self-care nursing is that clients are able to perform their own self-care without (or with only minimal) contact with health services on a long-term basis.

The Person as Client

In the traditional medical or illness model, people have a high level of passivity and allow health care providers to hold the majority of the responsibility and power. The health care is done "to" and "for" them, and the success or failure of that care depends on the skill of the health care provider. The term associated with the individual in this relationship is "patient."

In the self-care model, the individual has moved from a dependent relationship with the health care provider to functioning independently; the majority of the care is done "by" and "for" the client. The responsibilities involved in this approach are shown in Figure 1–2.

The term *client* will be used throughout the text to denote an individual in a collaborative relationship with a health care provider. (*Direct quotes that use the term* patient *have not been changed.*)

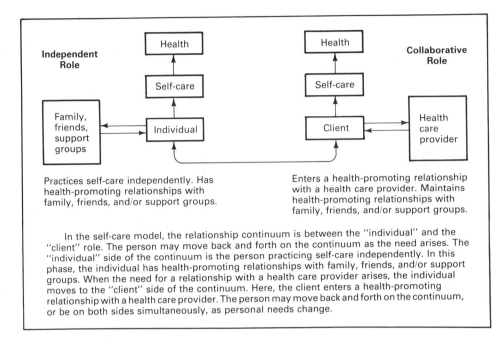

Figure 1–2. Individual–client continuum.

Theoretical Framework

Orem's *self-care deficit theory* (presented in Chapters 2 and 3) is utilized as the basic framework for integration of self-care concepts into daily nursing practice. The major focus of this text is on health maintenance and the promotion of normalcy. Some adaptations of Orem's theory have been necessary. Chapter 4 presents additional theories that are also relevant to self-care, including teaching/learning, communication, psychoanalytic, systems, developmental, stress/adaptation, biological, and nursing theories. Chapter 6 describes the ways in which these theories are integrated in self-contracting. The case presentations in Chapters 7–17 demonstrate integration of all of these theories in self-care nursing.

COMMONALITIES BETWEEN SELF-CARE AND OTHER HEALTH CARE BEHAVIOR

Self-care is often used synonymously with many different health care approaches in both lay and professional literature. A number of similar or overlapping behaviors exist in these areas, but each is also slightly different.

Activities of Daily Living (ADL)

Activities of daily living meet daily physical needs, such a eating, dressing, ambulating, and communicating. In the clinical area, the concept of ADL is frequently correlated with acuity. The terms *total*, *partial*, and *self-care* indicate the amount of physical care required by the client.

Another way of looking at ADL is to view a well person in an everyday environment; daily activities include personal hygiene, travel, nutrition, management duties, family relationships, and community activities. Although many of these activities could be classified as "self-care," they are often simply seen as routines that must be completed during the course of the day with little thought to how they affect health. Self-care involves making active choices about health care, not passively participating in activities that fulfill other needs and are completed without any health maintenance goal.

Stress Management

Increasingly, courses on stress management are being offered in a variety of settings. The content of these courses varies with the philosophy of the instructors and the needs of particular groups. Typical areas presented within the context of stress management are relaxation, meditation, visualization, exercise, biofeedback, communication, and assertion.

For the purpose of this text, stress management is viewed as a component of self-care. The entire practice of self-care is part of the effective management of stress. Self-care processes are synergistic in that work in one area frequently stimulates change in another. If a client is working on an intensive exercise program, nutritional improvement frequently follows. The exercise may also help the client to release frustrations accumulated throughout the day, in addition to providing many other benefits, such as improved cardiopulmonary efficiency, sleep, weight reduction, and increased self-esteem.

Patient Education

Patient education helps clients cope with an illness or specific condition by providing new knowledge or skills. Educational goals are usually set by the provider. The newly diagnosed insulin-dependent diabetic generally receives a standard set of instructions relative to insulin injections, urine testing, and diet.

Self-care education is related to patient education but focuses more on client goals than on provider goals. The purpose of self-care education is "to assist the client to achieve his desired outcomes in relation to which risks he chooses to avoid or not avoid."[26] Self-care education would assist clients to plan nutrition and exercise programs that would help them attain *their* goals of becoming physically fit.

Table 1–2 presents comparisons of the similarities and subtle differences between patient education and self-care education. Self-care education represents a major shift in philosophy from traditional patient education. The deci-

TABLE 1–2. PATIENT EDUCATION AND SELF-CARE EDUCATION COMPARISON

Points of similarity
  Learning theory: Utilized by both approaches.
  Resources: Both may use client alone, client and family, or client and friend/signifi-
    cant other.
  Setting: Both may be done in inpatient, outpatient, ambulatory care, or home setting.
  Purpose: Both processes are goal oriented.

Points of difference

	Patient education	*Self-care education*
Goals	Established by the health care provider or jointly with the provider and client.	Developed from the needs and preferences of the client.
Clients	"Patients" are usually sick and under the care of another.	Does not assume illness, client may be perfectly well.
Philosophy	Designed to help the patient cope with his or her disease, maintain health, or avoid a specific disease.	Anticipatory of health risk, directed at reducing client dependency on the health care provider.
Economic	Can generate income for the agency upon the decision of the provider.	Can generate income at the discretion of the client, but frequently generates no income.

(Adapted with permission from Levin, L.S. (1978). Patient education and self-care: How do they differ? *Nursing Outlook, 26,* 170–172.)

sion making and goals rest with the client; client dependency is consequently reduced.

Alternative Medicine
Ferguson describes alternative medicine as supplementing traditional physicians' tools and skills with those of other healing traditions.[27] In traditional medicine, pharmaceuticals, radiation, surgery, and laboratory tests are used to diagnose and treat diseases. Alternative medicine might utilize acupressure, acupuncture, yoga, exercise, shamanism, chiropractic, meditation, or nutrition to treat the same diseases.

Today, folk healers coexist with traditional health care practitioners. In some places, they are serving as paraprofessionals and are helping to close the communication and treatment gap between health care providers and clients.

Holistic Health/Wellness
"Holistic health is a system of care that is directed toward the integration and balancing of body, mind, and spirit. The goal of holistic health is to help the total person, rather than just to treat a disease."[28] Practitioners of holistic health often use techniques identical to or similar to those used in alternative medi-

cine, such as acupressure, kinesiology, or yoga. Self-care may also include any of these approaches.

This definition has many similarities to wellness, but, unlike wellness, holistic health is frequently focused on the healing of an illness or condition. Wellness practitioners frequently do not see clients who are "ill" but instead ask them to return when they are "well."

Self-Help

The self-help movement gained momentum in the 1970s. North Americans began to let go of institutional dependence and reclaim a sense of self-reliance.[29] Many professionals use the term *self-help* interchangeably with self-care. Generally, self-help refers to a process whereby laypeople organize in groups to meet mutually identified goals *without professional intervention.*

The groups *may or may not be health related.* The individuals may share a common problem, such as within a Weight Watchers group. Members might also organize to work on an issue such as the Equal Rights Amendment or be part of a women's consciousness-raising group.

Self-help may also refer to a process whereby individuals participate alone (in the same way that one could practice self-care alone). They might review a variety of health issues and use the information to solve problems, enhance health, or perhaps simply expand awareness.

ROLES OF SELF-CARE

Many professionals have conceptualized the scope of self-care in different ways. Fry defines four major self-care roles:

1. Health maintenance.
2. Disease prevention.
3. Self-diagnosis, self-medication, and self-treatment.
4. Participation in professional services.[30]

Examples of activities performed in each of these roles are presented in Table 1–3.

Health Maintenance

This component or role of self-care is the major focus of this text. Health maintenance is "any behavior or activity which results either in the prolongation of life expectancy or in an increase in the quality of life, whether or not this was originally intended as a main objective."[31] Health maintenance is not directed at a specific health care problem or disease, but at life-style and at health care practices that are generally beneficial.

TABLE 1–3. SELF-CARE SKILLS IN FRY'S FOUR SELF-CARE ROLES

Health Maintenance	Disease Prevention		
	Primary Prevention	Secondary Prevention	Tertiary Prevention
Consuming no alcohol or only in moderation	Familial history of diabetes: low weight, regular exercise, low sugar and decreased salt in diet	Breast self-exam PAP smears Stools for occult blood TB skin testing Blood pressure screening	Dialysis client: dietary/fluid management Post-myocardial infarction client:
Sleeping 7–8 hours per night			holter monitor
Eating three balanced meals per day at regular times	Familial history of hypertension: exercise, moderate weight, rest, decreased sodium intake, balanced work-play, relaxation skills	Idiopathic epileptic client: biofeedback Hypertensive client: limit caffeine Cardiac client: low fat, low sodium, low sugar dietary limitations	Post-mastectomy client: regular cancer screening Diabetic client: insulin regulation/ dietary management
Maintaining moderate weight			
Using no tobacco			
Exercising two to three times per week			
Practicing daily relaxation	Allergy history: no smoking and prevent contact with allergen		Asthmatic client: stress management program and limited contact with allergen
Wearing seat belts			
Maintaining relationships with family and friends	Familial history of emotional illness: develop relationships resources		
Playing regularly	Immunizations for specific diseases		
Having regular sexual activity	Fluoridation of teeth to prevent dental caries		
Providing for regular spiritual activity			

Figure 1–1 reviewed the variety of interdependent self-care skills that comprise health maintenance. A level of competence must be achieved in each of these areas to maintain an optimum state of health. Definitions, techniques, and practice guidelines are provided in subsequent chapters.

Disease Prevention

Disease prevention comprises "specific behaviors or activities which are intended to prevent either the experience or the spread of specific disease."[31] There are three types of disease prevention (see Table 1–3). In each, skills and practices have a slightly different aim:

TABLE 1–3 CONTINUED

Self-Diagnosis, Self-Treatment, Self-Medication	Participation in Professional Services
Self-diagnosis Doing self-vaginal exams Completing in home pregnancy test kits Learning to take blood pressure Recognizing danger signs and symptoms of illness Seeking professional help *Self-treatment* Low-sodium, low-cholesterol diet Selection of foods when eating out Weight control Exercise program Relaxation program Self-acupressure *Self-medication* Use of diuretic or antihypertensive medication Knowledge of Side effects of medication Interactions of medications with other medications, alcohol, or over-the-counter or "street" medication Danger signs and symptoms When to seek professional help	Seek consultation based on assets and limitations. Client may also continue to practice within self-care process. Examples include seeking consultation: For treatment of acute illness To learn new self-care skills, such as relaxation, acupressure, etc. For surgical intervention For childbirth

1. *Primary:* Avoiding a particular disease.
2. *Secondary:* Recognizing and treating a disease before major damage occurs.
3. *Tertiary:* Preventing further damage or disability as a result of disease.

Disease prevention also assumes continuance of all the health maintenance/ self-care skills identified in Figure 1–1 and Table 1–3.

Self-Diagnosis, Self-Medication, and Self-Treatment

These skills overlap with health maintenance and disease prevention skills. Skills relative to physical self-care predominate in this particular area. Sample activities performed in each of these areas are presented in Table 1–3.

People often practice in these areas independently. Many people feel perfectly comfortable in diagnosing their own coughs, colds, and sore throats and selecting over-the-counter medications to treat themselves. A study by Williamson and Danaher has shown that when people experience symptoms, 16 percent take *no* action, 63 percent use self-care *only*, 12 percent combine self-care with a visit to their general practitioners, 8 percent use a general practitioner only, and 1 percent use a hospital.[32] Thus, 75 percent of those in this study sample practiced self-care by diagnosing and treating their own symptoms.

This type of self-care is controversial. Concerns are expressed for client safety in relation to the increasing technical complexity of available health care. One argument is that the health care provider is significantly more knowledgeable than the client and is therefore better able to perform the functions of diagnosis, medication, and treatment.

Participation in Professional Services

Self-care does not exclude client use of professional health care services when required. Fry emphasizes development of the ability to seek assistance from health care providers at an appropriate time and in an appropriate manner. Self-care may continue simultaneously with client participation in professional services. (Table 1–3 and Fig. 1–2 further delineate this concept.) Participation includes careful selection of specific services and providers (see also Chapter 17).

FACTORS INFLUENCING CURRENT TRANSITIONS TO SELF-CARE

A transition from blind dependence on medical systems to a more balanced emphasis on the combined use of self-care models and traditional medical approaches involves many complicated factors. These include social, economic, and political issues.

Many believe that government has the role of choosing among policies and programs on the basis of their congruency with the public's interest. In spite of these clear statements from our federal government, operationalizing the goals in terms of reimbursement has yet to happen.

Evans refers to this process as "From Lifestyle Policy to Health Care Expenditure: Long Chain, Weak Links." He points out that this philosophy becomes vulnerable to attack because of the difficulty in validating the causal relationships that would ultimately prove preventive interventions are cost-saving strategies.[33]

For example, integrating healthy lifestyle habits that increase longevity also may increase the period of years a person spends in the high utilization period of health care services. The converse may also be true. Elevations in health status may extend years of good health and keep utilization rates low at any age. While reasons are unclear, however, utilization rates among Canadian elderly are rising and have been for a period of time.[34]

What Can Be Done?

In 1987, the Health Care Finance Administration reported 11.1 percent of the gross national product was spent on health care in the United States—more than in any other developed nation. Thirty-seven million Americans are without any health care insurance. Medicaid eligibility in some states has become increasingly difficult, with the maximum household income for a family of four set at $4248. Our social "safety net" is failing.[35]

Many national polls have indicated that the citizens of the United States favor the development of national health insurance. After the introduction of national health insurance in both Great Britain and Canada, per capita health expenditures average 20 to 70 percent less than in the United States; the age-adjusted mortality rates have sharply declined in both countries and are now slightly lower than in the United States.[36]

Dutton identifies the central dilemma as a lack of public accountability.[37] The imbalance in the political markets has been growing in recent years. For example, when Congress is funded by many special interest groups, it becomes increasingly difficult for Congress to adequately represent all members of society equally. Society must decide what health care services are needed, and how it will guarantee these services to all of its members.

Consumerism

Consumer and clients-rights groups have played an important role in the transition process. As people have become less dependent on institutions, they have initiated broad changes in the health care industry. Some of the consumer-related changes that influence the viability of self-care models include:

- The widely publicized "Health Bill of Rights."[38]
- Client access to personal medical records.
- Informed consent processes whereby the risks, as well as the benefits, of medical interventions are emphasized.
- New emphasis on the client's right to refuse treatment.
- Consumer participation in elimination of certain types of invasive or abusive treatments. (An initiative in Berkeley, California, has been introduced to ban the use of electroshock therapy.[39])
- Consumer and client pressure to allow fathers in delivery rooms and to provide more ready access to alternative birthing centers.
- Consumer and client pressure for industry to produce effective and inexpensive self-diagnostic home kits, such as in-home pregnancy testing and in-home PAP smears. (Medical suppliers are doing an ever-increasing percentage of business with the general public.[40])
- New emphasis on second opinions prior to surgical intervention. (In 1974, an estimated 2.4 million unnecessary surgeries were performed.[41] In one study of 1350 people supposedly requiring surgery, only 4 percent actually had surgery after a second opinion had been obtained.[42])
- An increasing prevalence of health maintenance organizations. These groups save cost through a variety of modalities including decreased utilization of inpatient services and encouraged utilization of preventive services.[43]
- Increasing deductibles and co-payments for acute care services (increasing the out-of-pocket expenses for this type of utilization).[44]

Popular Media

Radio and television programs have also significantly promoted self-care approaches by educating the public about the role of the individual in the health care system. Extensive lay literature covering such self-care topics as exercise, nutrition, relaxation, self-diagnosis, and the selection of professional providers is widely available.

Prevention and Cost-Effectiveness

The high cost of health care in this country is perhaps the single most important factor influencing a more widespread integration of self-care models. Government, other third party payers, and the general public have all become increasingly concerned about rapidly rising health care costs.

TABLE 1–4. A CONTEMPORARY FABLE: UPSTREAM/DOWNSTREAM

It was many years ago that villagers in Downstream recall spotting the first body in the river. Some old timers remember how spartan were the facilities and procedures for managing that sort of thing. Sometimes, they say, it would take hours to pull 10 people from the river, and even then only a few would survive.

Though the number of victims in the river has increased greatly in recent years, the good folks of Downstream have responded admirably to the challenge. Their rescue system is clearly second to none: most people discovered in the swirling waters are reached within 20 minutes —many in less than 10. Only a small number drown each day before help arrives—a big improvement from the way it used to be.

Talk to the people of Downstream and they'll speak with pride about the new hospital by the edge of the waters, the flotilla of rescue boats ready for service at a moment's notice, the comprehensive health plans for coordinating all the manpower involved, and the large number of highly trained and dedicated swimmers always ready to risk their lives to save victims from the raging currents. Sure it costs a lot but, say the Downstreamers, what else can decent people do except to provide whatever is necessary when human lives are at stake.

Oh, a few people in Downstream have raised the question now and again, but most folks show little interest in what's happening Upstream. It seems there's so much to do to help those in the river that nobody's got time to check how all those bodies are getting there in the first place. That's the way things are, sometimes.

Donald B. Ardell

(Reprinted with permission from Ardell, D.B. (1977). *High level wellness: An alternative to doctors, drugs and disease.* Emmaus, PA: Rodale Press, p. 6.)

There is no doubt that sophisticated medical and technological develop-ments have benefited many individuals. The ever increasing amount of finan-cial support these developments require has produced little change in the over-all health of the general population, however. There is no evidence that illness rates in our society have been affected by changes in physician–population ratio, technological improvements, or increases in the number of hospital beds.[45]

More than 70 percent of the billions of dollars allocated to health care supports hospitals, physicians, and the pharmaceutical industry, not preven-tive care efforts. The fable in Table 1–4 illustrates the futility of this approach. *Prevention*, including self-care, does seem to have an impact on the health of the general population. A sample of findings that support the crucial role of prevention and self-care are summarized below.

- Slight decreases in the incidence of heart disease since 1968 have been attributed to changes in self-care behaviors, such as decreases in smoking and dietary fat intake, rather than to increased technological advances or increased spending on medical care.[46]
- Reduction in mortality in automobile deaths has been specifically related to reduced speed limits, the use of seat belts, increasingly strict consequences for driving while intoxicated, and the higher cost of fuel, rather than to improved medical care and treatment.[47]
- A study by the University of Michigan found that pregnant teenagers had fewer perinatal complications than the national average after receiving coun-seling regarding self-care issues during the prenatal period.[48]
- Reduction in numbers of visits per client was achieved at Kaiser Permanente Hospital in San Jose, California, when an experimental client education program that dealt with the client's psychosocial risk factors was imple-mented *in addition* to traditional approaches.[49]
- An increase in life expectancy was documented by Belloc and Breslow for clients who practice six or seven of the following health care skills:
  1. Drinking no alcohol or only in moderation
  2. Eating breakfast every day
  3. Eating three meals a day at regular times
  4. Maintaining a moderate weight
  5. Refraining from smoking
  6. Sleeping seven to eight hours per night
  7. Exercising moderately two to three times per week[50]
- Stanford University researchers have documented a "substantial and sus-tained decrease in risk of cardiac disease" for subjects in a campaign that used television, radio, newspaper, and printed materials specifically aimed at smoking, exercise, and dietary changes.[51]
- Another project involving 299 beginning college students developed a cost-effective, modularized, and self-paced learning method for reducing stress. Results indicated that predicted illness rates may be decreased through knowledge of personal stress factors and stress-management self-care skills.[52]

These types of studies are slowly influencing public and private industry. Insurance companies are beginning to focus on new ways to encourage wellness as a way to reduce medical costs.

- Blue Cross/Blue Shield of Indiana "Stay Alive and Well" program saved $1.45 in health care costs for every $1.00 it invested in health promotion. Similar work-site wellness programs are run by Control Data Corporation, AT&T, and Johnson & Johnson.[53]
- One employer is offering a bonus to employees who stay healthy, with the result that employee health care claims have so far been reduced 60 percent.[54]
- Some life insurance policies provide special discounts for nonsmokers and people who exercise regularly.[55,56]
- Blue Cross/Blue Shield is supporting a variety of alternative programs, including an Ohio holistic cancer treatment program that combines traditional cancer treatment with helping clients feel better about themselves,[57] and a New York childbirth program that combines an in-hospital birth with postnatal home care.[58]
- Quaker Oats Company has decided that keeping its employees healthy is the right thing to do—for its bottom line. The company offers its workers the means to keep fit, tips on cutting medical costs, and cash bonuses to employees who stay healthy.[59]

These new approaches to health care raise a number of vital but unanswered questions:

- Will there be a decrease in the income and status of health care providers?
- Will costs shift from payment of the provider to cash outlay for self-diagnosis and self-treatment?
- Will self-care practices decrease hospital costs?

Nurses will certainly play an important role in the exploration of these issues during the next decade. As the appropriate use of self-care approaches with traditional medical models becomes more clearly understood and integrated into health care, the emotional and physical wellness of the nation will improve dramatically. This text is one effort in that direction.

SUMMARY

Self-care has been described by a variety of experts, including Orem, Ferguson, Levin, Sehnert, and Travis. Health, health behaviors, health as an investment, modeling of health care by health care providers, and the components and process of self-care were delineated as central to the philosophical focus of the text.

Self-care was compared and contrasted to other health care concepts, including activities of daily living, stress management, patient education, alternative medicine, holistic health and wellness, and self-help. Specific areas of commonality and difference were highlighted.

Self-care was described as a process having four particular roles: health maintenance; disease prevention; self-diagnosis, self-treatment and self-medication; and participation in professional services. *The focus of this text is on promotion of normalcy or the health maintenance role.*

Issues influencing self-care were discussed. Several factors that have an impact on the current direction of health care were emphasized, including consumerism, media, and economics.

STUDY QUESTIONS

Personal Focus

1. What are the self-care skills you personally practice?
2. Compare and contrast your personal philosophy regarding self-care with that of the text.
3. Describe your past experiences with self-care, both personally and professionally.

Client Focus

1. Interview two clients. Ask them what they see as their responsibilities in their relationship with you. What do they see as your responsibilities in the relationship? Compare and contrast their answers.
2. Select a client with whom you are currently working. Identify needs in each of Fry's four self-care areas.
3. Describe your clinical relationships as either nurse–patient or nurse–client. Are you practicing within the medical model or within the self-care model?

REFERENCES

1. American Nurses' Association. (1980). *Nursing: A social policy statement.* Kansas City, MO: Author, p. 5.
2. Orem, D. (1985). *Nursing: Concepts of practice* (3rd ed.). New York: McGraw-Hill, p. 31.
3. Bullough, V.L., & Bullough, B. (1978). *The care of the sick.* New York: Prodist Press, p.3.
4. Mora, G. (1975). Historical and theoretical trends in psychiatry. In A.M. Freedman, H.I. Kaplan, & B.J. Sadock (Eds.), *Comprehensive textbook of psychiatry* (Vol. I) (2nd ed.). Baltimore, MD: Williams & Wilkins, pp. 1–75.

5. U.S. Department of Health, Education and Welfare. (1975). *Forward plan for health: 1975–1981.* Washington, DC: U.S. Government Printing Office.
6. U.S. Department of Health, Education and Welfare. (1979). *Healthy people: The Surgeon General's report on health promotion and disease prevention.* Washington, DC: U.S. Government Printing Office.
7. U.S. Department of Health and Human Services. (1980). *Promoting health/preventing disease: Objectives for the nation.* Washington, DC: U.S. Public Health Service.
8. U.S. Department of Health and Human Services. (1981). *Strategies for promoting health for specific populations* (USDHHS Pub. no. PHS 81-501691). Washington, DC: U.S. Public Health Service.
9. World Health Organization. (1958). Constitution. In *The first ten years of the World Health Organization.* Geneva, Switzerland: Author, p. 459.
10. Stuart, K. (1984). Health for all: Its challenge for medical schools. *Lancet, 1,* 441–442.
11. La Lande, M. (1975). *A new perspective on the health of Canadians.* Ottawa, Canada: Minister of National Health and Welfare Information.
12. Naisbitt, J. (1982). *Megatrends.* New York: Warner Books, p. 134.
13. Orem. *Nursing: Concepts,* p. 90.
14. Ferguson, T. (1980). *Medical self-care.* New York: Summit Books, p. 18.
15. Levin, L.S., Katz, A., & Holst, E. (1976). *Self-care: Lay initiatives in health.* New York: Prodist Press, p. 11.
16. Levin, L.S. (1980). Power to the patient: A conversation with Lowell Levin. In T. Ferguson (Ed.). *Medical self-care.* New York: Summit Books, p. 26.
17. Levin. Power to the patient, p. 26.
18. Sehnert, K. (1980). Ten years of classes: A conversation with Keith Sehnert, M.D. In T. Ferguson (Ed.) *Medical self-care.* New York: Summit Books, p. 29.
19. Sehnert. Ten years, pp. 22–23.
20. Sehnert, K. (1986). *How to be your own doctor (sometimes).* New York: Putnam Publishing Group.
21. Sehnert, K. (1985). *Selfcare-Wellcare.* Minneapolis: Augsburg Fortress.
22. Travis, J. (1977). *Wellness workbook: A guide to attaining high level wellness.* Mill Valley, CA: Wellness Resource Center, p. 26.
23. Orem. *Nursing: Concepts,* pp. 92–93.
24. Watson, J. (1985). *Nursing: Human science and human care.* Norwalk, CT: Appleton-Century-Crofts, pp. 34–35.
25. Becker, M.H. (1977). The health belief model and sick role behavior. In Becker, M.H. (ed.), *Health belief model and personal health.* Thorofare, NJ: Charles B. Slack, p. 89.
26. Levin, L.S. (1978). Patient education and self-care: How do they differ? *Nursing Outlook, 26,* 171.
27. Ferguson. *Medical self-care,* p. 34.
28. Dossey, B.M. (1989). *Holistic nursing: A handbook for practice.* Rockville, MD: Aspen Publishers, p. 57.
29. Naisbitt. *Megatrends,* p. 131.
30. Fry, J. (1975, August 11–15), Role of the patient in primary health care: The viewpoint of the medical practitioner. Background paper for the Symposium on the Role

of the Individual in Primary Health Care, Institute of Social Medicine, University of Copenhagen.

31. Williamson, J.D., & Danaher, K. (1978). *Self-care in health*. London: Croon Helm, p. 109.

32. Williamson & Danaher. *Self-care in health*, p. 39.

33. Evans, R.G. (1984). *Strained mercy: The economics of Canadian health care*. Toronto, Canada: Butterworth's, p. 276.

34. Evans, R.G. (1983). We have seen the future and they is us. In T.W. Moloney & S.A. Scroeder (Eds.), *Proceedings of the commonwealth fund forum on the health care of the aged*. London: May 23–26, pp. 23–26.

35. Can you afford to get sick? (1989, January 30). *Newsweek*, pp. 45–46.

36. Himmelstein, D.U., & Woolhandler, S. (1986). Cost without benefit: Administrative waste in U.S. healthcare. *New England Journal of Medicine, 314*, 441–445.

37. Dutton, D.B. (1988). *Worse than the disease: Pitfalls of medical progress*. New York: Cambridge University Press, pp. 371–372.

38. Cron, T. (1970). A patient's revolt: Is it possible? *Hospital Progress*, Oct, 71.

39. Hager, P. (1982, August 17). Fate of electroshock therapy in Berkeley in voters' hands. *Los Angeles Times*, Sec. I, pp. 1, 18.

40. Naisbitt. *Megatrends*, p. 136.

41. House of Representatives, Committee on Interstate and Foreign Commerce. (1976). *Cost and quality of health care: Unnecessary surgery*. Washington, DC: U.S. Government Printing Office.

42. McCarthy, E., & Wioner, G. (1974). Effects of screening by consultants on recommended elective surgical procedures. *New England Journal of Medicine, 291*, p. 1331.

43. Feldstein, P.J. (1983). *Health care economics*. New York: John Wiley & Sons, pp. 326–355.

44. Feldstein. *Health care economics*, pp. 111–113.

45. Cochrane, A.L. (1974). Effectiveness and efficacy: Random reflections on health services. *British Medical Journal, 4*, 5.

46. Kristein, M., Arnold C.V., & Wynder, E.L. (1977). Health economics and preventive care. *Science, 195*, 457–462.

47. Cooper, B., & Rice, D. (1976). *Social Security bulletin*. Washington, DC: Social Security Administration

48. Nolan, G.H. (1977). Key to reducing risks of teenage pregnancy is psychosocial physician declares. *Behavior Today, 8*(41), 2–3.

49. Harrington, R,L., Koreneff, C., et al. (1977). Systems approach to mental health care in an HMO model (Project MH 24109). Washington, DC: National Institutes of Mental Health.

50. Belloc, N.B., & Breslow, L. (1972). Relationship of physical health status and health practices. *Preventive Medicine, 1*, 409.

51. Farquhar, J.W. Maccoby, N., & Wood, P.D. (1977). Community education for cardiovascular health. *Lancet, 30*. 1192–1195.

52. Hill, L., Smith, N., & Jasmin, S. (1981). Modularized stress management for reduction of predicted illness. *American Journal of the College Health Association*, 69–74.

53. McCormack, P. (1987, Dec 6). "Survivors of 'wellness epidemic': Exercise in the workplace bringing healthy returns." *Los Angeles Times*, part 6, p. 24.

54. Jacobs, J. (1980, July 6). Stay healthy, earn a reward. *San Francisco Sunday Examiner and Chronicle*, p. 1.
55. New York Life Insurance Co., 51 Madison Ave., New York, NY 10010.
56. Allstate Life Insurance Co., as advertised in *Time Magazine*, February 13, 1984.
57. Naisbitt. *Megatrends*, p. 138.
58. Naisbitt. *Megatrends*, p. 141.
59. Can you afford to get sick? (1989, January 30). *Newsweek*, p. 51.

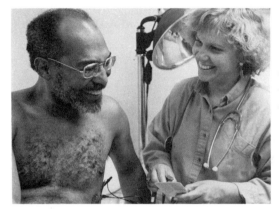

Treat people as if they were what they ought to be, and help them to become what they are capable of being.

Goethe

2 Self-Care and Nursing Practice

LEARNING OBJECTIVES

Upon completion of this chapter, readers will be able to:

1. Identify the current philosophy and focus of the American Nurses' Association regarding health care.
2. Describe the process of self-care using the following terms: self-care, self-care agency, self-care demand, self-care deficit, nursing systems.
3. Identify four types of clinical settings in which self-care is now integrated by nurses. Describe and discuss that integration.
4. Present a synopsis of Orem's self-care model.

DEFINITIONS

Self-Care Nursing   Self-care nursing is a specific approach to clinical practice that places primary emphasis on the client's ability to attain and maintain health. A major outcome of effective self-care nursing is that the client is able to perform self-care without (or with only minimal) contact with health care services on a long-term basis.

(Additional terms are presented in Table 2–3.)

INTRODUCTION

Nurses throughout history have taught self-care practices to clients. Nightingale promoted self-care by teaching soldiers in the Crimean War to care for and dress their own wounds. She viewed medicine's role as removing diseased parts, and nursing's role as putting the client in an environment that would allow the person to reach optimum health.[1]

In a more contemporary vein, Peplau considered nursing as a "significant therapeutic interpersonal process."[2] Her focus on joint identification of problems by the client and the nurse, with mutual goal setting, implementation, and resolution, has provided an ideal foundation for self-care practice.

Nursing has formally identified the need for self-care. The American Nurses' Association (ANA) has acknowledged that "individuals, families, and groups have considerable responsibility for their personal health."[3] In this light, the ANA recognizes nursing's ability to serve society's health needs by putting *health*, rather than illness, at the center of nursing's attention. Nursing is thus seen as the diagnosis and treatment of human responses to actual or *potential* health problems.[4]

Nursing specialty groups have also identified the need for nurses to become involved with preventive care and health promotion. International and national policy and trends were discussed in Chapter 1. Annual self-care conferences for nursing education and service have also been developed.[5,6]

Curran is a nurse who uses television to reach the public with simple messages about health maintenance. Her health segment series, "Alive at Five," is a 5-minute show on a local Milwaukee television news program that deals with such topics as exercise, nutrition, breast self-examination, and cancer treatments.[7] Using a similar approach, nurses across the country have begun to present workshops and seminars focused on self-care, wellness, stress management, time management, burnout, and so on. Modeling (by the nurse) of the health behaviors nurses ask clients to demonstrate is a concept integrated into many of these presentations.[8,9]

Nurse researchers have been creative pioneers in the self-care area and are studying ways to integrate self-care into clinical practice. Kearney and Fleisher have developed a scale (Table 2–1) that explores the crucial question of how to

TABLE 2–1. SELF-CARE AGENCY TOOL[a]

1. I would gladly give up some of my set ways if it meant improving my health.

2. I like myself.

3. I often feel that I lack the energy to care for my health needs the way I would like to.

4. I know how to get the facts I need when my health feels weakened.

5. I take pride in doing the things I need to do in order to remain healthy.

6. I tend to neglect my personal needs.

7. I know my strong and weak points.

8. I seek help when unable to care for myself.

9. I enjoy starting new projects.

10. I often put off doing things that I know would be good for me.

11. I usually try home remedies that have worked in the past rather than going to see a doctor or nurse for help.

12. I make my own decisions.

13. I perform certain activities to keep from getting sick.

14. I strive to better myself.

15. I eat a balanced diet.

16. I complain a lot about the things that bother me without doing much about them.

17. I look for better ways to look after my health.

18. I expect to reach my peak wellness.

19. When I have a problem, I usually want an expert to tell me what to do.

20. I deserve all the time and care it takes to maintain my health.

21. I follow through on my decisions.

22. I have no interest in learning about my body and how it functions.

23. If I am not good to myself, I believe I cannot be good for anyone else.

(Continues)

TABLE 2-1 CONTINUED.

24. I understand my body and how it functions.

25. I rarely carry out the resolutions I make concerning my health.

26. I am a good friend to myself.

27. I take good care of myself.

28. Health promotion is a chance thing for me.

29. I have a planned program for rest and exercise.

30. I am interested in learning about various disease processes and how they affect me.

31. Life is a joy.

32. I do not contribute to my family's functioning.

33. I take responsibility for my own actions.

34. I have little to contribute to others.

35. I can usually tell that I am coming down with something days before I get sick.

36. Over the years I have noticed the things to do that make me feel better.

37. I know what foods to eat to keep me healthy.

38. I am interested in learning all that I can about my body and the way it functions.

39. Sometimes when I feel sick I ignore the feeling and hope it goes away.

40. I seek information to care for myself.

41. I feel I am a valuable member of my family.

42. I remember when I had my last health check and return on time for my next one.

43. I understand myself and my needs pretty well.

aDirections for specific use of this tool can be found in the original article.

(Reprinted with permission from Kearney, B. & Fleischer, B. (1979). Development of an Instrument to Measure Exercise of Self-Care Agency. *Research in Nursing and Health, 2*(1), 28.)

measure and predict people's potential ability to care for themselves in a health-promoting way.[10] The Clark Health/Wellness Belief Scale presents a similar focus on the internal versus external orientation of client beliefs about health.[11]

SELF-CARE NURSING THEORY

Orem is the person most commonly associated with the integration of self-care into nursing practice. Her pioneering work has paved the way for a clearer delineation of the roles of the nurse, client, and physician in self-care approaches to health care.

Orem's work is utilized in many academic and clinical settings. Her major contribution to nursing thought centers on her interest in getting nurses to help clients learn to help themselves through the use of "deliberate and learned behaviors that purposely regulate human structural integrity, functioning, and human development."[12] Although this seems rather obvious, Orem is one of the first theorists in modern nursing to address this *formally.*

Orem sees one goal of nursing as providing help for people who are unable to help themselves. She also identifies helping people learn self-care skills to adapt to or recover from illness as a major nursing priority. In her model, nurses function as educators and consultants for clients. Education is the primary means employed to correct self-care deficits or problems in providing for one's own health needs. Table 2–2 presents a sample of one way in which Orem would help people begin to look at their actual and potential self-care skills. In Chapter 4, Orem's approach is compared and contrasted to other nursing theorists.

Synopsis of Orem's Self-Care Model

Although Orem's work has many different creative directions, in its simplest form her model is actually a statement of her basic beliefs about health and nursing. Orem believes that self-care is a learned, deliberate behavior that people perform to meet and maintain certain specific needs (*self-care requisites*), such as the need for exercise, pain control, relaxation, air, food, or water. At different times in each person's life, he or she (the *self-care agent*) has differing abilities or skills in practicing self-care (*self-care agency*).

When a self-care need is not met, a *self-care demand* is present. *Self-care deficits* exist when people are unable to meet their self-care demands. A nurse, family member, or friend (*dependent-care agent*) may be used in an educative or consultive relationship to help alleviate or correct the deficit. In health institutions, nurses perform this role and help people in three different ways. These are *supportive-educative, partly compensatory,* and *wholly compensatory* nursing systems.

Many nurses find Orem's work straightforward and easy to use but others

TABLE 2–2. DEVELOPING A CONCEPT OF SELF-CARE

1. Select an individual (a relative, friend, or associate or an inpatient or outpatient at a hospital) who has a chronic disease, has sustained an injury, has experienced an acute illness, or is pregnant for the first time.
2. In accordance with the individual's ability, interest, and willingness to comply with your request for information, ask the following questions (rephrase if desired) and record the answers.
   a. Since the occurrence of (name the conditioning factor, disease, injury, etc.), do you have to care for yourself differently than you did before its occurrence?
   b. What are some of your new activities or tasks? How did you learn about the need to engage in them?
   c. How do you fit the new tasks into the schedule of your daily activities?
   d. Can you do all of these new tasks for yourself? If not, who helps you?
   e. Did you know how to do these new tasks before the occurrence of (same as in all above)?
   f. How did you feel about learning to do the new tasks? How do you feel about doing them now?
   g. Of all the things that you know you should do, are there some things that you tend to forget or deliberately decide not to do? If so, why?

(Reprinted with permission from Orem, D. (1985). *Nursing: Concepts and practice* (3rd ed.). New York: McGraw-Hill, p. 37.)

find her framework and terminology difficult and confusing.[13] Although a *detailed* understanding of each of her concepts is unnecessary for the purpose of this text, some of her basic terms are utilized or adapted directly and are thus summarized in Table 2–3. An additional table (Table 2–4) presents a brief overview of Orem's division of three nursing systems.

CLINICAL APPLICATION OF SELF-CARE

Self-care models are at times criticized as being impractical for use in traditional health care settings. They are often considered a passing fad for those with "fringy" ideas, but not a part of mainstream clinical practice. In reality, there are many ways that self-care concepts have always been integrated by nurses, even though the term "self-care" might not be used. For example, nurses who work with cardiac clients on diet, exercise, and relaxation are actually

TABLE 2–3. OREM'S SELF-CARE TERMINOLOGY[a]

Term	Definition By Orem[b]	Use Within This Text	Example/Discussion
Self-care	A learned behavior, "the production of actions directed to self or to the environment in order to regulate one's functioning in the interests of one's life, integrated functioning and well-being." (1)	Use consistent with Orem's definition.	As a child, John learned to be careful around hot objects. This is a self-care behavior practiced by adults and children.
Self-care agency[c]	"The complex capability for action that is activated in the performance of the actions or operations of self-care." (1)	An assessment of each client's ability to provide self-care is addressed in each case presentation.	The ability to care for oneself involves many complicated issues, including motivation, knowledge, and skill. If John is only 3 months old, he probably does not yet have the skill, knowledge, or motivation to avoid hot objects. Until John learns that hot objects will hurt him, he will be unable to protect himself. Assuming that John is now old enough to practice the self-care activity of avoiding hot objects, he is the self-care agent.
Self-care agent[c]	"The person providing the self-care." (2)	Orem uses the term *patient* in discussing the self-care agent. This text uses *client*.	If John is too young to protect himself from danger, family members take on this role and become the dependent-care agents. If John were hospitalized, his nurse could be the dependent-care agent.
Dependent-care agent[c]	"The provider of infant care, child care, or dependent adult care." (2)	Nurses, friends, family, or other providers are dependent-care agents.	

33

Term	Definition by Orem[b]	Use Within This Text	Example/Discussion
Self-care requisites[c]	"Purpose or goals to be attained through the practice of self-care." Self-care requisites include universal, developmental, and health deviation aspects. (3)	The focus of this text is on universal and developmental requisites, although health deviation requisites are addressed in some of the case presentations.	John's basic needs (self-care requisites) are met through the practice of self-care. *Universal requisites:* include air, food, and water maintenance. *Developmental requisites:* include provision for his success in developmental tasks such as learning to walk. *Health deviation requisites:* include disease prevention, as in providing for John's immunizations. If John were very "accident prone," he would have a *need to develop more safety skills.* This would be his self-care demand. Other examples include the need to develop exercise skill, the need for adequate sleep, and so on.
Therapeutic self-care demand	"The measures of care required at moments in time in order to meet existent requisites for regulatory action to maintain life and to promote health and development and general well-being." (1)	In this text, the term *self-care demand* is used rather than "therapeutic self-care demand." The concept, however, remains the same. It identifies a need for self-care activity based on assessment of the client's assets and limitations. It is implicit that the client practicing self-care may or may not need the services of the nurse. People may meet their self-care demands on their own or with the aid of nursing services.	
Self-care deficit	"A relationship between self-care agency and therapeutic self-care demand in which self-care agency is not adequate to meet the known therapeutic self-care demand." (1)	This concept is used in the same way throughout this text. Some type of intervention is necessary when self-care deficits exist; that intervention may or may not include nursing services.	John has numerous accidents. His self-care deficit is: "Inability to provide for own safety without intervention due to lack of knowledge and skill."

| Nursing systems | "A continuing series of actions produced when nurses link one way or a number of ways of helping to their own actions or the actions of persons under care that are directed to meet these person's therapeutic self-care demands or to regulate their self-care agency." (1)

Table 2–4 presents Orem's three systems: supportive-educative, partly compensatory, and wholly compensatory. | Formal use of this concept occurs in only minor ways in this text. Focus is primarily on the supportive-educative system, although some case presentations include references to the other systems. | If John fractured a bone and it required open-reduction, during the surgery and the immediate post-operative period, he would be functioning within a wholly compensatory nursing system. While he was casted and began engaging in his regular daily activities, he would be in a partly compensatory system. When the cast was removed and initial physical therapy completed, he would be in a supportive-educative system. |

[a] Additional concepts relative to Orem's conceptualization of nursing process are presented in Chapter 3.

[b] Adapted from Orem, D. (1985). *Nursing: Concepts of practice* (3rd ed.). New York: McGraw-Hill, (1) p. 31, (2) p.84, (3)pp. 85–86.

[c] This term is not used formally in this text; however, its meaning and value remain the same and its use is implicit throughout.

TABLE 2–4. OREM'S THREE NURSING SYSTEMS

Nursing System	Nurse Action	Client Action	Clinical Example
Supportive-educative	Acts as a consultant or resource for client at his or her request.	Does own self-care, identifies own needs/goals. Seeks out resources needed to meet goals.	An individual identifies need for birth control. Seeks out nurse to get information. During consultation, becomes client. Makes choice based on information given. Individual practices self-care skill or birth control independently.
Partly compensatory	Assists client in performing some self-care skills when client unable to do so. Collaboratively identifies needs/goals with client for self-care performed by nurse.	Does own self-care within abilities. Needs assistance in some areas. Able to identify some needs/goals independently, some collaboratively.	Individual is at home postoperative colostomy. Has visiting nurse come to home daily. Is able to complete all self-care independently except ostomy care. In this area client has relationship with nurse to identify collaboratively needs/goals relative to ostomy. Nurse may assist in stoma care.
Wholly compensatory	Performs self-care for client, including identification of needs/goals.	Client does *not* perform any self-care skills, needs, or goal identification.	Client has post-trauma head injury. Is unconscious, maintained on ventilator and receives total parenteral nutrition. While providing wholly compensatory care for this client, the nurse may also provide supportive-educative care for the client's family/friends.

(Adapted from Orem, D. (1985). *Nursing: Concepts of practice* (3rd ed.). New York: McGraw-Hill, pp. 152–159.)

fostering self-care skills. Nurses who instruct clients in home dialysis are encouraging self-care within a partly compensatory system.

In recent years, numerous publications have documented the use of self-care by nurses in a variety of clinical settings. The following summaries are not exhaustive but provide an outline of the wide manner and range in which self-care concepts are currently being integrated in daily clinical practice.

Nursing Care of the Elderly

Changing health policy in the United States has meant that many elderly patients are being discharged "sicker and quicker" from acute care hospitals. This process can upset the balance for a senior who had been able to negotiate self-care demands with available resources prior to the hospitalization. Burnside talks about the need for careful evaluation of self-care skills, as well as dependent-care skills, when discharging elderly clients with complex needs—particularly when the client is leaving in the care of an elderly spouse.[14]

Many resources have been published that talk about the integration of the self-care model and the elderly.[15-18] Bower and Patterson reiterate this: "Orem's self-care model lends itself especially well to the nursing assessment and nursing care of elderly clients simply because self-care is *the* issue for the elderly."[19]

Acute Medical-Surgical Nursing

Self-care has traditionally been part of medical-surgical nursing. Hypertensive clients have been taught how to take their own blood pressures and to recognize important signs and symptoms. Clients with new stomas are taught skills for independent ostomy care.

Mullin believes that the self-care concept can be used in traditional medical-surgical systems. She practices with two primary assumptions:

1. Each individual's person belongs to himself or herself and only he or she has right over that person.
2. The nurse's relationship to that individual exists *only* to assist the person to maintain, restore, or increase the ability to provide his or her own self-care.[20]

Mullin asks, "Why am I doing this?" "How is this activity assisting the individual to be his or her own self-care agent?"[21] These questions focus nursing practice on the client, giving a client-oriented purpose to each activity, rather than making the activity simply a task to be performed. The second question helps to determine nursing accountability for actions and interactions and determines whether or not activities are oriented to self-care. Her approach to nursing process (Table 2–5) includes specific questions focused on client accountability.

Enterostomal therapy is a specific clinical area in which the self-care model is applied. Bromley discusses her use of Orem's three nursing systems in providing care to clients with ostomies.[22] In the initial postoperative stage, a wholly compensatory system is used with the nurse providing all of the care.

TABLE 2–5. SELF-CARE CONCEPT AND ACCOUNTABILITY

Plans for Implementation of Self-Care Concept to Determine Accountability[a]
Question: How is this nursing activity assisting the individual to be his own self-care agent?
Assessment
Did I include him in the assessment process?
Did I validate the assessment with him?
Have I considered his self-care rights and responsibilities?
Does he know how the nursing activity relates to his self-care activities at home?
Plan
Did I include him in planning?
Did I ask about and include his preferences?
Did I identify alternatives?
Did I let him establish the order of priorities?
Did I plan the sharing of information, attitudes, and skills so that he understands the nursing activity?
Did I ask him what support he needs?
Implementation
Did I do more than was necessary?
Did he do as much as was possible?
Did I cooperate with his plan?
Did I preserve his self-care rights and responsibilities?
Did I spend enough time so that he was comfortable asking questions?
Did I provide the support he needed to be able to do the nursing activity for himself?
Evaluation
Is he able to do the nursing activity for himself?
Is he able to tell me why he is not doing the nursing activity?
Is he able to relate the nursing activities to potential health needs experienced at home?
Conclusion
The nursing activity is assisting him by . . .
The nursing activity is not assisting him because . . .

[a]Lists are not complete and are intended only to illustrate the process.
(Reprinted with permission from Mullin, V. (1980). Implementing the self-care concept in the acute care setting. *Nursing Clinics of North America, 15* (1), 188.)

As the client progresses, a partly compensatory system is initiated with the client learning about and completing some stoma care. When discharged, the client is in a supportive-educative system, able to accomplish self-care and use the nurse as a consultant.

Obstetrics
Historically nurses have used self-care approaches by helping clients to practice skills in deep-breathing, breast preparation, pelvic strengthening exercises,

and numerous similar activities. Now hospitals have become more flexible in meeting client needs by providing alternative birth centers, prepared childbirth classes, rooming-in, father's unlimited visiting, and sibling visits. It remains difficult, however, to meet the self-care needs of clients who require cesarean sections.

Harris uses an educative self-care framework to increase the self-care agency (ability) of cesarean clients and their families.[23] She identifies self-care activities that can be carried out by either the client or her family. In planning these activities she assumes that significant others will be participating in the care. Harris has found that clients like to know what is happening to them and to be in control of their care. Although the process of self-care does not decrease the need for professional intervention, "it does mean that the focus of the visits may be changed to client teaching, client reporting, and physical monitoring."[24]

Endocrinology

Nurses play a major role in helping diabetics learn self-care skills for insulin injection, urine testing, diet therapy, and skin care. Fitzgerald sees modeling by the nurse as one way this is promoted.[25] Nurses must perform in ways consistent with what they teach.

Fitzgerald uses Orem's self-care framework to facilitate active participation in self-care and put clients in control of their health. She maintains a "view of the human being as capable of participating actively in health care."[26] She emphasizes that "health professionals should not relinquish their responsibility to use good judgment in helping individuals cope with diabetes and its medical management."[27]

Mental Health

Nurses have always played a significant role in helping mental health clients to understand and to manage problematic behaviors. Milieu therapy is one example of a process initiated and implemented by nurses that integrates self-responsibility and self-management with traditional psychiatric care.

Nurse clinical specialists have also begun to play a more formal role in mental health outpatient settings, where they teach clients to assess and monitor their own symptoms. Clients learn when to come into clinics for consultation or medication, but they also learn self-care approaches such as exercise, play, relationships, and nutrition that can be used in conjunction with medical approaches.

Underwood is one of the first nurses to write about formal integration of self-care concepts in psychiatric hospital settings. She recognizes that the client's disturbance in perception, thought, or motivation will affect his or her ability to meet basic biological and psychological needs. She believes that the self-care model "provides the nurse with a way of assessing and planning that supports the patient's own control over his daily living."[28] She feels that the "effects of institutionalization can be minimized or eradicated when the nursing goal of patient care is to promote the patient's ability to care for himself in day-to-day living."[29]

Ambulatory Care

Johnson-Saylor uses self-care concepts in her clinical practice at a university health service where the majority of clients are seeking contact for required physical examinations or for episodic complaints. She uses these contacts for health promotion through self-care education and practice. Her goals include: "(1) health maintenance based on risk and geared toward prevention of disease; (2) early detection; and (3) helping the client attain wholeness, balance, and optimum functioning in life."[30]

Although these health promotion goals are ideal, Johnson-Saylor recognizes that the "client's concern about the reason for the office visit must be met and attended to in a manner acceptable to him or her."[31] Problems with alcohol, smoking, stress, nutrition, and sexuality are major areas for intervention. Although the client's initial visit may have been for an exam or a specific complaint, the nurse emphasizes that the client need not have an illness to return and continue work on improving health care behavior.

School Nursing and Health Education

School nurses have traditionally provided first aid, child-health screening, and health education services for students. Many of these activities involve informal teaching of self-care skills such as dental hygiene or nutrition.

In a more formalized approach, Gantz describes the development of a project designed to supplement a required health education curriculum. Orem's self-care model was used to help sixty 10-year-old students:

1. Increase their knowledge about their bodies as holistic, integrated, responsive systems.
2. Learn and practice skills of observation, description, self-care, and management of common health problems.
3. Gain confidence in using a variety of methods and resources to pursue their interests and concerns.
4. Accept increasing responsibility for making health decisions.
5. Determine personal goals and actions to achieve them.
6. See health education as an active, stimulating experience appropriate and relevant to their needs and interests.[32]

Students identified what they wanted to learn. Typical topics included: "What makes urine yellow? What's an IV of D_5W? Where do fingernails come from? My friend said that if I played with my belly button, my legs would fall off." There were hands-on sessions with beef eyes and freeze-dried lung tissue. Interpersonal respect, teacher excitement, student ability to identify learning needs, and high-level interest in health subjects were among the outcomes of this program.[33]

In another elementary school setting, Lewis describes an experiential health care program in which children identify their health problems and what should be done about them.[34] The child's decision is used except when his or her choice "exceeds pre-existing standards as to what are acceptable dispositions for certain problems."[35] For example, a child would not be allowed to return to class with a high temperature, even if that were his or her choice.

Lewis describes this model as a "problem-oriented approach to team cure/care in which the patient is the most important member."[36] Although Lewis does not use the term self-care, she certainly describes a self-care process.

Alcohol Treatment

Increasing the self-care agency of adolescents was the focus of a clinical project by Michael and Simon-Sewall. They asked two questions: "How can a peer group, which encourages and supports sociability through the use of alcohol, foster and enhance responsible use of alcohol?" and "How can groups which are a material and forceful part of adolescence, serve as primary facilitators of positive change?"[37]

Group members were inpatients in an acute care center and met one hour daily for six weeks. The project utilized reality therapy in combination with Orem's self-care framework to develop a support system for adolescents. The group was responsible for identifying, evaluating, and modifying members' behavior. Contracts were used to emphasize commitment to behavior change. This process was found to be effective. Adolescent groups were able to exert enough peer pressure to control their members' drinking habits.

Hospice

The hospice provides a unique clinical setting for self-care. Walborn describes a model for a hospice program that includes both primary nursing and self-care. Self-care is chosen because of the increased opportunities for clients to exercise control and decision making over their care.[38]

Walborn discusses the use of a partly compensatory nursing system. In this system, both the nurse and the family perform some self-care measures for or with the client. Examples of self-care deficits for hospice clients include:

- Inability to assess pain and regulate doses of Bromptom's cocktail.
- Lack of knowledge and experience with death, dying, and grieving.
- Inability of family members to request assistance from friends and neighbors.[39]

Walborn's work has "individualized client care and facilitated the client's increase in self-care agency.[40]

Cardiac Rehabilitation

Cardiac rehabilitation programs have become increasingly sophisticated in using creative teaching/learning strategies to help clients attain and maintain healthy life-styles. Nurses have been actively involved in these programs together with other health care providers, such as nutritionists, exercise physiologists, and cardiologists.

Hoepful-Harris is one nurse who has written about her formal integration of self-care concepts into cardiac rehabilitation. Nurses at her agency use behaviorally-oriented strategies such as contracting to assist clients with the integration of new skills into their daily routines. Rewards are given for each small step or goal, for example, for each quarter-pound lost or lap jogged, improvements in percentages of body fat, improved vital signs, and improved functional capacity.[41]

Pediatrics

Pediatric nurses have traditionally promoted self-care activities through such means as preadmission hospital tours, play therapy, and breathing exercises for asthmatics.

Facteau focuses on the self-care abilities and responsibilities of the child and the role of a substitute self-care agent. She believes that "an important role for nursing is the assessment of a child's agency for self-care behavior and planning of specific intervention if deficits are found."[42] She identifies the child's self-care abilities as the result of a combination of factors: cultural background, cognitive and motor skills, and emotional developmental level.

Facteau points out that the substitute self-care agent varies with the developmental level of the child. During hospitalization, the self-care skills might be performed by the parent, nurse, or other health care provider, in addition to the client. In one typical example, a 4½-year-old female was admitted for a tonsillectomy. After the surgery, her mother continued to dress and wash her and brush her teeth, saying, "This is going to be our only child, so I guess I'm trying to keep her a baby forever."[43] The mother asked questions regarding normal abilities of preschool-age children and the nurse implemented a teaching plan based on identified self-care deficits.[43]

SUMMARY

This chapter described various ways in which self-care models and concepts have been integrated into clinical nursing practice. Specific applications of self-care in a variety of clinical situations, including nursing care of the elderly, medical-surgical, obstetrics, endocrinology, mental health, ambulatory care, school health, alcohol treatment, hospice, cardiac rehabilitation, and pediatrics, were presented. Orem's self-care deficit theory and terminology were discussed, and adaptations of her terminology for use in this text were explored.

STUDY QUESTIONS

1. Discuss the significance of self-care in your nursing practice.
2. Interview yourself by responding to the questions on self-care in Table 2–2.

Client Focus

1. Use the guidelines in Table 2–2 to interview a client regarding self-care.
2. Describe how self-care may be integrated into the nursing care of two clients with whom you are currently working.
3. Compare and contrast Orem's self-care model with the nursing model used by the health care agency where you are currently working.
4. Practice using Mullin's "Plans for Implementation of Self-Care Concept to Determine Accountability" in Table 2–5 by applying these questions to a client with whom you are currently working.

REFERENCES

1. Torres, G. (1980). Florence Nightingale. In J. George (Ed.), *Nursing theories: The base for professional nursing practice.* Englewood Cliffs, NJ: Prentice-Hall, p. 29.
2. Peplau, H.E. (1952). *Interpersonal relations in nursing.* New York: Putnam, p. 16.
3. American Nurses' Association. (1980). *Nursing: A social policy statement.* Kansas City, MO: Author, p. 5.
4. American Nurses' Association. *Nursing,* p. 9.
5. Veteran's Administration Medical Center. (1988). The self-care model of nursing: Coming of age. Palo Alto, CA: Author.
6. Third Annual Self-Care Conference for Nursing Education and Service. (1982). Self-care deficit theory: Curriculum and practice implementation. San Francisco: Author.
7. Connie Curran shares health tips on daily tv show in Milwaukee. (1982). *The American Nurse, 7*(14), 3.
8. Nurturing the nurse. (1982). San Diego, CA: Scripps Clinic and Research Foundation.
9. American Nurses' Association. (1982). Nurses as models of health: Self-care in perspective. Washington, DC: Author.
10. Kearney, B.Y., & Fleischer, B.J. (1979). Development of an instrument to measure exercise of self-care agency. *Research in Nursing and Health, 2*(1), 25–34.
11. Chambers-Clark, C. The Clark health/wellness belief scale. The Wellness Institute, 48 Johnstown Road, Sloatsburg, NY 10974. (Unpublished evaluation tool.)
12. Orem, D. (1985). *Nursing: Concepts of practice* (3rd ed.). New York: McGraw-Hill, p. 36.
13. Smith, S.R. (1981). "Oremization," the curse of nursing . . . baroque nursing theories couched in stilted pseudo-intellectual jargon. *RN, 44,* 83.
14. Burnside, I.M. (1988). *Nursing and the aged: a self-care approach.* New York: McGraw-Hill, p. 122.

15. Eliopolous, C. (1984). A self-care model for gerontological nursing. *Geriatric Nursing, 5*(8), 366–370.
16. Finnegan, T. (1986). Self-care and the elderly. *New Zealand Nursing Journal, 79*(4), 10–13.
17. Hankes, D. (1984). Self-care: Assessing the aged client's need for independence. *Journal of Gerontological Nursing, 10*(5), 27–31.
18. Hirschfield, M. (1985). Self-care potential: Is it present? *Journal of Gerontological Nursing, 11*(8), 29–34.
19. Bower, F., & Patterson, J. (1986). A theory-based nursing assessment of the aged. *Topics in Clinical Nursing, 8*(1), 22.
20. Mullin, V. (1980). Implementing the self-care concept in the acute care setting. *Nursing Clinics of North America, 15*(1), 183.
21. Mullin. Implementing the self-care concept, p. 184.
22. Bromley, B. (1980). Applying Orem's self-care theory in enterostomal therapy. *American Journal of Nursing, 80*(2), 245–249.
23. Harris, J. (1980). Self-care is possible after cesarean delivery. *Nursing Clinics of North America, 15*(1), 191–204.
24. Harris. Self-care is possible, p. 193.
25. Fitzgerald, S. (1980). Utilizing Orem's self-care nursing model in designing an educational program for the diabetic. *Topics in Clinical Nursing, 2*(2), 57–64.
26. Fitzgerald. Utilizing Orem's model, p. 58.
27. Fitzgerald. Utilizing Orem's model, p. 64.
28. Underwood, P. (1980). Facilitating self-care. In P. Pothier (Ed.), *Psychiatric nursing.* Boston: Little, Brown, p. 116.
29. Underwood. Facilitating self-care, p. 125.
30. Johnson-Saylor, M. (1980). Seize the moment: Health promotion for the young adult. *Topics in Clinical Nursing, 2*(2), 10.
31. Johnson-Saylor. Seize the moment, p. 11.
32. Gantz, S.B. (1980). A fourth-grade adventure in self-directed learning. *Topics in Clinical Nursing, 2*(2), 29, 30.
33. Gantz. A fourth-grade adventure, pp. 33–36.
34. Lewis, M.A. (1974). Child-initiated care. *American Journal of Nursing, 74*(4), 652.
35. Lewis. Child-initiated care, p. 654.
36. Lewis. Child-initiated care, p. 655.
37. Michael, M., & Simon-Sewall, K. (1980). Use of the adolescent peer group to increase the self-care agency of adolescent alcohol abusers. *Nursing Clinics of North America, 15*(1), 157–158.
38. Walborn, K.A. (1980). A nursing model for the hospice: Primary and self-care nursing. *Nursing Clinics of North America, 15*(1), 206.
39. Walborn. A nursing model for the hospice, p. 207.
40. Walborn. A nursing model for the hospice, p. 214–215.
41. Hoepfel-Harris, J.A. (1980). Improving compliance with an exercise program. *American Journal of Nursing, 80*(3), 449–450.
42. Facteau, L.M. (1980). Self-care concepts and the care of the hospitalized child. *Nursing Clinics of North America, 15*(1), 145.
43. Facteau. Self-care concepts, p. 153.

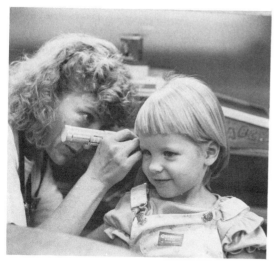

The true measure of the value of nursing service rests in the degree to which it modifies the health behavior of others.

R. B. Freeman, *Techniques of Supervision in Public Health Nursing*, 2nd ed. (Philadelphia: W. B. Saunders, 1949).

3 Self-Care and the Nursing Process

LEARNING OBJECTIVES

Upon completion of this chapter, readers will be able to:

1. Define nursing process.
2. State the purpose of the nursing process.
3. List three advantages of an organized nursing process.
4. Describe two ways in which the nursing process parallels the self-care process.
5. Describe the nursing process format that will be utilized in this text.
6. Summarize the focus of each of the four nursing process phases integrated in this text: assessment, diagnosis, plan, and evaluation.

DEFINITIONS

Nursing process "Labels a concept involving a pattern of observation and logical thinking that is the basis for formulating the nursing care plan."[1] The nursing process provides an organized, deliberate, and systematic approach to nursing practice.

Behavioral Objectives Specific statements of outcomes that can be clearly measured and observed. Objectives are stated so that outcomes must occur within a specific time. These types of detailed statements are helpful in determining whether actions taken toward a specific end have been successful.

Phases of the Nursing Process

Assessment The deliberate, systematic collection of data, together with the assignment of meaning to the input received. Emphasis is on assessment of the educational needs of the client as well as specific assets and limitations related to self-care skills.

A statement of a *self-care demand* is made following a comprehensive assessment. That statement indicates a specific set of self-care actions needing to be performed in order to meet human needs;[2] an example would be "need for adequate sleep."

Diagnosis A statement of each real or potential self-care deficit for each self-care need that the client is unable to meet without assistance. *Self-care deficit* statements parallel diagnostic statements; they simply state the self-care area in which the client is unable to meet some specified self-care need because of inadequate motivation, knowledge, or skills;[2] for example, "inability to provide for adequate sleep due to low motivation."

Plan This phase of the nursing process includes setting objectives as well as carrying out specific nursing and client actions that lead to the attainment of objectives. This phase is sometimes labeled "intervention" or "prescription and implementation" (Table 3–1). In this text, the planning phase of the nursing process is divided into two sections: (1) setting objectives and (2) reaching objectives.

Evaluation Summary statement of client responses to personal and nursing actions taken to reach a specific objective. This includes an ongoing assessment of alteration in knowledge, motivation, and skill regarding specific self-care behaviors.

INTRODUCTION

Social workers, psychologists, physicians, and all health care providers have some sort of conceptual framework or basic approach to their work and a

TABLE 3–1. COMPARISON OF TERMINOLOGY UTILIZED BY FIVE DIFFERENT AUTHORS IN DESCRIBING BASIC PHASES OF THE NURSING PROCESS

Orem[a]	Alfaro[b]	Yura and Walsh[c]	Little and Carnevali[d]	Hill and Smith (format for this text)
Diagnosis and prescription (ends with statement of self-care deficit)	Assessment	Assessment (ends with analysis of data and making conclusions)	Assessment	Assessment (based on self-care demands)
	Diagnosis		Diagnosis	Diagnosis (statement of self-care deficit)
Designing and planning	Planning	Planning	Prescription (setting goals)	Plan A. Setting objectives B. Reaching objectives (client and nurse actions)
Producing and managing care Initiation Conduction	Implementation	Implementation	Implementation (nursing actions)	
Control (evaluation)	Evaluation	Evaluation	Evaluation	Evaluation

[a]Orem, D. (1985). *Nursing: Concepts of practice* (3rd ed.). New York: McGraw-Hill, pp. 222–237. [b]Alfaro, R. (1986). *Application of nursing process: A step-by-step guide.* Philadelphia: J.B. Lippincott. [c]Yura, H., & Walsh, M. (1983). *The nursing process* (4th ed.). New York: Appleton-Century-Crofts. [d]Little, D., & Carnevali, D. (1983). *Nursing care planning* (3rd ed.). Philadelphia: J.B. Lippincott.

systematic way to communicate with each other and their clients. Although individuality and creativity are utilized within that basic structure, professionals still establish some consistent way of carrying out their specific functions in the health care system. Without this structure, health care would be chaotic and haphazard.

Nursing process identifies the way in which nurses structure and guide their practice. "Nursing process labels a concept involving a pattern of observation and logical thinking that is the basis for formulating the nursing care plan."[1]

Stevens points out that the focus of each phase of the nursing process differs from that of a medical model process, although the same basic phases are followed in both:[3]

Medical Model Term	**Nursing Process Term**
Client examination	Client assessment
Diagnosis	Nursing diagnosis
Prognosis	Goal setting
Prescription	Nursing care plan
Therapy	Nursing intervention
Evaluation	Evaluation

Nursing process is "alive," dynamic, and continual, not static. It forms the basis for communication within the nursing profession and with other health care providers. Nursing process also:

1. Provides a structured approach that facilitates client involvement in care.
2. Facilitates data collection for research purposes.
3. Easily parallels the self-care model of nursing practice.
4. Parallels the self-care process which the client may be practicing simultaneously (see Fig. 3–1).

Terminology and Nursing Process

Nursing process provides a basic approach to professional practice. *The process remains the same even if the words describing each phase of the process are slightly different.* Table 3–1 presents a summary of five labels for nursing process. A combination of these terms (or even different terminology) may be used in any specific nursing curriculum or clinical setting. In each example consistent phases are followed, and nurses continue to think about interactions with clients in the same basic way. Table 3–2 compares Orem's conceptualization of nursing process with that of this text.

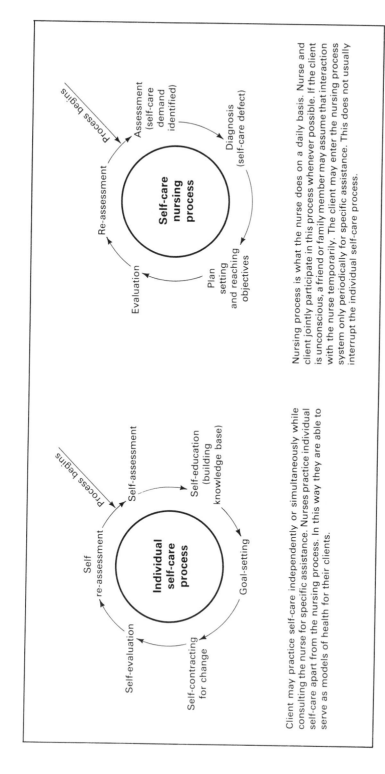

Figure 3–1. Comparison of the individual self-care process and the self-care nursing process.

TABLE 3–2. COMPARISON OF OREM'S NURSING PROCESS CONCEPTUALIZATION WITH THAT OF THIS TEXT

Hill and Smith (format for this text)	Orem[a]
Assessment Assessment based on self-care demand of the client. Assets and limitations are reviewed. Self-assessment is a major focus. Goal is for client to learn to complete self-assessment without assistance. Learns to identify need for professional intervention.	*Diagnosis and prescription* *Assessment* should focus on obtaining answers to five crucial questions (see p. 51). Initial determination of why (if at all) person needs nursing care. *Diagnosis:* nursing judgment about the client's existing health care situation and decisions about what can and should be done. Self-care demand (see p. 31). Self-care deficit (see p. 31).
Diagnosis Statement agreed on by nurse and client. Reflects an inability to meet a self-care demand without assistance. Self-care deficit may result from inadequate knowledge, motivation, or skill.	*Designing and planning* Nursing care is *designed* to contribute to client's achievement of health goals. System may help family and friends to provide temporary care for client. *Planning* specifies roles, resources, activities. Time, place, and frequency of performance of activities by the client, the nurse, and others are considered.
Plan Setting Objectives Clear, behavioral statement of what the client plans to accomplish. Can be observed and measured within a certain time. Reaching Objectives Specific statements of actions that will be taken by the client or the nurse to reach the objective.	
Evaluation Statement that objectives were or were not met. A nonjudgmental, dynamic process. Leads to further self-assessment and alterations in self-care plans. Follow-up focus: changes in thoughts, feelings, actions; changes in knowledge, motivation, and skill.	*Producing and managing care* Initiation, conduction, and control of nursing action to: 1. Compensate for self-care limitations and facilitate adaptation. 2. Overcome self-care limitations of client and/or family so that future health needs can be met more effectively. 3. Foster and protect client's current self-care abilities and prevent the development of new self-care limitations.

Orem, D. (1985). *Nursing: Concepts of practice* (3rd ed.). New York: McGraw-Hill, 222–240.

BASIC PHASES OF THE NURSING PROCESS

Pre-process Issues

Certain issues, though often not clearly labeled within the nursing process, are vital to successful interactions with clients. Some of these issues or needs are:

1. Establishment of a degree of trust between client and nurse.
2. Definition of the role the nurse will play in the client's care [and the role the client will play in his or her own care*].
3. An opportunity for the client to voice initial fears, release pressing questions, and begin to feel a degree of comfort in the client role.
4. A positive environment which permits successful pursuit of the nursing process.[4]

The more these needs are initially met, the more easily the nursing process can be pursued. The use of nursing process within a self-care model raises an additional important issue. In order to be helpful, nurses must have some knowledge, motivation, or skill in the area of self-care the client is pursuing. All nursing interactions are influenced by the modeling process.

- self-care demand
- assets
- limitations

With all approaches to nursing process, the first step is to make a complete assessment. In a variety of ways the nurse asks, "What is going on here?" or "What exactly is happening or has happened?" By working with the nurse to answer these questions, the client learns self-assessment skills, which are crucial to the assessment process. Nurses must have assessed their own health behavior in order to help clients learn this important skill.

Various assessment tools provide a format for organized information gathering. Each nurse eventually chooses a favorite assessment style and adopts a specific format. Table 3–3 presents a number of key assessment points in outline form. *It is assumed that nurses will complete an extensive physical screening process with clients before addressing the self-care issues discussed in this form and explored in each of the self-care-focused nursing care plans throughout this text.*

Assessment is not limited to the client's presenting physical or emotional problem. It must also include the client's perception of the problem (subjective data) as well as other significant objective data. A nursing data base includes a

---

*Author's addition.

TABLE 3–3 SELF-CARE FOCUSED NURSING PROCESS

Client statement of purpose for consultation:

Assessment

A. Data collection
   1. Self-assessment tools completed
   2. Client clarification of reason for consultation relative to self-assessment process
   3. Developmental stage (e.g., adolescent, retirement)
   4. Recent life changes/current life stress (e.g., pregnancy, divorce, job change)
   5. Physical and emotional health status
   6. Sociocultural orientation (e.g., past, present values relative to culture)
   7. Economic issues (resources available for self-care practice)
   8. Support systems (e.g., current family, friends, community support)
   9. Models (past and current for self-care skills in general and specific to reason for consultation)
   10. Cognitive level/language skills (ability to read, understand materials) Learning style (e.g., visual, auditory, tactile)
   11. Coping style (past and current, e.g., drugs, exercise, prayer)
   12. Current knowledge, motivation, skill regarding self care
   13. Current life-style, values, and self-care practices (e.g., time, energy, etc., to practice self-care)
   14. Client and nurse joint summary of assets and limitations relative to presenting issue (congruence of objective and subjective data)
   15. Other
B. Self-care demand: summary statement of self-care need
C. Referrals
   Is the demand within the scope of the nurse and the agency?
   Nurse's ability to model the needed behavior?
   Nurse's knowledge in this area?
   Need for referral *before* continuing?

Diagnosis

A. Self-care deficit: statement of each deficit (real or potential) for each self-care demand
B. Due to inadequate knowledge, motivation, or skills
C. Differential diagnostic considerations (self-care in *conjunction* with skills from other health care providers?)

Plan

A. Setting objectives
   1. Client's objective (first priority, stated behaviorally)
   2. Realistic objective (re: time, money, setting, baseline, safety)
   3. Reevaluation date set
B. Reaching objectives
   1. Steps taken by nurse and client to reach specific objective
      Client assumes major responsibility for self-care behavior changes
      Nurse acts as educator, consultant, and supervisor when needed
   2. Actions focus on correcting deficits in knowledge, motivation, and/or skill
   3. Based on previous success and/or failures in self-care behaviors
   4. Other

Evaluation

A. Were the objectives met?
B. If not met:
   1. Unrealistic (insufficient knowledge, motivation, skill)?
   2. Specific revisions needed?
C. Client evaluation of process
   1. Feelings about the process?
   2. Found most helpful and least helpful?
   3. Family reaction to the self-care change?
   4. Change in self-care strengths (able to identify needs, initiate plans)?
   5. If contracting utilized, were rewards actually given?
D. Nurse evaluation of process
   1. Maximum responsibility given to the client?
   2. New teaching strategies needed?
   3. Nurse served as model during interactions? Provided adequate feedback for client?
   4. Precautions carried out? Safety incorporated into the plan?
   5. Follow-up timing and process regularly identified?

comprehensive view of the client's body, mind, and spirit, not simply specific medical problems.[5] This focus on the total person is also known as *holistic nursing.*[6–8] Certain factors may greatly facilitate or limit the person's self-care practices. These include culture, economic and social conditions, family relationships, developmental level, and environmental stress.

For example, the nurse gathers data related to Mr. Peter's hypertension by actual measurement of his blood pressure, but extensive data are also gathered related to his life-style, family relationships, ability to express his feelings, and so on. Mr. Peters plays an active role in this process.

Nurses utilizing self-care models pay particular attention to an assessment of the client's *educational needs* in relation to his or her current health state and self-care abilities. Orem cautions nurses against gathering extensive information that cannot be used in any practical way with clients. She believes that assessment should be aimed at answering *only* five crucial questions.

1. What is the client's self-care need now? At a future time?
2. Does the client have a deficit for engaging in self-care to meet that need?
3. What is the nature and reason for that deficit?
4. Should the client be helped to refrain from self-care or to protect already developed self-care capabilities?
5. What is the client's potential for engaging in self-care in the future? Gaining new knowledge? Learning new self-care techniques? Improving motivation?[9]

Both nurse and client assess the self-care abilities (or self-care agency) of the client. Assessment focuses on the client's *knowledge* about that self-care area, *motivation* to perform self-care, and overall self-care *skills*. In the assessment phase, clients learn to recognize their own self-care demands, assets, and limitations.[10]

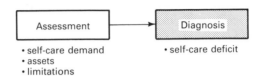

In the second phase of the nursing process problems are identified and labeled in order of priority. For example, the nurse recognizes that Ms. Walters has a problem with respiration and provides prescribed oxygen before talking with her about her additional problems—fear of death and anxiety about hospital procedures. Diagnostic statements flow logically from data gathered during nursing assessment.

Orem's model utilizes the term "self-care deficit" to refer to the inability of the client to perform self-care because of a lack of knowledge, skill, or motivation, or some combination of the three.[11] Orem views diagnosis as an "investigative operation that enables nurses and clients to make judgments about the [client's] existing health care situation and decisions about what can and should be done."[9] In her model the nursing diagnosis (of self-care deficit) is seen as the final component of the assessment phase and precedes the second phase of actual nursing planning (see Tables 3–1 & 3–2). The nursing diagnosis is a concise and simple statement of each (real or potential) self-care deficit for each self-care demand that the client is unable to meet. (Table 3–3 describes the focus of the diagnostic phase that will be utilized throughout this text.)

While nursing diagnoses have become the model, the approved list of nursing diagnoses have been criticized because it contains only alterations or impairments from normal health.[12] Clients with strengths in specific areas or clients who are at risk for the development of particular self-care deficits are not included. The North American Nursing Diagnosis Association meets every two years, and the authors look forward to the development of nursing diagnoses that meet criteria for clients who are primarily healthy.[13]

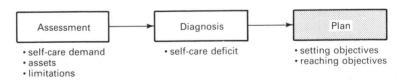

All nurses go through some sort of planning phase as they work with clients. In self-care nursing, the plan includes a determination of what the client would like to change in improving his or her self-care abilities as well as the actions that will be taken by the client, the nurse, or both. The plan involves establishing objectives, judging priorities, and designing methods to resolve problems.[14] Clients, family members, and a number of different health care providers may be involved in this process.

In this text the planning phase of the nursing process is divided into two sections: (1) setting objectives and (2) reaching objectives. In some models this planning phase may be labeled in slightly different ways. Orem divides this phase into two steps: (1) designing and planning, and (2) producing and managing nursing care. This division is adapted and integrated in clinical presentations within this text. Table 3–3 presents a synopsis of data relevant to this phase of the nursing process.

Setting Objectives

Orem identifies this phase as the designing component of the nursing process.[15] She specifies a number of considerations that take place in relation to:

1. Protecting developed self-care skills.
2. Bringing about new development in self-care ability (acquiring new knowledge, motivation, skills).[16]

In this step the nurse and client jointly identify what is to be accomplished in promoting self-care or correcting specific self-care deficits. Specific and realistic objectives are identified after considering factors of time, money, setting, and safety. Objectives are planned in relation to a realistic baseline; plans are built upon the client's *current* self-care skills (not on past or future skills).

Behavioral objectives. Objectives are most helpful when they are stated specifically and identify a clear outcome that can be observed and measured. Time frames describing when an outcome must have occurred (e.g. within one hour, one week) help in determining that actions taken toward a specific end have been successful. Objectives that are written in this way are called *behavioral objectives.* They clearly state:

1. Who will do an action.
2. What that action will be.
3. When it will be done.
4. Where it will be done (if appropriate).
5. How well or to what extent it will be done.

For example:

1. David will
2. Complete a 10-minute relaxation exercise
3. At 10 P.M.
4. At home
5. On three out of seven days during each week for one month.

At any point David (or his nurse) can measure the success of his self-care plan. This is quite different from a vague statement such as "David will learn to be more relaxed."

At times, nurses expect clients to perform behaviors that were never clarified. Statements surrounding "compliance" are frequently vague. They often mean that clients should not annoy nurses but do not clearly describe what they should do. When objectives are stated behaviorally, both nurse and client are more apt to focus clearly on specific plans for success.

Goal Versus Objectives. Most clients and many nurses use the terms *goal* and *objective* interchangeably. Professionals disagree about whether the differences in these two terms should be a crucial issue in clinical settings. In academic and administrative nursing the differences are strictly recognized and "proper terminology" is often demanded. Briefly, goals are considered *broad* statements of intent or outcomes; they do not describe the process necessary to reach the goal[17] (e.g., "have low staff turnover"). Objectives, unlike goals, can be quantified and measured[18] (e.g., "each nurse will have two mental health days off with pay in every six-month period"). Objectives contribute to meeting goals—if the nursing staff is less stressed, there will perhaps be less turnover.

Both terms are integrated within this text. When clients complete self-contracts, *goal* is used because it is generally more familiar and less mysterious. An attempt has been made to use the more specific term objective when plans are being considered by the nurse. There may, of course, be some overlapping of these two terms when the nurse and client are jointly discussing self-care plans.

Regardless of the specific term utilized, there are several key guidelines that are integrated into setting self-care objectives and goals.

1. Plans for behavioral change are clear, specific, measurable, realistic, nonpunitive, and safe.
2. Breaking long-term objectives into small steps is incorporated into all plans for self-care.
3. Objectives must be carefully selected to provide enough of a challenge to give satisfaction yet not be so challenging as to be impossible to reach.
4. Objectives are *written.* This process in itself helps to clarify issues of planning and commitment to self-care.
5. Objectives are set, clarified, and reevaluated *with* clients, not *for* clients.

(Specific steps for clients to use in setting self-care goals are presented in Appendix B.)

Reaching Objectives

In Orem's model, once a direction for action has been determined, the nurse moves from designing to planning care. In a separate phase care is then actually provided and managed.[16] In this text the process of reaching objectives includes actions taken by both the nurse and client to meet specific objectives. It includes specific actions of intervention or implementation. This use overlaps with Orem's third phase (Table 3–1), in that it includes provision of actual nursing care.

Orem discusses a number of issues that merit consideration in the planning and production of nursing care (e.g., timing, setting, and supplies). The major theme of all interactions with clients, however, is the primary concern for helping people to develop and maintain an ever-increasing ability to care for themselves. This issue guides all steps taken by both the nurse and client. Orem presents a comprehensive list of potential client and nurse actions taken during this phase.[16] They all address the primary themes of maintenance or enhancement of self-care. Family members and friends are identified as playing an important role in supporting self-care accomplishments.

The planning phase begins when the nurse and client identify priorities, consider various alternative actions, and select those most suitable to achieve the objectives. These actions may be carried out by the nurse, the client, the family, or other helping people. As part of this phase, predicted consequences of any plan are pointed out to clients and family members.

Client and nurse actions typically focus on a number of areas. The roles and responsibilities of the nurse and the client (and family members) generally remain the same regardless of the specific deficit being addressed.

Themes of Client Actions	**Themes of Nursing Actions**
Initiate self-assessment	Model health and self-care
Identify priorities	Provide education (teach self-assessment and self-contracting)
Make action plan	
Follow through with each step, e.g.:	Help client build knowledge base
Make phone calls	Manipulate environment as needed for safety, privacy
Alter environment	
Buy equipment	Provide for ongoing consultation
Enlist support systems	Provide support, encouragement
Initiate self-evaluation	Reduce stumbling blocks
Identify new needs	Facilitate ongoing evaluation process

Factors that facilitate or impede stated plans are considered and dealt with. Resources, motivation, and family support in the self-care process are continually assessed.

Rationale for nursing actions is based on a variety of theoretical approaches. Since client education regarding behavioral change is a major focus of self-care nursing, integration of teaching/learning theory is central to many nursing actions. The planning phase of the nursing process is finished after objectives are identified, client and nursing actions are completed, and the actions are recorded by the nurse, the client, or a family member.

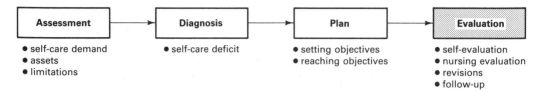

Evaluation serves as a beginning point for further assessment, planning, and intervention and provides for continued appraisal of the client's behavioral changes (see Table 3–3). When behavioral objectives have been established, it is relatively simple to assess if each specific objective was met. It is more difficult, however, to identify and analyze factors that have either facilitated or blocked attainment of objectives. The evaluation process frequently leads to recognition that additional behaviors need to be changed before initial objectives can be achieved.

Orem does not distinctly identify an evaluation phase of the nursing process. She does, however, address crucial evaluation issues in her production and management phase of nursing care. Evaluation steps taken during this phase include:

1. Helping clients to monitor themselves to determine the effectiveness of self-care measures.
2. Making nursing judgments about the sufficiency and efficiency of self-care.
3. Reviewing the meaning of alterations in self-care behavior.
4. Making recommendations for client or nurse role alteration to meet self-care needs.[16]

Self-care nursing models utilize self-evaluation extensively. In this approach the nurse does not perform an evaluation separate from ongoing interactions with the client. The client and the nurse complete the evaluation jointly and review each objective, current status of identified goals, effectiveness of each action, data adequacy and accuracy, data interpretation, and so on. The client asks: "Has my self-care behavior changed?" and "If not, why not?" The nurse asks ways in which he or she has facilitated or impeded the change process for the client. Feedback from clients regarding specific nurse and family actions is vital.

Effective follow-up provides for continuity of the self-care process and ensures that the client does not become "lost" in the health care system. Will the client need assistance a month from now from another health care provider? A return appointment in 2 weeks? Telephone follow-up on progress at regular intervals? Specific formats exist for gathering this information (see Fig. 3–2).

SUMMARY

This chapter described the way in which Orem's self-care approach to nursing process is adapted and integrated within this text. The basic phases of nursing

---

SAMPLE EVALUATION FORM

(To be completed by client before next session)

1. What was your goal(s)?

2. How have you done so far?

3. List the steps you took to reach that goal:

4. What and/or who was most helpful in reaching your goal?

5. What major problems did you have?

6. List your questions for the nurse and other health care providers:

7. What type of specific help do you need from the nurse now?

Figure 3–2. Sample evaluation form.

process were reviewed. Concepts of self-assessment and self-evaluation were emphasized. Important parallels between the nursing process and the self-care process and how they can be used simultaneously were also discussed.

STUDY QUESTIONS

Personal Focus

1. Review the ways in which the nursing process parallels the self-care process. Evaluate your ability to initiate and complete the self-care process. How does this influence your personal and professional life?

2. A self-care approach to nursing practice is built on client–nurse collaboration. Nurses cannot tell clients what to do but must work *with* them. Talk to your peers about this approach. Are there any aspects of it that you find difficult?

3. Write a behavioral self-care objective for yourself. Discuss it with a peer.

Client Focus

1. Role play a situation with a peer in which you describe the nursing process to a client. What would you say? What aspects would you emphasize?

2. How would you describe the nursing process to a physician or other health care provider? What aspects would you emphasize?

3. Assume that your new client tells you that he or she would prefer that *you* set the objectives for behavior change since he or she does not have your knowledge. What would you say? What would you do?

4. Describe a clinical situation in which a client has a relationship with a nurse but is also simultaneously practicing self-care.

REFERENCES

1. Little, D.E., & Carnevali, D.L. (1983). *Nursing care planning* (3rd ed.). Philadelphia: J.B. Lippincott, p. 222.
2. Orem, D. (1985). *Nursing: Concepts of practice* (3rd ed.). New York: McGraw-Hill, p. 31.
3. Stevens, B. (1979). *Nursing theory.* Boston: Little, Brown, p. 93.
4. Yura, H., & Walsh, M. (1983). *The nursing process* (4th ed.). New York: Appleton-Century-Crofts, p. 131.
5. Dossey, B. (1981). Nursing diagnosis. *Nursing 81, 2*(6), 34.
6. Blattner, B. (1981). *Holistic nursing.* Englewood Cliffs, NJ: Prentice-Hall.
7. Swinford, P.A. & Webster, J.A. (1989). *Promoting wellness: A nurses handbook.* Rockville, Md: Aspen Publications.
8. Dossey, B., Keegan, L., Guzzetta, C., & Kolkmeier, L. (1989). *Holistic nursing: A handbook for practice.* Rockville, Md: Aspen Publications.
9. Orem. *Nursing concepts,* p. 225.
10. Sacco, L., & Joseph, L.S. (1980). Self-care and the nursing process. *Nursing Clinics of North America, 15*(1), 140.
11. Sacco & Joseph. Self-care and the nursing process, p. 27.
12. Popkess-Vawter, S. (1984). Strength-oriented nursing diagnoses. In M.J. Kim G. McFarland, & A. McLane, (Eds.), *Classification of nursing diagnosis.* St Louis: C.V. Mosby, p. 443.
13. North American Nursing Diagnosis Association. (1987). *Classification of nursing diagnoses: Proceedings of the seventh conference.* St. Louis: C.V. Mosby.
14. Self-evaluation report. (1976). Report submitted to National League for Nursing. Dayton, OH: Wright State University, School of Nursing, p. 96.

15. Orem. *Nursing: Concepts,* p. 231.
16. Orem. *Nursing: Concepts,* p. 237–240.
17. Bailey, J.T., & Claus, K.E. (1975). *Decision making in nursing.* St. Louis: C.V. Mosby, pp. 34–35.

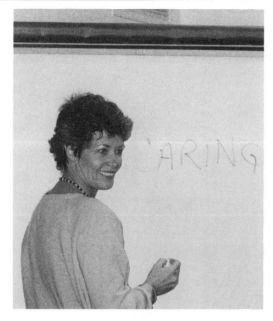

Give me a fish and I will eat for a day. Teach me to fish and I eat for a lifetime.

Chinese proverb

4 Theoretical Approaches to Self-Care

LEARNING OBJECTIVES

Upon completion of this chapter, readers will be able to:

1. List four theoretical approaches (from other disciplines) that provide a basis for self-care nursing.
2. Discuss the significance of self-care in the following nursing models: Orem, Watson, Hall, Roy, and Blattner.
3. Identify two theories relevant to self-care nursing and describe clinical use of these theories.

DEFINITIONS

Systems   A set of interrelated, interdependent parts or units. Systems may be open or closed. All living systems are open systems.

Adaptation   The person's response to the environment that promotes general goals, including survival, growth, reproduction, and mastery.

(Additional terms are defined in Table 4–1.)

INTRODUCTION

Some theoretical framework forms the basis of all professional nursing actions. Many nurses, however, may not be able to identify and verbalize their theoretical approaches to other nurses and health care providers. Nurses all too frequently use habit, tradition, or guesswork as the only basis for making nursing decisions.[1]

Although nurses need to understand the theoretical framework for their clinical actions, many view discussions of theories and models as mysterious and intimidating. Their anxiety stems from a belief that theory is the realm of academic nurses and is not relevant to daily clinical practice.

Wilson states that although theory is often considered "magical" by many nurses, it really is nothing more than an effort to describe, explain, and predict the outcome of nursing actions.[2] One way in which this is done is through identification of ongoing interrelationships in practice.[1] These significant interrelationships include those between nurses and clients and between nurses and other health care providers. When these interrelationships are clearly stated, approaches to nursing practice are also clarified.

In self-care nursing, a number of different concepts, theories, and models relate to each other and together form a theoretical framework (Table 4–1). In all clinical situations, nurses base their assessments, assumptions, and actions on a *synthesis* of various theoretical views from other disciplines (*borrowed knowledge*)[3] as well as from nursing. The models and theories reviewed in this chapter are presented in Figure 4–1. They are significant to self-care nursing practice but are not intended as an exhaustive survey of all the theories that could apply to this clinical approach.

Clinical Application

The following clinical situation demonstrates the ways in which theories are integrated into nursing practice. A case presentation is provided first. Table 4–2 then summarizes the ways in which a number of theories and models would be utilized with this family. Following this example, each theoretical approach is briefly reviewed.

TABLE 4–1. RELATIONSHIP OF CONCEPTS, THEORIES, AND MODELS

	What They Are	What They Do
Concepts	Symbols that represent a set or series of common attributes.[a] Thoughts that promote certain images. Common concepts in nursing are: humanity, health, society, patient/client/nursing.[b]	Form the basis for nursing theory. Vehicles of thought that involve images.
Theory	A broad comprehensive set of statements developed from concepts that describe, explain, and predict a particular phenomenon.[c] A statement of "how and why" something works.	They are not "magic,"[d] Theories describe, explain, and predict outcomes of situations (e.g., Bandura's "social learning theory" describes how people learn through modeling and imitation).
Model	Often used interchangeably with theory; however, models are more broad and general.[e] They are abstractions that represent symbolically the structure or skeleton of an original system (e.g., as in an architect's model of a nursing station in a hospital).	Use concepts to develop a symbolic structure that represents the actual system. Identifies the essential components of nursing practice [e.g., (1) who receives the nursing care, (2) the goal or purpose of nursing, and (3) the role and activities of the nurse].[f] Can be used to develop theory.

Concepts generate principles. Relationships between these principles generate theories which eventually are used (in a predictive manner) to solve problems. Theories are always subject to testing; the strength of a theory is dependent on how it stands the rigors of testing. Thus theories are always subject to modification. Theories generate models. (At times, models also lead back to development of new theories or refinement of current theory.)

[a]Torres, G. (1980). The place of concepts and theories within nursing. In J. George (Ed.), *Nursing theories: The base for professional nursing practice.* Englewood Cliffs, NJ: Prentice-Hall, p. 105.
[b]Torres. The place of concepts, p. 2.
[c]Torres. The place of concepts, p. 4.
[d]Wilson, H. (1982). Magic Words. San Francisco: Third Annual Self-Care Conference for Nursing Education and Service.
[e]Roy, C. & Roberts, S. (1981). *Theory construction in nursing: An adaptation model.* Englewood Cliffs, NJ: Prentice-Hall, p. 23.

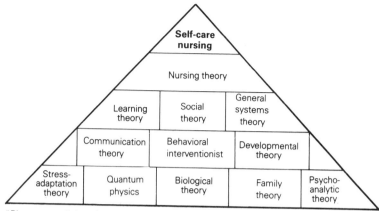

*Placement of theories on the diagram does not imply order of importance.

Figure 4–1. Theoretical approaches to self-care nursing.

Case Presentation

Fred and Ellen Hansen are both 65 years old. Their sixth and youngest child left home a month ago to attend college. Two weeks ago, Fred retired after more than 30 years in a successful administrative position with a local furniture company.

The Hansens have suddenly become aware of how much their lives had revolved around those of their children and grandchildren. All of their six children now live in different parts of the country and only occasionally visit the Hansens' small, rural community.

Since Fred's retirement, both he and Ellen are home much of the day. They are unaccustomed to this intense contact with each other and feel that "there is nothing much to talk about." They had not prepared for retirement or their recent change in life-style.

During the last month the Hansens have each had approximately five contacts with their nurse practitioner for a variety of complaints, such as colds, sore throats, back pain, and insomnia. Fred reports that he needs a hernia operation and would like to schedule it immediately. They have not been adequately caring for themselves. They find it hard to "buy food and cook only for two—so we often don't have dinner."

During contacts with the nurse, the Hansens eventually began to talk about some of their feelings of sadness over the loss of their familiar roles. They also explained how anxious they were about forming a new relationship with each other. Table 4–2 presents examples of the ways in which theoretical material could be helpful for nurses working with this couple.

TABLE 4–2. SAMPLE APPLICATION OF THEORIES AND MODELS

Theory and Model	Potential Application
Teaching/learning theories Operant/reinforcement Gestalt/cognitive Humanistic Social learning	A combination of many teaching/learning theories will form a basis for educational interventions with the Hansens. They may need to be taught new self-care skills relative to their recent life-style changes (e.g., maintaining good nutrition even though there are no children at home). Their thoughts and feelings about aging, perceived loss of their children, and changes in their personal relationship will also be explored. Recognition of their unique experiences will occur; they will also be taught the normal, expected experiences during this phase. The nurse will serve as a model of health and demonstrate self-care skills.
Communication theories	Effective communication will form the core of all interactions between the Hansens and the nurse. The nurse will serve as a model for clear and assertive communication and will help the couple develop skills in this area.
Systems theory Family systems Social systems	Nursing diagnosis and interventions are partially based on recognition that Fred and Ellen Hansen's behaviors have an impact on each other. Aging and illness of their parents will have an impact on the Hansen children.
Developmental theories	"Normal" emotional and physical development during this phase of aging or maturity will be explained to the Hansens. The nurse will be aware of developmental tasks for this life period. The Hansens' progress with these tasks will be assessed and discussed.
Stress/adaptation theory	The Hansens have experienced four major changes in the last few months. This stress leads to wear and tear on the body. Their recent physical illnesses may be seen as a reflection of their high stress levels. They will be taught to limit life changes and plan effectively for those that cannot be avoided.
Psychodynamic theory	The Hansens may be helped to explore individually their deeper feelings about loss and aging. In a nondirective way the process of development of insight will be facilitated. Focus will be on the meaning of these recent changes and how that relates to past experience.
Biological theory	Ongoing physical assessment will be a component of contact with this family. Their physical health status will be continually reevaluated. Physical factors associated with their current anxiety and sadness will be considered (e.g., anemia, cardiac difficulty).
Nursing models Orem's self-care model Hall's care-core-cure model Roy's adaptation model Blattner's holistic model Watson's theory of human care	In all five nursing models, helping the Hansens to develop and maintain new self-care skills will be one focus of intervention. Education regarding predictable maturational stress during this life phase will take place; ways to manage this stress will also be taught. In each model the Hansens will play an active role in assessing their problems and setting goals for new behavior.

A META-THEORY FOR SELF-CARE: GENERAL SYSTEMS THEORY

We know that working with self-care requires the utilization of information, models, and theories from a variety of disciplines. How can this information, each with its own set of jargon, be integrated in some useful and meaningful way?

The founder of general systems theory, Bertalanffy described its objectives in five points[4]:

1. There is a tendency toward integration of concepts and principles among the basic and behavioral sciences.
2. The integration reflects a core belief in an overall general theory of systems.
3. This general systems theory helps to identify theory in non-physical fields of science.
4. General systems theory also helps to unify scientific concepts and theory by developing and identifying concepts and principles that run vertically through the individual sciences.
5. Adoption of these ideas can help to further scientific education.

Kramer and de Smit see two purposes for the utilization of systems thinking:

1. Development of a common language.
2. To give insight into methodology inherent in the systems approach—the holistic approach.[5]

A system is a set of interrelated, interdependent parts or units. Systems theory describes and predicts the way in which these sets function to maintain equilibrium. Systems may be open or closed. All living systems are open systems. A system is assumed to have a tendency to achieve balance among the various forces operating within and on it. *Equilibrium* or *steady state* are two terms that describe this phenomenon. Another major assumption of this model is that change in one part of the system will effect change in all other parts of the system—just as moving one part of a delicately balanced mobile will cause all parts of the mobile to move.

Systems theory supports the concept of holism. A whole is different from and more than a summation of its individual parts. Each client is seen as an integrated system with relationships among its parts. The nurse is interested in all of these parts and not just one of them. Use of general systems theory helps the nurse to understand and synthesize information from a variety of disciplines. The "borrowed" theories and models that are most relevant to self-care nursing are presented below. This brief review is not intended as a comprehensive discussion of each formulation. It is presented only to support potential applications to self-care nursing.

Teaching/Learning Theory

Learning is a relatively permanent change in behavior that occurs as the result of experience.[6] Learning theories deal with how and why people learn and change behavior. Clients usually need to learn how to practice self-care; they also need to learn ways to motivate themselves on a regular basis.

The nurse plays a major role in helping clients to correct knowledge deficits in specific self-care areas. To do this, the nurse must base clinical practice on sound theories of learning.

Four major learning theories are utilized in self-care approaches to nursing. They are operant conditioning/reinforcement theory, gestalt/cognitive field, humanistic, and social learning theory.

Operant Conditioning/Reinforcement Theory

Operant conditioning refers to the fact that behavior can be altered through stimulus–response pairing (for example, a pigeon will learn to peck a certain number of times to achieve food). Insight and the meaning of behavior are not relevant in this theory of learning. Behavior modification is a form of operant conditioning.

Reinforcement theory explains the development as well as the management of behavior and thus forms the basis of behavior modification. It identifies the fact that reinforced behaviors tend to be repeated. Nurses regularly use reinforcement techniques. The use of praise and feedback while helping women to focus and deep-breathe during labor and delivery provides an example of this.

Punishment is also a form of operant conditioning. For example, Antabuse is used as an aversive stimulus (punishment) with alcoholics. Schick smoking clinics utilize mild electric shock as a deterrent to smoking. These techniques sometimes provide rapid improvement, but behavior change is generally not maintained over time.

As clients learn new self-care skills, praise and reinforcement facilitate and maintain these new behaviors. Self-assessment, self-monitoring, and self-contracting are used to help people learn and practice self-care. The framework for all of these approaches is taken primarily from operant conditioning and reinforcement theory (see Chapter 6).

Gestalt Learning/Cognitive Field Theory

In this learning model, biological and social factors within one's environment are seen as intertwined in important ways. A basic assumption of this theory is that people do the best they can for themselves relative to their unique perceptions.[7] This assumption is particularly relevant to self-care nursing. Clients perceive the psychological aspects of their personal, physical, and social worlds in unique ways. They then act on these perceptions and beliefs. Self-care education often involves the process of correcting false beliefs that have led to repetition of poor health care practices.

With cognitive approaches the first step is to point out that only practice and hard work will correct irrational thoughts and beliefs. Self-defeating behavior (for example, smoking, overeating, failure to use seat belts) are seen as related to antecedents and understandable causes. Ellis' rational emotive model (Chapter 6) utilizes cognitive learning theory and also applies to self-care nursing.[8,9]

Humanistic Learning Theory

This learning theory places major emphasis on the "whole person" and the meaning of the experiences and resulting behavior of each person. Humanists focus on the emotional components of behavior and place less emphasis on cognitive aspects. A major assumption of this model is that behavior is directed toward achieving increased personal adequacy and ability to cope with life. Self-evaluation and self-criticism foster independence, creativity, and self-reliance.[10,11]

The relationship between student and teacher (like that of client and nurse in self-care nursing) is also significant in the humanistic learning process. This approach views learning as being enhanced by the warmth, acceptance, and continued encouragement of the teacher.

Social Learning Theory

Bandura defines social learning as the process of learning new behavior or modifying undesirable behavior through a process of imitation or role taking. This type of learning can be conscious or unconscious and can occur with or without reinforcement for the imitative behavior.[12] This model is popular, in part, because it blends cognitive, humanistic, and reinforcement models of learning.

A major aim in nursing is enhancing the client's knowledge, motivation, and skills to perform self-care. Modeling of health and self-care behavior is a primary way of accomplishing this goal. Clients tend to imitate the behavior of their nurses. Chapter 5 presents a more detailed exploration of the role of the nurse as a social model of self-care.

Table 4–3 presents some of the major principles of teaching/learning derived from these four learning theories. These principles are integrated in all approaches to teaching clients about self-care.

Behavioral Interventionist Model

During the last several years, there has been significant growth in the field of behavioral medicine. This particular model recognizes that behavioral and environmental interventions to promote lifestyle change can have major impact on quality of life and life expectancy.

There are four key assumptions in this model: (1) The interventionist influences the participant by encouraging responsibility assumption; (2) the interventionist offers pathways to new behaviors; (3) the ultimate decision for behavior change rests with the participant; and, (4) therefore, only the participant can change his or her behavior.[13]

TABLE 4–3. TEACHING/LEARNING PRINCIPLES: APPLICATION TO SELF-CARE NURSING[a]

Operant Conditioning/ Reinforcement Model	Gestalt Learning- Cognitive Field Model	Humanistic Learning Model	Social Learning Model[b]
Clients should learn by "doing," not by being passive. Clients need to repeat and practice new self-care skills. Rewards should be built into new learning activities. Reinforcement is essential. Initially, reinforcement should be given immediately following the desired behavioral response. Once the desired response has been learned, intermittent reinforcement maintains positive behaviors most effectively.	Many sense experiences should be used when learning new skills (e.g., touch, sight, smell, etc.) Direction of learning should be from simple to complex. The *meaning* of self-care in the whole context of the client's life is important. Clarity as to these relationships will enhance learning of new skills. Goals should be set by clients. Clients should continually restate their beliefs and perceptions. Creative thinking should be encouraged.	Anxiety level may add or detract from new learning. Interventions to lower anxiety may be of first priority. Different types of learners respond best to different types of environments. The learning atmosphere will influence the outcome of teaching. The client's first concerns must be satisfied before other issues can be dealt with.[c] Nurses need to help clients feel that they are capable of coping with new learning tasks.[c]	Clients learn by observing their nurses. Family members need to pay attention to the impact that they have on each other's health behaviors. Self-care is learned most effectively by imitation of the health care provider's health behavior.

[a]Hilgard, E.R. & Bower, G.H. (1975). *Theories of learning* (4th ed.). Englewood Cliffs, NJ: Prentice-Hall, pp. 608–609. © 1975.)
[b]Additional implications for this model are presented in Chapter 5.
[c]Jenny, J. (1979). Humanistic strategy for patient teaching. *Health Values: Achieving High-Level Wellness, 3,* 175-180.

It is the nurse's responsibility to create a climate for change and intervention. In establishing a therapeutic relationship with a client, it is necessary to create a high level of involvement including joint decision making, achievement of internal commitment, and exploration of the pitfalls occurring during the process.

The nurse needs to recognize that the assumption of responsibility by the client to change behavior is essential for this model to work. Responsibility avoidance by the client sabotages the process. Contracting and modeling, as well as many other techniques, can also play major roles.

Communication Theory

All communication has a denotative (what the words actually say) and a connotative (more subtle meaning of the words, including nonverbal communication) level. Ideally, these two levels would match as messages were sent back and forth between the senders and receivers. Then people would not feel misunderstood and become frustrated in efforts to express their feelings and needs. In reality, perfect matching between what is said and what is understood by the receiver rarely occurs.

Accurate communication is particularly relevant to self-care nursing. Nurses must be able to communicate clearly and assertively. As nurses help clients identify their self-care needs, it is crucial to be sure that as much distortion as possible is removed from their interactions (e.g., "guessing," "reading into what the person says," "ignoring nonverbal clues").

Psychoanalytic Theory

One of the major assumptions of self-care theory is that people are interested in making positive health decisions on their own behalf.[14] At times it appears that clients are not capable of this. People often do not act in their own best interest, but rather perform repetitive, self-destructive behaviors without awareness or ability to change or control their actions (for example, drug abuse, smoking, alcoholism). Deficits in the area of motivation to perform specific self-care practices exist in these instances.[15]

Psychoanalytic theory forms one basis for understanding these deficits in motivation. All psychological models incorporate, in at least some way, Freud's discovery and labeling of the conscious and unconscious. The psychoanalytic model places emphasis on the attainment of conscious control of behavior. Interventions are focused on strengthening the personality and thus helping the person to achieve a satisfying adjustment to reality.[16]

Self-care nursing, like psychoanalytic models, also places emphasis on conscious control of behavior. Deficits in motivation to practice self-care are acknowledged. Nurses help clients to see the role that the past had and still has in the formation of current self-care deficits.

Family Systems Model

Families are open systems. A change in one family member affects all family members. Just as any one physiological system (for example, the endocrine system) or any one family member strives for equilibrium, family units also strive for balance and homeostasis. When a client has a heart attack, change occurs in the whole family. The client's eldest daughter may have to quit college and get a job. The spouse may have to spend long periods of time at the hospital and have trouble getting off from work. Young children may miss both parents. The family system will strive to reduce this tension and reach some adaptive state. New individual and joint resources will be utilized in this effort. For some families, dissolution is the most adaptive state and provides optimum tension reduction. Nurses use knowledge of family systems in helping families to predict and manage responses to stress.

Social Systems Model

In addition to being part of a family, clients are also parts of other social systems, such as work, school, neighborhood, and so on. In a simplified sense, social systems function in ways that are most likely to reduce tension and maintain equilibrium. Ways in which power is lost, gained, and maintained within institutions are described in this model. Change is particularly difficult for some people and in some social settings. A very traditional hospital system, for example, may find it particularly difficult to allow fathers to observe and participate in cesarean deliveries. Nurses need to acknowledge the power of social systems to enhance or block efforts to develop self-care programs within institutions.

Developmental Theories

Development is often used to refer to both growth (actual increase in size or complexity) and maturation (a sequential unfolding at fixed rates). Humanistic and holistic models of nursing use the term "development" in a broad sense that includes elements of both personal growth and maturation.

Erikson, Freud, Piaget, Sullivan, and Kohlberg each has developmental models that assume change is part of life. These models focus on processes of growth and maturation. "Developmental models postulate that the system under scrutiny—a person, small group, interpersonal interaction, an organization, a community or a society—is going 'somewhere,' that the changes have some direction."[17]

These directional changes may be identified as "stages," "levels," or "phases." Each stage or phase of life has characteristic tasks that must be completed for further development to occur. Each individual follows *predictable* phases in development. Personal styles of development can coexist within these predictable phases. Although all individuals go through certain phases, their behavior in each phase may vary. Each person reacts in slightly different ways to adolescence, childbirth, or death.

Nurses include a developmental perspective in all work with clients. The knowledge that clients will experience certain kinds of stress at each developmental phase provides one basis for health education and other nursing interventions.

Stress/Adaptation Theory

Certain illnesses, such as headaches, heart attacks, colitis, diabetes, backaches, and arthritis, are commonly linked to stress.[18] Theories that describe physiological and psychological reactions to stress help the nurse predict how clients may respond in particularly stressful situations. Differentiating between typical and atypical reactions in these circumstances is central to appropriate diagnosis and effective interventions.

Selye, the "grandfather of stress theory," identifies stress as a universal phenomenon that occurs with all changes, regardless of desirability of the change and degree of control of the situation.[19] Stress requires a series of physical and emotional adaptations.

Both positive (eustress) *and* negative (distress) changes are stressful to people and elicit the same physiological response. People react to stress differently depending on the amount and the specific meaning it has for them in their family and social environment.

Selye has described specific emotional, physiological, and cognitive changes that occur at different phases in reacting to stress. He points out that each person needs to find his or her own natural predilections and stress levels—the best level that promotes personal growth and health and prevents illness.[20]

Stress is needed for growth and survival; the goal is not to eliminate it but to reduce unnecessary sources and maintain healthy and adaptive responses when it does occur.

Levels of stress and the impact of stress on daily life are acknowledged in the self-assessment process. Assessment tools such as the Holmes and Rahe Social Readjustment Rating Scale (see Appendix A) help clients recognize the number of stressful changes they experience.[21] Extensive changes in personal, family, and work life are positively correlated with a higher potential for illness. Clients can use this information in practicing self-care—a client who has had a new baby, changed jobs, and moved to a new house will learn that she needs to limit any further life changes and pay particular attention to her health for the next six months in order to decrease her potential for becoming ill.

Lazarus and Folkman have added significantly to this body of knowledge through looking at stress appraisal, coping, and adaptational outcomes.[22] Their work utilizes a transactional model to view the person and the environment in a mutually reciprocal, bi-directional relationship. They view stress as a "relationship between the person and the environment that is appraised by the person as taxing or exceeding his/her resources and endangering his/her well-being."[23]

Biological Theory

Biological theory includes extensive scientific formulations concerning the physiological components of illness. Elaborate classification systems categorize the signs and symptoms observed by the nurse, physicians, other health care providers, and the client. Clinicians sometimes assume that disease is the result of genetic or physiological factors, so they place less emphasis on the emotional and psychological condition of the client. This has been the major focus of the traditional medical model.

Nurses in every setting incorporate biological theory into practice. Nurses are aware of the functioning of body systems in health and illness. Holistic assessments require attention to the physical status, somatic symptoms, manifestations of organic disease, metabolic disturbances, and so on, as well as psychosocial history of the client. The ability to understand the interrelationships between physical *and* psychosocial factors in health and illness is vital.

Biological theory cannot be ignored in self-care nursing. All self-care skills are facilitated when clients are able to see connections between their physiological and psychological states.

Quantum Physics Theory

Quantum physics deals with the movements and changes of matter and energy at the levels of atomic and subatomic matter. This new approach underpins all functions of the body: moving, breathing, eating, building, minding, healing, and transforming. It offers new insight into physical processes, consciousness, health, and disease.[24]

Through quantum physics, "one can see that the mind begins to emerge as evidence of the ancient 'soul'—that which governs the body, both consciously and unconsciously."[25] Consciousness, in its quantum role as observer, alters the body, enabling each bodily function to occur.[26]

NURSING MODELS AND SELF-CARE

Nursing models are also used as a framework for self-care practice. Orem has outlined a basic approach for application of self-care concepts in nursing. Her specific structure and ideas are presented in Chapters 2 and 3 and are not repeated here. There are many other nursing theorists who utilize self-care concepts that may be labeled in slightly different ways. Orem sees the major goal of nursing as helping people learn to sustain life and health, recover from disease or injury, and cope with their effects.[27] Other nursing models have very similar goals.

For many years the work of Henderson, Orlando, Weidenbach, and many others has influenced nurses to help clients learn to care for themselves more effectively. While self-care is a part of most nursing models, only four contemporary nursing models have been selected for discussion in the interest of space and simplicity. The remaining part of this chapter briefly presents the nursing models of Watson, Hall, Roy, and Blattner and discusses the ways in which these overlap or differ from Orem regarding the concept of self-care. For consistency, the term *client* will be used in presenting all models.*

Watson: Theory of Human Care

Watson looks at nursing within a human science and art context. Her values point to a deep respect for the individual's ability to change and grow. She sees nurses facilitating the person's growth toward gaining increased self-knowledge, self-control, and self-healing within health and illness. The nurse's role is one of a co-participant in change through the human care process.

Major goals are identified as a preservation of harmony with mind-body-soul and maintenance of human dignity and integrity. These goals are associated with finding meaning in existence and experience, mental and spiritual growth, and potentiating instances of transcendence and self-healing.[29]

Hall: Care-Core-Cure

Hall has developed a theory of nursing based on the concepts of "care," "core," and "cure." Her approach places emphasis on self-care, although she does not use this specific term. Her *care* component of nursing involves the nursing contacts relevant to a laying-on of hands. She specifically perceives this as bodily care and translates it as the nurturance component of practice.

The *core* component, on the other hand, refers to the therapeutic use of self in all nonphysical contacts with clients. In this context the nurse helps the client to express feelings about the disease process. Self-healing and improvements in self-esteem are seen to follow this process. Hall's assumption is that the "motivation and energy necessary for healing exist within the patient rather than in the health care team."[29]

The *cure* component comprises specific interventions based on physical prescriptions. This element, which often includes delivery of medical care rather than nursing practice, most closely involves other members of the health team.

Hall's theory of nursing was specifically implemented for a rehabilitation setting. She has identified it as appropriate for adult clients who are not in acute phases. Her model has been criticized as being too restrictive and limited, but Hale and George have pointed out that applications in a number of settings are possible.[30]

---

*Except when using direct quotes.

In Hall's model clients are explicitly viewed as in control of their health. Data collection is for the benefit of the client and not the nurse. Its focus is to increase client self-awareness. The nurse works with the client and family to help them understand and implement health plans. Client-made decisions are continually supported. Changes in outward behavior are seen as a reflection of growth in self-awareness. This model is essentially an insight-oriented approach to nursing practice and emphasizes psychodynamic principles.

Hall places an emphasis on client responsibility for personal health and growth. This is consistent with Orem's self-care model. Orem's model, however, places more emphasis on active reeducation of clients. Hall views teaching of clients in a more nondirective and permissive sense. Reflection is used as a primary, nondirective tool in helping clients to acknowledge and alter internal feelings and motivation.

Hall's teaching methods potentially take much longer (perhaps because she worked with clients on a long-term basis) than the more active approaches advocated by Orem. In reality, clinicians probably utilize a combination of both of these approaches. In some instances, actively teaching a client about vital health information is appropriate to facilitate the client's abilities to gain that information in his or her own way over longer periods of time.

Roy: Adaptation Model of Nursing

Roy's adaptation model utilizes a systems theory framework. Although she does not use the specific term "self-care," the concept is central to her formulations. Roy has pointed out that she views the client holistically and is striving to develop a theory of the holistic person as an adaptive system.[31]

Roy's early work identifies the client as an individual. Her later writings extend the meaning of "client" to a family, group, community, or society.[31]

Roy views the nurse as a "promoter of client adaptation." She describes four primary adaptive modes: physiological needs, self-concept, role function, and interdependence.[31] Roy's view is similar to Orem's in that the nurse's role is to help the client learn and practice self-care, an adaptive activity. The client is respected as an active participant in all health care. This is also true in the Hall and Blattner models.

Clinicians practicing from Roy's model manipulate stimuli in the client's environment. (e.g., reducing excessive light or noise may be necessary to promote sleep.) Clients may need assistance in increasing, decreasing, or modifying both internal and external stimuli to promote adaptation.

Both client and nurse are actively involved in the assessment of specific needs and the plans to alter these stimuli. In cases where clients are completely incapable of participating in this type of process, nurses are seen as *temporarily* assuming this role for the person.[31] This parallels Orem's differentiation of circumstances in which "wholly compensatory care" is needed (see Chapter 2).

In Roy's model, health teaching is seen as a central nursing intervention and as an activity that promotes adaptation. This again parallels the emphasis on education in the Orem, Watson, Hall, and Blattner models.

Blattner: Holistic Nursing

Blattner has developed a holistic nursing model that closely incorporates many of the ideas and concepts of Orem's self-care model. The goal of her model is "to use preventive, nurturative, and generative activities to assist clients toward achieving their own high-level wellness."[32]

Preventive nursing activities are those that maintain and promote health and prevent health disruption, as in teaching prenatal nutrition classes.[33] *Nurturative* activities involve caring, comforting, supporting, and sustaining, such as providing support for the family of a dying relative. This aspect of Blattner's model parallels parts of both the care and core components of Hall's model.[33]

Her third type of nursing activity is *generative*. These are creative and innovative healing techniques that encourage client, family, and community self-care and self-help.[33] Helping participants of a senior citizens' center establish self-care groups is an example of this. This is a much wider focus than that of Hall's model, which pertains primarily to individual clients. Blattner's focus on generative nursing activities is closer to Orem's concept of self-care nursing. Both emphasize building and supporting the clients' and community's abilities to manage and maintain health.

Teaching self-care skills is clearly one focus of her model. Blattner conceptualizes three areas in which the processes of her nursing model are focused: (1) intrapersonal areas, (2) interpersonal areas, and (3) community systems.

Self-awareness and self-responsibility are the cornerstones of holistic health nursing.[33] They are also central in the Orem and Hall models. In all of these models, clients bear active responsibility for their own behavior and responses in health or illness states. Table 4–4 compares the four models discussed in this section.

SUMMARY

This chapter described the way in which nursing theories and models provide a basis for all nursing actions. General systems theory was used as a meta-theory to provide a framework for understanding and synthesis of interdisciplinary theories utilized in nursing intervention. Clinical utilization of this material was demonstrated in one case presentation.

This chapter presented an overview of theories relevant to self-care. Included were: teaching/learning, behavioral interventionist, communication,

TABLE 4–4. COMPARISON OF NURSING MODELS

Nursing Model	View of Client	Goal of Nursing	Nurse's Role: Focus of Intervention	Comments
Orem's self-care model, 1959	Client and environment form an integrated system. The person is a unity, functioning biologically, symbolically, and socially. Clients are responsible for performing actions on their own behalf.	To provide help for individuals unable to help themselves. Help client learn self-care actions to sustain life and health as well as recover from disease and cope with its effects.	Consultant and teacher. Assesses if and why client needs help. Education is major intervention to correct self-care deficits. Interventions may be partly or wholly compensatory or supportive-educative.	Focus on education of clients. Model not originally defined for use with out-patients.
Hall's care-core-cure model, 1960	Motivation and energy for healing are within the client. Client is in control and is the best person to set goals and priorities.	To help the client reach the core of the problem. Change in behavior follows understanding.	Advocate for clients. Provides alternative choices for clients. Reflection leads to insight, a major intervention. Permissive, nondirective teaching.	Originally designed for rehabilitative nursing. Client seen as center for health. More psychodynamic than behavioral in orientation.
Roy's adaptation model, 1969	The person is a "whole being" in constant interaction with the environment. Adapts to change through different modes to maintain integrity. Client plays active role in the health care process. Sets goals with the nurse.	To promote adaptation through adaptive modes. Help clients to adapt by manipulating the environment.	Assess adaptation or maladaptation with clients. Attempts to manipulate environment by either increasing, decreasing, or altering stimuli in the environment to assist adaptive behavior.	Sees client as active in the process of health care. Education is central to nursing intervention.
Blattner's holistic nursing model, 1980	Client is responsible for own body and mind. Can choose sickness or health. Client is a very active participant in the health system.	To use preventive, nurturative, and generative actions to assist clients toward achieving their own high-level wellness.	Uses nine life processes to prevent illness, nurture health, and generate new ways of healing. Holistic model used for self-growth as well as for clients.	Places emphasis on preventive as well as more traditional actions. Self-help valued. Self-awareness in both nurse and client emphasized. Nurse is a model for self-responsibility.
Watson's theory of human care, 1985	Individual patients are viewed as agents of change. Allows self to be healed through both internal and external means. Has a commitment to preservation of harmony with mind-body-soul.	Mental–spiritual growth for self and others. Finding meaning in one's own existence and experience, discovering inner power and control, and potentiating instances of transcendence and self-healing.	Nurse can be co-participant in change through human care process. Utilizes interventions which are referred to as carative factors.	Perspective is spiritual–existential and phenomenological while drawing on eastern philosophy.

psychoanalytic, systems, developmental, stress/adaptation, quantum physics, and biological theories. The nursing models of Watson, Hall, Roy, and Blattner were discussed relative to their perspectives on self-care and were compared with Orem's model.

STUDY QUESTIONS

Personal Focus

1. Identify the theory that has (or theories that have) most influenced your perspective of self-care.
2. Review Table 4–3; identify the ways that are most effective in helping you learn a new skill.
3. Which approaches to self-care have you found most helpful in working with your family? Friends?

Client Focus

1. Identify the nursing model or models utilized in your educational or clinical setting. Discuss this model or models with your peers. Summarize the goal, role of the client, and role of the nurse in this model.
2. Choose a client from your current practice. Identify the major theories and models that you use or will use in being helpful to this client.
3. What is the relationship of life stress to illness? Describe your current clients who have diseases labeled as "psychosomatic." What stresses did they have in the weeks or months before the onset of their illnesses? How could you teach these clients about limiting life changes?

REFERENCES

1. Torres, G. (1980). The place of concepts and theories within nursing. In J. George (Ed.), *Nursing theories: The base for professional nursing practice.* Englewood Cliffs, NJ: Prentice-Hall, p. 4.
2. Wilson, H. (1982). Magic Words. San Francisco: Third Annual Self-Care Conference for Nursing Education and Service.
3. Johnson, D. (1968). Theory in nursing: Borrowed and unique. *Nursing Research,* 17(3), 206–209.
4. von Bertalanffy, L. (1956). General systems theory; *Foundations, development, applications.* New York, G. Braziller. p. 21.
5. Kramer, N.J.T.A., & de Smit, J. (1977). *Systems thinking.* Leiden, Netherlands: Martinus Nijhoff Social Sciences Division, p. 6.
6. Lefrancois, G.R. (1972). *Psychological theories and human learning: Konger's report.* Monterey, CA: Brooks/Cole, pp. 7–8.

7. Bigge, M.L. (1971). *Learning theories for teachers.* New York: Harper & Row, pp. 204–210.

8. Ellis, A. (1973). *Humanistic psychotherapy: The rational-emotive approach.* New York: Julian Press/McGraw-Hill.

9. Ellis, A. (1979). Rational emotive therapy. In R. Corcini (Ed.), *Current psychotherapies.* Itasca, IL: F.E. Peacock, p. 185.

10. Rogers, C. (1961). *On becoming a person.* Columbus, OH: Charles E. Merrill.

11. Rogers, C. (1969). *Freedom to learn.* Columbus, OH: Charles E. Merrill.

12. Bandura, A. (1977). *Social learning theory.* Englewood Cliffs, NJ: Prentice-Hall, p. 22.

13. Benfari, R.C. (1987). Behavioral models and methods for preventive health programs. In H.F. Vanderschmidt, D. Koch-Weser, P.A. Woodbury (Eds.), *Handbook of clinical prevention.* Baltimore, MD: Williams & Wilkins, pp. 93–121.

14. Levin, L.S. (1976). The layperson as the primary health care practioner. *Public Health Reports, 91*(3), 209.

15. Orem, D.E. (1985). *Nursing: Concepts of practice* (3rd ed.). New York: McGraw-Hill.

16. Ford, D.H., & Urban, H.B. (1963). *Systems of psychotherapy.* New York: John Wiley & Sons.

17. Chin, R. (1980). The utility of systems models and developmental models for practitioners. In J.P. Riehl & C. Roy (Eds.), *Conceptual models for nursing practice* (2nd ed.). New York: Appleton-Century-Crofts, p. 30.

18. Siegel, B. (1989). *Peace, Love, and Healing.* New York: Harper & Row.

19. Selye, H. (1976). *The stress of life* (rev. ed.), New York: McGraw-Hill.

20. Selye, H. (1981). Foreword. In B. Blattner, *Holistic nursing.* Englewood Cliffs, NJ: Prentice-Hall, pp. vi–vii.

21. Holmes, T.H., & Rahe, R.H. (1967). The social readjustment rating scale. *Journal of Psychosomatic Research, II,* 213–218.

22. Lazarus, R.S., & Folkman, S. (1984). *Stress, appraisal, and coping.* New York: Springer, p. 325.

23. Lazarus & Folkman. *Stress, appraisal, and coping,* p. 21.

24. Wolf, F.A. (1986). *The body quantum: The new physics of body, mind, and health.* New York: Macmillan, p. xviii.

25. Wolf. *The body quantum,* p. xxi.

26. Wolf. *The body quantum,* p. xxv.

27. Orem. *Nursing: Concepts,* pp. 24–47.

28. Watson, J. (1985). *Nursing: Human science and human care, a theory of nursing.* Norwalk, CT: Appleton-Century-Crofts, pp. 73–74.

29. Hall, L.E. (1966). Another view of nursing care and quality. In K.M. Straub & K.S. Parker (Eds.), *Continuity of patient care: The role of nursing.* Washington, DC: Catholic University of America Press, pp. 47–66.

30. Hale, K., & George, J.B. (1980). Lydia E. Hall. In J. George (Ed.), *Nursing theories: The base for professional nursing practice.* Englewood Cliffs, NJ: Prentice-Hall, p. 42.

31. Roy, C., & Roberts, S. (1981). *Theory construction in nursing: An adaptation model.* Englewood Cliffs, NJ: Prentice-Hall.

32. Blattner, B. (1981). *Holistic nursing.* Englewood Cliffs, NJ: Prentice-Hall.

33. Blattner. *Holistic nursing,* p. 25.

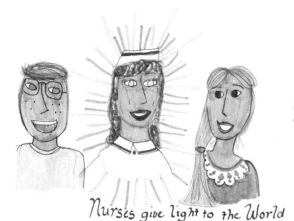

Nurses give light to the World

Example is not the main thing in influencing others, it is the only thing.

Albert Schweitzer

5 Modeling

LEARNING OBJECTIVES

Upon completion of this chapter, readers will be able to:

1. Describe the significance of social learning as related to nursing practice.
2. Identify ways in which health and self-care behaviors are learned.
3. Identify both positive and negative ways in which nurses model health.

DEFINITIONS

Model   A person who teaches by demonstrating new ideas, skills, and behavior.
Social Learning   The process of learning new behavior through imitation.
Imitation   The act of copying behavior from another person.

Identification   A process that occurs when the subject takes on the values or qualities of the model.

INTRODUCTION

Modeling defines the way in which people learn by *observing* others. Long ago Aristotle said, "Man is the most imitative of all living creatures, and through imitation learns his earliest lessons."[1] According to Bagehot, "Modeling is undoubtedly one of the strongest and most enduring elements of human nature."[2]

Modeling is a phenomenon that is easy to observe within the animal kingdom. Lorenz has written about his discovery of "imprinting" in the animal world.[3] At certain developmental points newly hatched goslings follow any moving object and believe it to be their mother. In natural situations, it is the mother's behavior that becomes imprinted on its baby. Most animals learn to find food and to seek safety and shelter by observing and imitating the behavior of mature models. Without the ability to learn by observation, they could not survive.

In the same way, children prepare for life by imitating behaviors modeled by their parents, grandparents, brothers, and sisters. Acquisition of language provides a simple example. Children learn to talk by imitating sounds. Usually they receive praise, even if their imitation is only a rough approximation of an actual word. This praise helps children learn, and they continue to copy the language of their adult models.

Parents are often chagrined by the fact that children imitate the language of their models even *after* learning to speak. ("We use those 'four-letter words' at home when we are mad, but *you are not* to use them at school or at Grandma's.")

Modeling of sex-role behavior is another example of the way that people learn by observing and copying the behavior of others. Baby girls watch their mothers and pretend to cook. Boys watch their fathers drive off to work and pretend to do the same. As roles change, so does this play acting: boys cook and girls grab a briefcase.

Significance of Modeling in Learning and Maintaining Health Behavior

"During the socialization process, children adopt many health-related habits and practices which will permanently influence their adult behavior."[4] The child learns this self-care from daily observation of models. Brushing teeth, eating, sleeping, and exercising are examples of these basic practices. If children see their parents exercise every day, they will probably do the same. In school, children learn health promotion skills and ways of handling illness from the school nurse and their teachers.

Health-enhancing activities learned in childhood are carried on throughout adult life. Unfortunately other values and behaviors are also learned. When a girl is told that menstruation is a "curse," and that she should not exercise during this time, she may hold this belief throughout her life. Learned attitudes and behaviors are very difficult to change.

It is *difficult* to help people learn to value and practice positive health behavior if they have had no early models for that behavior. It is still *possible*, however, and it does occur. Even for adults, modeling is one of the primary ways through which changes in values and behavior can occur.

Some of these models—Jack LaLanne, Charles Atlas, Joe Bonomo, and Richard Simmons—have had national followings. Through their "fitness fads" they have provided excellent health models for adults. Jane Fonda has become a health and fitness model of unprecedented scope. Adults imitate her behavior (and that of popular Jazzercise or aerobic dance instructors on television) in the same fashion that children imitate the health behaviors of their parents.

MODELING: SOCIAL LEARNING THEORY

Bandura's social learning theory has been briefly discussed in Chapter 4. His primary belief is that learning new behavior, modifying current behavior, and extinguishing unwanted behavior all occur in the social-learning context of group interactions. He believes that behavior patterns are most effectively learned through two primary factors[5]:

1. Influence of social models (such as parents, teachers, television heroes, nurses)
2. Differential reinforcement (such as praise or reward) being predictably associated with the behavior[5]

It can be inferred that these two factors are of primary importance in the learning and maintenance of self-care health behaviors.

Imitation is a concept central to social learning theory; it is the act of copying a model or example. Bandura says that imitation of behavior by *observing* others is the basis of human learning.[5] Both children and adults, for example, sing the songs and jingles of television commercials. As in sports or art, the behavior or skills of others are often copied with great conscious effort. At other times, learning through modeling may not involve conscious thought. The little boy who struts after seeing an Arnold Schwarzenegger film is probably not aware that he is recording or displaying Schwarzenegger's movements.

Identification is another concept that is central to social learning theory. This term refers to the way in which children "become the same" or take on the same qualities and values of their models, usually their parents. This behavior become an enduring part of the individual's personality and life-style.

Identification occurs when imitation has already been present for a prolonged period of time. Attitudes about life, health, religion, money, and politics occur through the process of identification.

The ultimate goal in modeling health care behavior is not merely to encourage temporary imitative action but to *promote long-lasting life changes*. When health values are incorporated through the process of identification (that is, not merely imitated), long-term health behavior change will occur.

Bandura and his colleagues have refined their social learning theory. Their work has specific applications to the learning and maintenance of self-care health behaviors.[5,6] Findings of particular relevance to self-care nursing include the following:

- Clients will practice self-care in the context of the *value* placed on it in their culture. It may take some time for clients to imitate health behaviors modeled by nurses if they are from different cultures.
- Clients will more readily imitate nurses whom they perceive to be *similar* to themselves in terms of values, race, social class, culture, and so on.[7]
- Clients who are *praised* for imitating specific health behaviors are more likely to copy a number of other health behaviors modeled by the nurse.
- If nurses are perceived as having status and *prestige* within health care systems their behavior will be more readily modeled.
- Clients will be more likely to repeat behaviors of models who have been *rewarded* rather than punished for behaving in that way. For example, if a nurse is reprimanded for "taking too much time" in teaching a health behavior to a client (rather than praised for those efforts) the client will often place less value on the new health skills.
- Clients who perceive the nurse as warm, *empathic,* and open will be more likely to model the nurse's health behavior.[8]
- Clients are usually in *vulnerable* states when interacting with nurses. This vulnerability makes it more likely that the client will be more susceptible to modeling the nurse's behavior. For example, in a pediatric emergency parents can learn (through imitating the nurse) to speak in a soft, low voice to their children and breathe slowly and deeply. This occurs even if these behaviors have not been formally taught by the nurse.
- Most clients find *group support* helpful when changing health behaviors. Peer pressure to exercise, stop smoking, avoid sugar, and so on is helpful in initiating new health behavior. Clients model each other in this process.
- *Live models* are imitated most readily. Clients often learn best with personal teaching sessions. Film and cartoon models are also highly effective.

NURSES AS MODELS OF SELF-CARE

In nursery and postpartum areas, parents can see nurses holding, bathing, and feeding newborns. They learn to care for their own children by observation. In pediatrics, the calm demeanor of the nurse with an ill or injured child reassures both the parents and the child.

These opportunities to model supportive care help parents in unfamiliar circumstances. Conversely, if nurses are anxious or uncomfortable, stressed parents will model that behavior as well. Such imitation will inevitably affect the child in a subtle, negative manner.

These simple modeling behaviors are often enough to change the behavior of clients, family, and friends. Although it has seldom been specifically addressed, this process has traditionally been recognized throughout nursing education and practice. It has consistently been integrated as a conscious teaching strategy.

In the past, the consequences of modeling were recognized in many ways. Stringent admission requirements for nursing students included parameters for weight and hairstyle and strict regulations on smoking, drinking, uniforms, and general health status. It was believed that the appearance and health habits of these nurse candidates would one day affect client self-care. Instructors were careful to assign good "role model" nurses to work with students in clinical courses.

In nursing literature, the importance of modeling has been directly addressed. In one text, *Modeling and Role-Modeling: A Theory and Paradigm for Nursing*,[9] extensive recommendations for clinical usage of modeling concepts are offered. Today, even if the word modeling is not used, a major part of nursing literature speaks to the personality, health, and "self-awareness" of the nurse as being crucial to health care.[10–12]

"It is becoming increasingly clear that the most important *instrument* in the health care system is the health professionals themselves."[13] Siegel has emphasized that the *relationship* between the client and the nurse or doctor is often the primary healing factor. The ability of the staff to provide love, care, and hope for severely ill clients does often produce miraculous recoveries.[14]

The Nurse's Own Health

The well-being of nurses does affect their ability to deliver quality care.[15] Nurses and other health care professionals are often not given adequate preparation and support for self-care skills to enable them to practice well-being in their personal and professional lives.

It is ironic that the professionals who are supposed to teach about health and assist sick clients often have a difficult time doing just that for themselves. Problems of burnout, substance abuse, and suicide among health professionals are increasingly recognized. There is new emphasis on teaching self-care skills in health professional training, to ensure that the individuals who are trained will continue to be available to serve those who need them.

As Americans have learned of the benefits of positive self-care, interest and activity in this area have risen dramatically. This phenomenon has penetrated the nursing profession as well, resulting in new workshops and programs encouraging nurses to focus on meditation, acupressure, nutritional guidance, and other self-care techniques. Within clinical agencies, aerobic dancing and Jazzercise programs are offered at change of shifts. More specific seminars deal with problems of burnout and the effect of stress on personal and professional behavior.

Professional nursing organizations have begun to respond directly to nurses' needs for health and self-care. Many local and national conventions address these issues. Employee assistance programs are becoming more common in nursing. For example, the American Nurses' Association encourages employers to offer health treatment options for substance abuse *before* disciplinary action is taken.

These programs not only encourage nurses and other health care providers to focus on their own health but generate support systems and models within peer groups. These developments help to create positive images of nurses, both inside and outside the profession.

Nursing Images

When the word *nurse* is mentioned, an image comes to mind. For many people the image comes from the memory of a nurse who has cared for a family member. Usually this image is distorted, with nearly all women in white identified as nurses, not distinguished from each other as RN's, LVN's, or nursing assistants. This condition is also complicated by infighting within the profession. Sometimes even nurses are perplexed about who and what nurses are— and what their responsibilities may include. The present severe shortage of nurses is often, at least partially, attributed to the poor image that nursing has with the public.

Stereotypical nursing images can be both positive and negative. Positive images and media portrayals present nurturing nurses who are warm, intelligent, and competent. A less flattering image is of a mindless handmaiden carrying a bedpan or the tyrannical, harsh Nurse Ratchett of *One Flew Over the Cuckoo's Nest*. Besides these images there is that of the "real-life" one-to-one nurse: a friend, neighbor, parent, spouse, or health care provider.

What are the health care behaviors of these real-life nurses? How do clients perceive them? How do they see themselves? Whatever the stereotyped images may be, people *watch* nurses. Thus, the nurse has a significant opportunity to influence people in positive or negative ways. Many nurses are interested in the impact that Kaye Rafko (Miss America of 1988—a nurse) will have on the public image of nurses. Some fear that the image of the *cute* but not too clever handmaiden may be reinforced. Others feel that she will be able to use her title and exposure to promote nursing.[16]

Are nurses' practices and values congruent with the messages they give their clients? If nurses drink alcohol to excess or do not exercise, what happens when they counsel clients in these areas? A client may imitate unhealthy behaviors as well as healthy ones. The client may receive a "do as I say, not as I do" message. This communication is difficult for the client, friend, family, or peer. Healthy behaviors may even go unrecognized in the presence of such mixed messages.

Nurses are not perfect models. When nurses acknowledge that clients are imitating their behavior, it can precipitate anxiety and defensiveness. A critical care nurse might respond: "My technical skills are excellent. I'm certified nationally. What difference does it make if I'm 50 pounds overweight?" For many nurses, competency in technical skills has taken precedence over their own self-care. Although the need for technical competency is certainly recognized, the need for nurses to model positive health behaviors is also important.

Individual health behaviors are the result of past learning and conscious and unconscious attempts at self-care. Family traditions and cultural background play important roles. Understanding this concept enables nurses to look at their roles as models in a nonpunitive, tolerant way. Nurses cannot expect either their clients or themselves to change overnight.

The struggle to become a good model of self-care is a long but rewarding one. Nurses need to give themselves permission to start, fail, start over again, anf finally succeed at developing positive self-care behaviors. Developing these behaviors is a slow process, taken in small steps. Remembering to be patient, supportive, and nonpunitive is the best way to ensure success.

Self-assessment is often the first step in the modeling process, encouraging nurses to become more involved in personal self-care. If nurses choose to integrate positive self-care choices in their lives on a regular basis, this will be reflected in their own health status—and be recognized (and modeled) by clients. Figure 5–1 is an example of a self-assessment tool examining several health care areas in which modeling is important. There are additional self-assessment tools in Chapters 7 through 17.

SUMMARY

In this chapter social learning theory was used as a basis to explain the process of learning by imitation. Variables that influence social learning—including culture, reward, prestige, similarity to self, warmth and empathy, susceptibility, and proximity—were discussed. The role of nurses as health models for clients, family, friends, and peers was emphasized. Nurses can help clients to imitate, and eventually integrate, health behavior in daily life through the process of identification.

STUDY QUESTIONS

Personal Focus

1. How has social learning influenced your nursing practice?
2. Give two examples of ways in which you have learned health care behaviors.

Directions: Circle the numbers below which are most true for you.

	Almost never	Seldom	Often	Almost always
1. I know the state of my health.	1	2	3	4
2. I have regular check-ups, including B/P, PAP, and dental checks.	1	2	3	4
3. I am a nonsmoker.	1	2	3	4
4. I drink in moderation or not at all.	1	2	3	4
5. My weight is within established norms for my height.	1	2	3	4
6. I limit my intake of salt, fat, and sugar.	1	2	3	4
7. I get adequate amounts of sleep.	1	2	3	4
8. I get adequate amounts of aerobic exercise (three times a week for 30 minutes).	1	2	3	4
9. I cope with stress effectively.	1	2	3	4
10. I know the relaxation response and practice it.	1	2	3	4
11. I take time for my family and friends.	1	2	3	4
12. I play at least four times a week.	1	2	3	4
13. I attend to my spiritual needs.	1	2	3	4
14. My sexual life is satisfying.	1	2	3	4
15. My environment is safe and pleasant.	1	2	3	4

Awareness questions:
1. How do you rate yourself as a model of health?
2. How would you like this self-assessment to look in six months? What steps could you take to meet that goal?
3. Congratulate yourself for the ways in which you are a good health model.

Figure 5–1. Do I model health?

3. Identify two ways in which you model positive self-care behavior.
4. Ask one colleague his or her perception of your modeling of self-care skills.
5. Complete the assessment questions in Figure 5–1.

Client Focus

1. Interview two clients. What are their perceptions about nurses as models of self-care behavior?
2. Discuss why the concepts of imitation and identification are important to nursing practice.
3. Identify three of Bandura's concepts that have particular relevance to your work with clients.
4. Help one client discuss the way in which he or she has learned health behavior from significant family, peer, and professional models.

REFERENCES

1. Aristotle. (1941). As attributed to in N.E. Miller & J. Dollard, *Social learning and imitation*. New Haven, CT: Yale University Press, p. 311.
2. Walter Bagehot. (1941). As attributed to in Miller & Dollard, *Social Learning*, p. 291.
3. Lorenz, K. (1952). *King Solomon's ring* (M.K. Wilson, Trans.). New York: T.Y. Crowell.
4. Rosenstock, I. (1977). The health belief model and preventive health behavior. In M. Becker (Ed.), *The health belief model and personal health behavior*. Thorofare, NJ: Charles B. Slack, p. 52.
5. Bandura, A. (1977). *Social learning theory*. Englewood Cliffs, NJ: Prentice-Hall.
6. Bandura, A., & Walters, R. (1963). *Social learning and personality development*. New York: Holt, Rinehart & Winston, p. 108.
7. Bandura. *Social learning theory*, pp. 40–48.
8. Francis, V., Korsch, B.M., & Morris, M.J. (1969). Gaps in doctor–patient communication: Patient's responses to medical advice. *New England Journal of Medicine, 280*, 535–540.
9. Erickson, H.G., Tomlin, E., & Swain. M.A. (1983). *Modeling and role-modeling: A theory and paradigm for nursing*. Englewood Cliffs, NJ: Prentice-Hall.
10. Swinford, P.A., & Webster, J.A. (1989). *Promoting wellness: A nurse's handbook*. Rockville, MD: Aspen Publications.
11. Dossey, B., Keegan, L., Guzzetta, C., & Kolkmeier, L. (1988). *Holistic nursing: A handbook for practice*. Rockville, MD: Aspen Publications.
12. Taylor, C., Lillis, C., Lemore, P. (1989). *Fundamentals of Nursing*. Philadelphia: Lippincott, p. 29.
13. Scott, C.D., & Hawk, J. (1986). *Heal thyself: The health of health care professionals*. (New York: Brunner/Mazel, p. xvii.
14. Siegel, B. (1986). *Love, medicine, & miracles*. New York: Harper & Row.
15. Scott & Hawk. *Heal thyself*.
16. (1987). Miss America's an R.N. Will it make a difference? *R.N., 50*, 35–37.

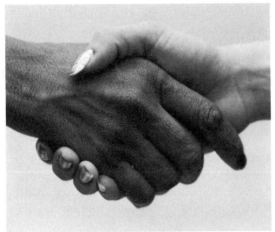

It's supposed to be a professional secret, but I'll tell you anyway. We doctors do nothing. We only help and encourage the doctor within.

Albert Schweitzer

6 Self-Contracting

LEARNING OBJECTIVES

Upon completion of this chapter, readers will be able to:

1. Define self-contracting.
2. Describe the theoretical framework of self-contracting.
3. List nine steps in the contracting process (see Appendix B).
4. List three advantages of self-contracting.
5. Identify three special considerations related to the contracting process.
6. Discuss the role of follow-up in the self-contracting process.
7. Complete a personal self-contract (see Appendix B).
8. Help one client to complete a self-contract.

DEFINITIONS

Self-contract   An agreement that an individual makes with himself or herself, with or without the assistance of a support person. It is used to improve self-care health behavior.

Self-talk   "A set of evaluating thoughts that you give yourself about facts and events that happen to you. Self-talk results in various kinds of emotional reactions."[1]

INTRODUCTION

Self-contracting is an effective clinical tool. It provides a formally structured, written format for clients and professionals (individually or jointly) to use to improve self-care skills. A sample of one self-contracting format is presented in Figure 6–1.

Self-contracting builds on the high value society places on self-control and self-management. In educational settings children and adults develop and complete individualized learning plans. Self-contracting is particularly relevant in nursing education where independent learning is becoming more the norm than ever before.

Informal use of this approach is found in many nonclinical as well as clinical settings and in many professions. It is becoming increasingly popular.[2–6] Table 6–1 presents examples of the use of the contracting process in a variety of settings. Appendix C presents samples of contract forms.

THEORY AND TECHNIQUE

All self-contracting approaches are based on the *theory and principles of behavior modification*, a model of behavior change built on operant conditioning/reinforcement principles. *Behavior therapy* is a specific approach that aids behavior modification by effectively combining reinforcement, cognitive, humanistic, and social learning theories.[7] In behavior therapy clients are actively "reeducated" in a supportive relationship with a helping person. A major focus is on individual control and responsibility.

Reinforcement (reward) of any specific behavior increases the likelihood that the same behavior will occur again.[8] Usually initial reinforcement comes from others, but in ideal situations health behaviors become self-reinforcing. Often the pleasant feelings of health and well-being alone are enough to maintain healthy behavior.

Other theories presented in Chapter 4 are also integrated; communication,

SELF-CONTRACT

MY GOALS:

Short-term — by the end of six weeks I will . . . *Walk for 20 minutes 4 x a week*

Long-term — by the end of six months I will . . . *walk/run for 30 minutes 5 x a week*

ENVIRONMENTAL PLANNING: (all the steps I will take to reach my goal)

1. Buy good walking shoes.
2. Set my alarm clock 30 minutes early.
3. Set out my exercise clothes the night before.
4. Find pretty place to walk in.
5. Keep a calendar on my refrigerator (star for each day I meet my goal).

THOUGHTS AND ACTIONS

Helpful thoughts:	Helpful actions:
I really do sleep better when I exercise like this.	Get a friend from work to walk with me.
Non-helpful thoughts:	**Non-helpful actions:**
It's more important that I get my rest today.	Eating a heavy meal before my planned exercise time.

MY REWARD   (if I meet my goal) *My sister will clean my apartment for me.*

THE COST: (if I fail to meet my goal) *I will clean my sister's apartment for her.*

REEVALUATION DATE: 6 weeks — 7/30
                                        6 months — 11/13

I agree to help with this project: I agree to strive toward this goal:

___*Janet*_____   ___*Eve*_____   __6/3__
(Support person)   (Your signature)   (date)

Figure 6–1. Self-contract. Format adapted permission from Baldi, S., et al. (1980). *For your health: A model for self-care.* South Laguna, CA: Nurses Model Health, p. 47.

TABLE 6–1. SELF-CONTRACTING IS USED IN MANY SETTINGS

Education	Facilitates use of self-directed learning; emphasizes autonomy and shared responsibility.
Health Education	Promotes active involvement in self-care. Examples include: Parent Effectiveness Training Premarital counseling Alcoholics Anonymous Weight Watchers Reach to Recovery.
Clinical Nursing	Facilitates self-care. Examples include: Postoperative clients: "I will cough and deep-breathe five more times and then I am going to relax." Hypertensive clients: self-management of weight, exercise, salt intake, and smoking. Severely depressed clients: make contract agreements with nurse psychotherapists to call before suicidal feelings become intense.

In all of these situations nurses facilitate and support the contracting process, but the actual work is self-management by the client.

psychoanalytic, systems, developmental, stress/adaptation, and biological theories play significant roles in helping clients change behavior through self-contracting.

There are specific techniques that may be used to facilitate self-contracting. Some of these behavioral techniques follow.

Assertion Training

Assertion training helps people learn to communicate in a clear, nonpassive, nonaggressive manner. To meet specific self-contracting needs, clients must communicate assertively. The person may need to learn to say *no* effectively and without guilt (for example, a self-care plan may require going home from work on time in order to exercise, instead of working overtime to maintain a poorly staffed institution). See Chapter 8 on psychological self-care for specific techniques.

Behavioral Rehearsal

Behavioral rehearsal is a structured approach in which the client "practices" for an event perceived as frightening until the anxiety associated with the event decreases.[9] This role-playing method has been used successfully in a variety of educational and therapeutic settings. Psychodrama is one type of behavioral rehearsal that helps clients prepare for predictable situations in which friends or family members discourage change. For example, a client who is learning new eating patterns may want to rehearse saying no *before* going to a family holiday celebration. In this way it will be less difficult to resist reverting to old patterns.

Behavioral rehearsal helps clients learn assertive responses for problematic interactions. Clients learn to abandon old ways of behaving and to practice new adaptive habits. Expressing self-praise and focusing on one's strengths and past successes is another means of increasing self-confidence.

Disputing Irrational Beliefs/Self-Talk [1]

Figure 6–2 presents a Rational Self-Help Form. Based on work by Ellis, this worksheet addresses his belief that problematic behaviors are correctable through a process of rational thought.[10] Self-talk helps clients acknowledge the power of the "self-fulfilling prophecy." Negative thought patterns can be altered and replaced by more positive thoughts and actions.

For example, if clients have a belief that they will never be able to inject their own insulin, it is likely that they will continue to resist acquiring that skill. Their perceived inabilities will reinforce the belief that they are truly incapable. A rigid resistance to learning this and other self-care skills will then occur.

Incompatible Responses

Practicing activities that are incompatible with problematic behaviors also facilitates change. Problematic behaviors are eliminated more quickly if settings are arranged so that rewards are given for behaviors incompatible with the undesired behavior.[11] A person cannot smoke and perform a relaxation exercise *at the same time.* If a person is rewarded for repeating a relaxation exercise when an urge to smoke is felt, the smoking behavior will decrease and eventually end.

ADVANTAGES OF SELF-CONTRACTING

There are a number of major advantages of self-contracting. A discussion of each point follows.

Reduces Client Passivity and Dependency

Active involvement in the health care process is a central focus of self-contracting. Self-contracting places responsibility on the client at every age level. Lewis has demonstrated that even grade-school children can effectively initiate and manage their own self-care needs.[12] Children often complete self-contracts to eat fresh vegetables, do ten push-ups, and so forth.

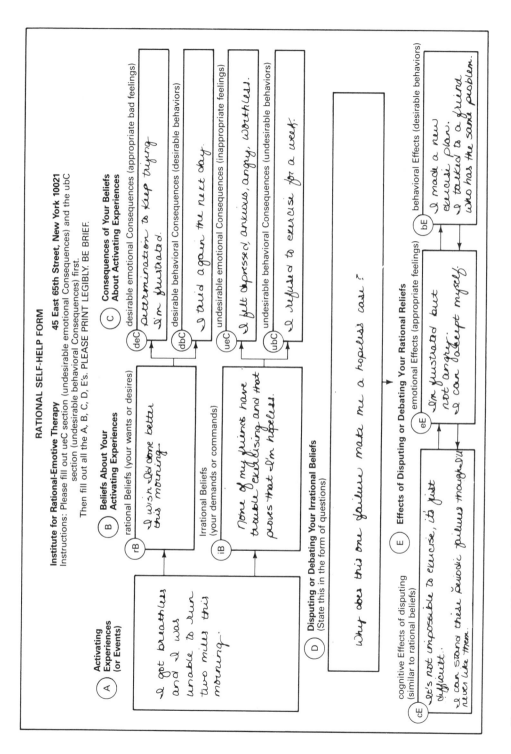

Figure 6–2. Rational self-help form. (Used with permission from Institute for Rational-Emotive Therapy. 46 E. 65th Street, New York, NY 10021.)

Parallels the Nursing Process and Self-Care Models

Self-contracting provides clarity and structure for clinical practice and is consonant with nursing process. The way in which nurses organize their thoughts is consistent with the way clients are taught self-assessment and self-contracting. Table 6–2 compares the two processes.

Provides a Direct and Simple Approach to Self-Care

Self-contracting approaches are easily learned and are applicable in a large variety of settings. Lengthy or expensive courses are unnecessary. After a client has demonstrated an initial success with this method, it will quickly be applied to other health concerns as well. Family members and friends frequently begin to experiment with these simple methods. Brief, descriptive workbooks can be used to distribute this information effectively to large numbers of people at minimal cost (see Appendix B).

Focuses on Specific Objectives

A major advantage of the self-contracting process is that it demands clear identification of objectives and goals.* Although this need for specificity can enlighten the client and nurse, it requires much patience and work. Client goals often do not match the goals that a health care provider would set for the client. One example of this is a hypertensive client who smokes or maintains a high-sodium diet. An extreme example is a client who demands the right to commit suicide.

As consumers become active providers of their own health care, these subtle and complex philosophical questions are intensified. Many nurses are shocked by the wide divergence that can exist between nurse and client goals. The self-contracting process provides a structure through which these differences can be identified and discussed.

Some nurses may feel a loss of authority as clients gain new control. They must remember that clients have *always* possessed this control; clients have *always* been able to refuse medications or other specific health care regimens. During the process of self-contracting, these clients decisions may be directed in a specific, positive fashion.

In most cases collaboration through contracting will actually give the nurse new feelings of control and clarity. When behavioral objectives are clarified, roles are delineated, and the nurse may feel a greater sense of self-esteem and professionalism.[13] The vagueness and confusion that often accompany evaluation of care are decreased.

Facilitates Compliance

The process of negotiating a self-contract can clarify the issues that make it difficult for the client to modify his or her life-style and behavior. The problem

---

*In this chapter "goals" and "objectives" are used interchangeably.

TABLE 6–2. COMPARISON OF THE PHASES OF SELF-CONTRACTING AND THE PHASES OF THE NURSING PROCESS

Self-Contracting[a]	Nursing Process[b]
1. *Assessment:* Client completes self-assessment tools. Utilization of peer assessment and consultation with nurse.	1. *Assessment:* Data collection utilizing client self-assessment as well as nursing assessment. Assets and limitation relative to self-care needs are reviewed.
2. *Problem identification:* Client summarizes and analyzes assessment data with assistance as necessary. Major areas for change are identified and listed in order of priority.	2. *Diagnosis:* Client and nurse identify self-care limitations or deficits in specific areas; may be related to lack of knowledge, motivation, or skill.
3. *Goal setting, environmental planning, and reinforcement choice:* Client identifies a specific goal, plans how to accomplish that goal, predicts potential interference, and chooses rewards for success and costs for failure.	3. *Plan, setting and reaching objectives:* Nursing and client objectives are set. Nursing actions and client actions are initiated. Factors that facilitate or impede goal achievement are addressed.
4. *Reevaluation:* Dates regularly set, program altered as necessary with ongoing assistance from partner.	4. *Evaluation:* At regular intervals nurse and client evaluate outcome pertinent to specific objectives. New self-care skills are reviewed.

[a]See Figure 6–1.
[b]See Chapter 3.

of noncompliance (i.e., a person's informed decision not to adhere to a therapeutic recommendation)[14] can be seen in a different perspective. The individual may desire to comply but is prevented from doing so by certain factors. The person may attempt to alleviate anxiety about his or her hospitalization or illness by refusing to participate in the health care regimen. Other stressors such as financial concerns, family, work, and personal relationships can contribute to noncompliance.[15] Discussing and solving problems related to negative side effects of prescribed treatment can increase the rapport and feelings of satisfaction between the nurse and client. Collaboration with the client also increases the nurse's awareness of the client's knowledge deficits regarding schedules, medications, follow-up care, and community resources.

Facilitates Open Communication

When people complete contracts with partners, they must talk about their hopes, needs, and past experiences with success and failure. Communication channels between the client and nurse and between the client and family members are invariably opened during the self-contracting process.

Facilitates Personal Experimentation by Nurses

A final advantage of the self-contracting model is that it can be easily tested and used personally by nurses. Self-contracting provides a ready method for nurses to integrate self-care skills into their personal and professional lives.

Firsthand contracting experience is invaluable, assuring that nurses are not asking clients to "do as I say, not as I do." From this essential experimentation nurses will develop their own personal adaptations of specific contracting techniques.

SPECIAL CONCERNS REGARDING SELF-CONTRACTING

As in any health change process there are specific concerns that must be addressed.

Is Self-Assessment Reliable?

Self-assessment and self-monitoring tools are major elements of the contracting process and are presented in Chapters 7 through 17. Friends and family may also be helpful during the assessment process. Farquhar has indicated that important learning takes place when clients compare assessments by their peers with their own self-assessments.[16]

The phenomenon of clients giving "socially desirable responses" is also a concern. Some nurses feel a need to prove or validate client self-assessment independently. In actuality there is a high level of agreement among self-monitored, peer-monitored, and independently observed assessment.[17]

These concerns over the accuracy of self-assessment are lessened when the nurse acknowledges that he or she plays a *secondary* role in the total change process. Self-contracting encourages each person to effect behavior change for himself or herself—*not* for the nurse or partner.

Regardless of its accuracy the assessment process is helpful to clients. An independent "therapeutic effect" has been reported. Self-assessment is a "reactive" process. As clients assess their behavior, they cannot avoid both overt and covert reactions. Even inaccurate self-monitoring begins the self-regulatory process.[18] New personal awareness, introspection, and behavior change often accompany client record keeping and assessment.[19]

Is It Too Time Consuming?

Many nurses erroneously believe that contracting consumes an inordinate amount of time and is therefore not cost effective. Research has indicated that this is not the case. Steckel noted that the average amount of staff time devoted to contracting was 11 minutes.[3]

The initial phase of the contracting process, involving a complete assessment *is* time consuming. Once completed, however, the client is usually committed to the self-care process. Problems with noncompliance are frequently avoided when clients set their own goals. A major percentage of nursing time is saved when nurses no longer have to convince or coerce clients to comply with goals set by others.

Will It Be Used Punitively?

Some people inadvertently set unattainable goals. In these instances the negative experience of inevitable failure may lower client self-esteem and decrease the likelihood of future contracting success. Nurses may blame their clients or themselves; clients may also blame themselves. These types of punitive experiences must be avoided. Contracts should always be initiated on a trial basis only; periodic reevaluation is essential. Failure is viewed as a means to facilitate learning and growth ("try and try again"). It is not considered a terminal statement of client inadequacy. Nurses and other support partners must be particularly patient and supportive.

Is the Follow-Up Process Adequate?

No matter how zealous a client is, the importance of professional follow-up cannot be overstressed. Clients benefit from objective reevaluation and suggestions from nurses. An emphasis on follow-up can help avoid the unfortunate fragmentation of traditional health care delivery ("See the doctor only when sick" or "Take this medication only as long as symptoms persist"). Follow-up without professional contact is also important and can be built into self-care plans. Clients can report progress or difficulties to family members, peers, ministers, and others.

As in any change process, potential problems or complications must be anticipated during self-contracting. Some of these potential difficulties are addressed below.

Assessment of Knowledge Base. Nurses and clients require a sound knowledge base in all areas of self-care for the implementation of any self-contract. For example, clients may attempt to lose weight without knowledge about nutrition or the dangers of rapid weight loss. When nurses are unable to supply this information, they must acknowledge their limitations and use additional resources. Ongoing assessment of the client's knowledge base is an important part of the follow-up process.

Effects of Rapid Behavior Change. Ideally, self-contracting will lead to *gradual* changes in client behavior. Sometimes the changes may be rapid and upsetting, neglecting client feelings or unleashing them too quickly.

Health professionals sometimes express concern that clients will be "psychologically" harmed by rapid behavior change. A sudden surge into awareness (flooding) of repressed conflicts can occur; it is imperative that nurses be aware of this possibility. With preparation the nurse can help clients manage this crisis and refer them to specific resources when necessary.

Other complications may occur when immediate but superficial behavioral improvements divert attention from more basic problems and feelings. A person may exercise obsessively to avoid dealing with an unhappy marriage, for example. Symptom substitution, another phenomenon, refers to the replacement of one symptom with another. Nurses are familiar with clients who experience rapid headache relief but soon return to emergency rooms with low-back pain or other complaints. Clients are often concerned that positive change in one self-care area will precipitate problems in another. Openly discussing this phenomenon with clients can eliminate many of these fears.

Therapeutic Prediction. This may diminish some of the potential difficulties of self-contracting. A dialogue using therapeutic prediction might begin like this:

> "Last time you tried this you got discouraged after two weeks. That might happen again. Let's talk about plans to try to avoid that."

or

> "Are you thinking that you might want to return to heavy smoking like you did the last time you tried to lose weight?"

A positive relationship ensures that this type of comment is not perceived as criticism. "Brainstorming" helps the client discover feelings and actions that might inhibit successful change. Clients who are contracting to stop smoking, lose weight, exercise regularly, or perform any new health behavior, need to be constantly encouraged to assess their behavior and what it may mean to their life goals, their needs to fail or succeed, and the reactions of family and friends. When difficulties are discussed and reevaluated with warmth and humor, the likelihood of their occurrence is decreased.

Impact on Family and Friends. Partners usually "change" together. Accommodating this process, nurses can use systems theory to involve all members of a family in positive change. A couple trying to lose weight provides an excellent example of resistence to change. When one partner successfully begins to lose weight, the other partner often encourages the spouse to break their diet, avoiding the threat of change and the possible end of the relationship ("Just one piece of pie won't hurt you"). Self-contracting with family partners provides an excellent way to ease this conflict and promote positive health change.

Use of Support Groups. The use of follow-up groups and community self-help groups is of primary importance in self-contracting. A natural outcome of the self-care movement may be an increase in the number and quality of community support groups such as Parents Without Partners, Weight Watchers, prepared childbirth classes, ileostomy and colostomy clubs, diabetic clubs, bereavement groups, and so on. Some nurses may find that they need to help clients form these groups if there are none already existing.

SUMMARY

In this chapter the basic theory and technique concerning the process of self-contracting was presented. It was designed to be read with Appendix B, which provides a simple and concise nine-step approach to contracting. It is designed for use by both nurses and clients. Appendix B presents samples of various self-contracting forms to use with clients, families, friends, and peers.

The many advantages as well as special considerations of self-contracting were discussed. Skills in self-assessment and the importance of the follow-up process were emphasized.

STUDY QUESTIONS

Personal Focus

1. Choose one area of self-care and complete a self-contract with a peer or family member as your partner (see also Appendix B).
2. How did the contracting process work for you? What did you have trouble with? Could you get help from a peer in this area?
3. Did you find that associated changes occurred in your life when you began self-contracting?
4. What are the typical ways in which you sabotage or help yourself change behavior?

Client Focus

1. Identify two clients from your current clinical practice with whom you might use self-contracting. Assist them in selecting one behavior to use in completing a self-contract.
2. Assume that a client comes to you for a third contact and is very disappointed in his or her rate of success. What would be your first reaction? What would you do?
3. Describe how you would teach a client about the importance of follow-up in the contracting process.
4. Plan how you would work with a client who could identify no rewards. What would you do first?
5. Describe nursing interventions for clients who set unrealistic goals (see also Appendices B and C).
6. See if any client on your unit has a nursing diagnosis of "noncompliance." Introduce the idea of contracting to this client.

REFERENCES

1. Zastrow, C. (1979). *Talk to yourself: Using the power of self-talk.* Englewood Cliffs, NJ: Prentice-Hall, p. 60.
2. Dossey, B., Keegan, L., Guzetta, C.E., & Kolkmier, L.G. (Eds.). (1988). *Holistic nursing: A handbook for practice.* Rockville, MD: Aspen, pp. 370–376.
3. Steckel, S. (1982). *Patient contracting.* Norwalk, CT: Appleton-Century-Crofts.
4. Jasmin, S., Hill, L., & Smith, N. (1981). Keeping your delicate balance—the art of managing stress. *Nursing 1981, 11,* 52–57.
5. Cassey, J.L. (1985). The suicide prevention contract. *Perspectives of Psychiatric Care, 23* (23), 99–103.
6. Brykezynski, K. (1982). Health contracting. *Nurse Practitioner 7,* 27–31.
7. Rim, D., & Masters, J. (1985). *Behavior therapy, techniques and empirical findings.* Orlando, FL: Harcourt, Brace, Jovanovich, p. 234.
8. Hergenhahn, B.R. (1982). *Introduction to theories of learning.* Englewood Cliffs, NJ: Prentice-Hall, p. 110.
9. Meichenbaum, D., & Cameron, R. (1974). The clinical potential of modifying what clients say to themselves. In M.J. Mahoney & C.E. Thoreson (Eds.), *Self-Control: Power to the Person.* Monterey, CA: Brooks/Cole, pp. 263–290.
10. Ellis, A. (1962). *Reason and emotion in psychotherapy.* New York: Lyle Stuart.
11. Rim & Masters. *Behavior therapy, techniques and empirical findings.*
12. Lewis, M.A. (1974). Child-initiated care. *American Journal of Nursing, 74,* 652–655.
13. Brunner, L., & Suddarth, D. (1986). *The Lippincott manual of nursing practice* (4th ed.) Philadelphia: Lippincott.
14. Carpenito, L. (1987). *Nursing diagnosis, application to clinical practice* (2nd ed.). Philadelphia: Lippincott, p. 408.
15. Miller, J. (1984). *Coping with chronic illness: Overcoming powerlessness.* Philadelphia: F.A. Davis.
16. Farquhar, J.W. (1988). *The American way of life need not be hazardous to your health.* New York: W.W. Norton, p. 61.
17. Plutchik, R., & Conte, H. (1989). Self-report scales for the measurement of depression. *Psychiatric Ann. 19* (7), 367–371.
18. Broden, M., Hall, R.V., & Mitts, B. (1971). The effect of self-recording on the classroom behavior of two eighth-grade students. *Journal of Applied Behavior Analysis, 4* (3), 191–199.
19. Kazdin. Self-monitoring and behavior change, pp. 220–231.

Part II: Self-Care Primarily Associated with the Mind

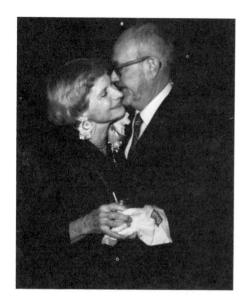

Friends can be good medicine.

California State Department of Mental Health,
"Friends Can Be Good Medicine," 1981

7 Relationships

LEARNING OBJECTIVES

Upon completion of this chapter, readers will be able to:

1. Identify and describe the significance of relationships to human development.
2. Identify three personal qualities that lead to the ability to communicate effectively.
3. Describe the connection between interpersonal relationships and health, wellness, longevity.
4. Identify self-care steps that build and maintain relationships.
5. Complete a self-care plan for improvement of personal relationships.
6. Assist a client in completing a self-contract to improve relationships.

DEFINITIONS

Relationship   A connection between people. A relationship may be peaceful, loving, antagonistic, or characterized by disinterest.

Alternative relationships   A term used to signify contacts with social support groups, community causes, pets, or objects on a temporary or permanent basis, which substitute for or augment relationships with significant family members and friends.

Intimacy   A state of relationship usually characterized by warmth, mutual sharing, and understanding. Relationships based on conflict may also be intimate.

Therapeutic or professional relationships   Relationships for a specific purpose such as nursing, medical, psychological, or spiritual care. The nature of these relationships is often governed by rules or conventions regarding fees, time arrangments, and specific obligations.

Support system   A person's social community or network of relationships; to whom a person can go or rely on in times of stress or need, including friends, relatives, neighbors, church members, professional organizations, unions, and so on.

Loneliness   A painful feeling caused by the absence of positive relationships; emotional isolation from others.

Aloneness   The state of being separate or apart from others. Aloneness may be a welcome state and does not necessarily imply loneliness.

Caring   A stance, attitude, and commitment to the welfare of another person. A self-transcending and creative act of conscious intention toward the other.

INTRODUCTION

"Man is not meant to live alone." The common sense of this Biblical precept is generally recognized. Many people are lonely and regret their isolation and lack of love relationships. Yet the importance of relationships for health continually remains underrated. Relationships are often taken for granted or assumed to be out of a person's direct control. ("It's hard to meet people." or "I just haven't met the *right* person.")

All developmental theorists recognize the importance of relationships. Sometimes this recognition is overt. For example, Mahler's theory of separation–individuation specifically deals with the child's changing relationship to its mother.[1] Other theorists suggest the importance of relationships in a more subtle way. Freud's theory of oral, anal, and phallic stages of development implies the presence of a caretaker who nurtures the infant, implements toilet training, and so on.[2] Of all the developmental theorists, Erikson has perhaps most directly emphasized the crucial rule that relationships play in each developmental period.[3] He describes the process of growth, from birth to death, as intimately linked to the quality of one's interpersonal relationships at each life phase. Developmental tasks are successfully accomplished only when feedback and support from others are available on a predictable, consistent basis.[4] A person becomes a person by encountering others and in no other way.[5]

CHARACTERISTICS OF RELATIONSHIPS

People value and desire different qualities in their friendships. In one study, characteristics were ranked "important" or "very important," reflecting what many find valuable in close friendships. The three most valued characteristics were: the friend keeps confidences, is loyal, and gives warmth and affection.[6] All close relationships have several features in common. The following is a description of some the major qualities of a relationship.

Trust
Perhaps the most important quality of a relationship is trust. People involved in a friendship are comfortable with one another; they can share both good and bad times. Generally, the basis for this trust is that each partner feels listened to, understood, and accepted.[7]

> A friend is one
> to whom one may pour
> out all the contents
> of one's heart,
> chaff and grain together
> knowing that the
> gentlest of hands
> will take and sift it,
> keep what is worth keeping
> and with a breath of kindness
> blow the rest away.
> Arabian proverb

Comfort and Support
Friendships consist of mutual experiences in which the needs of both persons are recognized. Each individual shares personal feelings, abilities, and attitudes. A major aspect of all friendships is the ability of both parties to tolerate disappointment and crisis, even to fight or disagree while still maintaining trust, closeness, and caring.

One of the most important but subtle gifts given in a relationship is simply the gift of being close. Friends share different types of activities. The process of "just being together" seems to be more important than the activities themselves. Skills acquired and feelings experienced with one person can be transferred in positive and useful ways to other relationships.

Communication

The art of communication is openness and a willingness to enter the other person's point of view and explore it until it is familiar territory. When the other person's perspective is understood and valued, then a true dialogue has occurred.[8]

Many problems in relationships stem from difficulties in communication. Relationship self-care involves learning to speak clearly, to state one's own needs in an open and honest way, and then to negotiate when difficulties and conflicts occur. The ability to communicate clearly is not a skill that comes naturally. Deficits in communicating and problematic early relationships may lead to blocks that can create difficulties throughout life. A child raised by an unpredictable adult may have difficulty trusting what anyone says. Some people may need to learn new communication and negotiation skills to function comfortably in close relationships.

A communication skill that is frequently undervalued is listening without offering advice. Many people feel pressured to give advice when sought out by a friend with a problem. Many times simply listening empathically, "being with" the person, is most helpful.

Empathy

Empathy occurs when one can "stand in the other person's shoes" and understand the other's feelings. Empathy is not sympathy where one is feeling *for* the other person; rather it is an expression of feeling *with* someone.[9] Children can only learn to have empathy for their family and peers if they have received empathy as infants and toddlers.[10] Relationships can only be developed and maintained through "rough spots" if both people have the capacity for tolerance and empathy for each other.

Genuineness and Acceptance

Genuineness refers to honesty and openness in self-expression, letting the other person know one's thoughts and feelings. It is that ability to "be yourself" in an interaction with someone else. Although no one reveals all of his or her personal life and feelings to every person, the ability to be genuine is vital to a good relationship.

Acceptance, respect, and regard for others "just as they are" are also crucial aspects of healthy relationships. A sense of good will and nonpossessiveness are part of this type of acceptance. A need to change the other person creates primary difficulty in many relationships.

Intimacy and Caring

The need for intimate relationships is deeply rooted in human values. The ultimate in human interaction is intimate one-to-one relating and caring. True intimacy is a self-initiated, self-sustaining process that requires continual nourishment and attention to the relationship.[11] Intimacy occurs when an individual allows another to see his or her truth. Many people feel that "if people knew who I really was I would lose their love." Intimacy is a key to emotional freedom. Caring for others is contagious and creates intimacy for all involved.

Love

Love is a feeling of happiness and joy that emanates from, to, and through the heart. It is the greatest healing force and is the highest expression of communication between two people. Knowing what love is can be confusing because people mix love with many other types of human experience.

In the *Art of Loving*, Fromm defines love as the overcoming of human separateness, as the fulfillment of the longing for union.[12] He describes four basic elements common to all forms of love. These are care, responsibility, respect, and knowledge. Mature love includes wanting the other person to grow and helping the other person achieve his or her fullest potential. This act of love toward another leads the individual to discover and love his or her own true self.

Touch

Although touch may not be a component of *all* relationships, it is often a spontaneous, nonsexual, integral aspect of many human contacts. Widows and widowers often state sadly that the thing they miss most is "just someone to hold my hand once in a while." Isolated hospital clients also complain about the lack of touch in their lives. This is a particularly crucial need for AIDS patients. The need for human touch (as a vital part of relationships) is recognized in nursing practice.[13]

Developmental Phases of Relationships

All relationships have a beginning, middle, and end. While these phases are obvious in long-term relationships, they also occur during very brief interactions.[14] In the beginning people are strangers. They slowly share aspects of themselves. Each may "test" the other and withhold sensitive issues until he or she feels comfortable, understood, and accepted.

The middle phase begins when trust has been established, and people have begun to learn more about each other and develop a sense of caring and support. The awareness that one may turn to the other when a problem arises is a vital ingredient. This phase presents a possibility for the development of an even closer relationship. For example: two women work side by side in an office typing pool. Each morning they have a pleasant coffee break together. At first their conversations are general, "small talk." After several weeks one of them has car trouble. The other offers to pick her up and drive her to work while the car is in the shop. The friendship is strengthened by this act of caring and other more personal contacts are generated.

Every relationship has an end, a final phase. A job change, a dying parent, or a friend moving away can all be examples of this. In many instances there is time to prepare, so that goodbyes and closure can be a valuable experience for both people. The relationship can be summarized. Conflicts and misunderstandings can be resolved and set aside. Memories and gratifications can be reviewed. Anger at being abandoned may be ignored, discussed, or joked about. Gifts or photographs are often exchanged.

DIFFICULTIES IN RELATIONSHIPS

People want to be close to others; yet there are numerous obstacles to establishing and maintaining meaningful relationships. Each person's unique history, cultural and family background, beliefs, and expectations contribute to the compatibility or incompatibility of a friendship. A history of child or sexual abuse, alcoholism in the family, abandonment, or emotional or mental disturbances make it difficult to know what a healthy relationship is or how to build rapport and trust with another person.

There is a tendency to repeat family patterns by having relationships with or marrying people who will stimulate early, unresolved childhood conflicts that can be reenacted within the relationship and hopefully, resolved eventually. This desire to "right old wrongs" and win love is often the unconscious motivation behind falling in love.[15] The person is trying to get what he or she never got as a child—love, approval, acceptance—from a person similar to the parent who withheld these basic needs. This destructive pattern of behavior often results in addictive relationships that reinforce the underlying fear of being unlovable and unworthy of having a better life.[16]

The use of defense mechanisms to alleviate anxiety can interfere with healthy relationships. For example, displacement of feelings onto another can sabotage peaceful co-existence. A wife who has been criticized by her boss at work may vent her anger on her husband, who in turn vents it onto their child. *Projection* is another psychological defense mechanism that operates in most relationships. Love and hate can be the expression of projections. When a person becomes alienated from some quality he or she despises in himself or herself, the person projects that quality onto others and hates them. Conversely, when a quality that he or she would like to experience but does not is alienated, he or she projects it onto others and loves them. The people hated or loved are targets for his or her projections.

Difficulties in intimate relationships sometimes result from failed expectations. Some disappointment and anger are normal in any ongoing relationships. Many people, however, have consistently unrealistic expectations of relationships, fostered by saccharine images of marital and family life in the media ("Someday My Prince Will Come" or "The Waltons").

Self-exploration can help to put the past in the past and to experience the present in the present. Popular magazines are filled with articles on "How to Make Your Marriage Work" and "How to Make More Time for Your Mate." Best sellers provide an array of self-help books—such as *Intimate Partners: Patterns in Love and Marriage,*[15] *The Struggle for Intimacy,*[17] and *How to Break Your Addiction to a Person*[16]—that offer excellent suggestions and ideas for working on relationships.

NURTURING RELATIONSHIPS

People can practice specific self-care actions that nurture relationships. Just as a garden needs water and sunlight, satisfying, lasting relationships need tending. Table 7–1 presents specific ways to provide this nourishment. Table 7–2 presents self-care actions that can help reduce the potentially damaging effects of conflict. (Also see Chapter 8 on psychological self-care.)

Conflict resolution is a well-known concept in business. Similar rules can be adapted to personal relationships for the purpose of settling disagreements, reaching compromises, and deciding on fair and loving courses of action. The bargaining rules are as follows:

TABLE 7–1. WAYS OF BUILDING AND MAINTAINING RELATIONSHIPS

1. Mark a calendar with your own "red-letter days"—anniversaries, birthdays, special occasions. Celebrate them with those close to you.
2. Decide to add some new holidays to your calendar: the beginning of fall, the end of a semester. Consider celebrating "Christmas" once a month!
3. Set a goal of meeting and talking with one new neighbor, classmate, or co-worker each week.
4. Send a note or card to someone you are close to just to say "hello."
5. If you live in a family, have dinner *together* at least twice a week. Be sure that the television set is off!
6. Have "family meetings" regularly to discuss plans and problems.
7. Make it a habit to invite a friend to dinner once a month.
8. Explore your community. Learn about and become active in at least one club, organization, or service group.
9. Send acknowledgments of sympathy cards, flowers, and presents.
10. Call one friend on the first of each month; let him or her know that you are thinking about the nice times you have had together.
11. Celebrate job promotions.
12. Call a friend who is ill; offer to help.
13. When you try a new recipe, save a portion of it for a neighbor.

TABLE 7–2. SELF-CARE ACTIONS DURING RELATIONSHIP CONFLICT

During conflict, explore these helpful actions:

1. "Time out": a cooling-off period of variable length (minutes to weeks). This may lead to a new perspective on the problem.

2. Assertiveness training: helps a person communicate needs clearly and minimizes passivity and aggression.

3. Negotiation: with the help of a third party (e.g., family, member, friend, teacher, minister, or other person whom both people respect).

4. Review expected behaviors for the life stage of the persons concerned. For example:
   Toddlers have tantrums
   Adolescents are unpredictable
   New siblings and step-children cause stress
   Midlife crises challenge relationships
   Aging parents provoke guilt and grief

5. Practice self-care in all areas. People with healthy self-esteem maintain relationships more easily than do those with poor self-images. Self-care in the areas of nutrition, exercise, sleep, and so on, leads to enhanced self-esteem.

6. In addition to other self-care efforts, professional consultation for individual, couple, or family counseling may be useful.

1. Prepare your agenda ahead of time.
2. State clearly and matter-of-factly what you want without "shoulds" or demands.
3. Listen to your partner's requests. Carefully review and consider his or her point of view. Validate with him or her that you understand what it is that is expected of you.
4. Take nothing for granted. Make all issues explicit. Ask all questions you can think of.
5. Remember that nobody has an a priori right to anything. Rights are established by agreement.
6. Be willing to give up something in order to gain something else. No one can expect to get everything that one wants.
7. Never agree unless you feel that you are getting a satisfactory deal.
8. Once a decision is agreed upon, stick to your part of the bargain.

The Magic of Support Groups

Support groups can be a source of nourishment, encouragement, and information for people in relationships. Groups for "grief work," adult children of alcoholics, cardiac rehabilitation, and weight-loss support are a few examples of the many available resources. Organized groups provide ongoing support for people during times of change and crises.[18] Support groups serve the purpose of:

- Satisfying the longing to be connected
- Offering bonding through adversity
- Turning stigma into honor
- Transforming the helpless into helpers
- Eliminating customary barriers
- Offering "back fence" knowledge and wisdom
- Allowing powerful emotions to be expressed[19]

CHANGES IN RELATIONSHIPS

The need to share life with others is pressing in today's fast-paced society. The traditional extended family with the built-in companionship of grandparents, aunts, and uncles has been replaced by the nuclear or one-parent family. More and more adults are living as single persons. According to the U.S. Census Bureau, about 41 percent of all adults of marriageable age (15 and older) are single.[20] More than one million children are raised by their fathers alone and even more are raised by single mothers. The numbers are so high that people have begun to accept the idea of nontraditional households as being normal.

People may be making the traditional choice in opting for a family in the 1980s and 1990s, but they are doing it in nontraditional ways and with nontraditional partners.[21] Blended families (with stepchildren) are very common. Some women are choosing to have babies without a committed partner. Couples who have chosen career over family are now having children at a later age. Age-old stereotypes are being ignored as older women and younger men and women with higher incomes than men are establishing partnerships. Homosexual relationships are becoming more acceptable in society.

Economic strains on families leave less time for relationships. More than 70 percent of American women with children under the age of 18 work outside the home. Lack of sufficient high-quality child care is a major problem in the United States. The stress on both men and women of maintaining careers, child care, and home management often leaves little time for relationships with family and friends. High mobility also decreases the opportunity for lasting relationships and feelings of belonging to a community. People move and change jobs as frequently as every two or three years. Many people do not know their neighbors and are unaware of basic community resources. Communal living arrangements, babysitting cooperatives, and church outreach programs all can be helpful.

The AIDS epidemic has contributed to less sexual experimentation and more monogamous relationships. The pendulum is swinging back to a more traditional, conservative movement.[21] Both single and married people have been spending more time at home "cocooning" rather than going out for entertainment, parties, and food. People are eating at home, watching rented videos, reading, and conversing in the comfort and privacy of their homes. Single people find it more difficult than ever to meet people and have turned to computer dating services, personal ads, and support groups to find connections and kinship.

RELATIONSHIPS AND HEALTH

Relationships are important for good health. Infants need human warmth and contact to survive and grow. If cuddling with a mothering person is not available, babies fail to thrive and sometimes die, even if there is adequate provision of food, cleanliness, and temperature control.[22,23] Harlow found that monkeys raised without physical contact with a mothering figure were socially withdrawn and acted in a bizarre manner. Immature monkeys preferred to stay near dolls (surrogate mothers) made of cloth that did not give food rather than near dolls (surrogate mothers) made of wire that did.[24]

Nurses intuitively know the value of touch and human contact in soothing clients of all ages. Nurses in pediatric units may carry infants in Snugli bags while performing other duties. Therapeutic touch is being used in many clinical settings. Nurses are acknowledging the importance of family visits to patients in intensive care and are allowing more flexible visiting hours.

Hospitalized clients generally seem more relaxed and comfortable after short visits from staff and family members. Straightening out a bed or chatting for a few minutes can have a reassuring effect. Hospices help clients face death by providing human contact.

Highlights of research on the link between relationships and physical and mental health are listed below.

Mortality

- Socially isolated persons have two to three times the overall risk of dying than do people who maintain supportive relationships. This is true regardless of self-reported health status and risk factors such as smoking, drinking, lack of exercise, and obesity.[25]
- Terminal cancer strikes divorced persons of both sexes more frequently than it does people who are married.[26]
- Cardiac death rates were two to six times lower for Irishmen who remained

in Ireland (and thus did not disrupt their social ties) than for their siblings who immigrated to the United States.[27]

- Death from malignant tumors and suicide was more likely for physicians who had initially (25 years prior) reported more interpersonal difficulties and loneliness than their classmates.[28]
- The death rate from cardiovascular disease is 2.5 times greater for divorced men than for married men of the same age (age 40).[29]
- The death rate from myocardial infarction was less than one-half of the predicted rate in Roseto, Penn., where the Italian-American population clung to close family and neighborhood ties, despite other risk behavior such as obesity and smoking.[30]
- Death from coronary thrombosis and arteriosclerotic heart disease is strikingly high among recently widowed men age 55 and older, who as a group have a 40 percent higher death rate within the first six months of widowhood than do married men of the same age.[31]

Health Deterioration

- Pregnant women under stress and without supportive, confiding, personal relationships have three times the number of complications experienced by women undergoing similar levels of stress but who maintain such relationships.[32]
- A loss of a major relationship prior to the first symptoms of cancer has been consistently reported.[33]
- People experiencing multiple life changes have a higher chance of becoming ill in the following year than people without multiple life changes. The life changes consistently rated as most stressful all have to do with personal relationships, including death of a spouse, divorce, and marital separation.[34]
- Men who are forcibly unemployed but with high levels of social support have significantly fewer mental and physical health problems than do those with low levels of social support.[35]
- In an Australian study, 28 percent of widows compared with only 4.5 percent of married women reported nervousness, nightmares, panic, depression, blurred vision, chest pains, shortness of breath, infections, and headaches.[36]
- Coronary heart disease is three to five times higher among Japanese men acculturated to Western ways and least integrated into their own culture (independent of traditional risk factors such as diet, cholesterol levels, blood pressure, or smoking) than among Japanese men who maintain strong ties with their own culture.[37]

Depression and Mental Illness

- Rates of psychiatric hospitalization are roughly five to ten times greater for separated, divorced, and widowed persons than for married people.[38]
- The existence of an available confidant confers significant protection against the development of depression.[39]
- Men and women in Edinburgh, Scotland, who had confidants and friends

had significantly fewer psychological and physical symptoms than did those who lacked confidants and friends.[40]

How Does Social Contact Prevent Disease?

The high correlation between lack of social contact and illness strongly suggests a causal relationship. Exactly how this happens is unclear. Berkman and Syme suggest the following:

1. The socially isolated person may be more likely to adopt self-destructive health practices.
2. Social isolation may lead to depression, which might—in turn—predispose people to accidents and suicide.
3. The absence of social networks may produce physiological changes in the body that increase susceptibility to disease; whereas the presence of social support systems may actually decrease physical susceptibility.[25]

Millon's studies with men infected with the AIDS virus found that individuals with strong commitment and a willingness to face challenges have greater numbers of certain immune-system cells. He suggests this is because they seem more likely to gather friends around who offer emotional support and cheer them up.[41]

ALTERNATIVE RELATIONSHIPS

The benefits to relationships do not result only from direct contacts with friends or family. The feeling of being competent, necessary, and productive can also be achieved from a variety of alternative relationship activities which may include caring for pets or personal belongings (e.g., boats), pursuing hobbies, or working for social causes.

Alternative relationships can also involve people. "Foster Grandparents," "Big Brothers," and "Parents Without Partners" provide alternative relationships with other human beings. Volunteerism by young, upper-class professionals has markedly increased in the last few years. Volunteers and participants in these human resource programs have the opportunity to share love and feel vital to the lives of others.

Relationships with Pets

Pets fulfill a human-like companionship and social support role for people of all ages. Stroking animals and talking to them may stimulate the production of endorphins.[42] This sensory input does seem to enhance health and promote healing in a number of different clinical settings.[43]

Contemplating fish in tanks has been found to reduce stress reactions as measured by blood pressure in both normotensive and hypertensive individuals.[44] Many dentists have large aquariums near their dental chairs to reduce client anxiety and fear. Sales of pet fish and aquarium equipment have risen dramatically in the last few years.

Huntington Memorial Hospital in Pasadena, Calif. employs two full-time labrador retrievers (and their pet therapist/owner) to provide comfort and support for oncology patients.[45]

Research documents this important role of pets in clinical practice:

- Mentally ill clients who received three-hour visits from puppies once a week showed significantly higher levels of confidence, competence, and decreased depression at an eighth week follow-up. The control group had received visits from the handlers but not the puppies.[46]
- Eighty percent of hospice residents in one setting have reported that one-hour visits from pets from an ASPCA shelter once a week for ten weeks made them feel less lonely and isolated.[47]
- Widowed pet owners have been shown to have less health decline and less anxiety about their own death (following the death of their spouse) than widows without pets.[48]
- One study showed that giving an elderly group a pet bird resulted in happier, healthier clients.[49]
- Young clients who participated in "petting sessions" with kittens and puppies were found to be more cooperative and to respond better to therapy than did a control group.[50]
- In a state hospital for the criminally insane, there were fewer medication requirements, less depression, fewer suicides, and fewer violent episodes in the wards in which clients were allowed to have pets.[50]
- A study at the University of Maryland found that blood pressure, stress, and tension were consistently reduced when clients had pet dogs.[51]

PROFESSIONAL RELATIONSHIPS

Nursing theory has consistently emphasized the *relationship* between nurse and client as a primary healing factor. Many consider this the essence of nursing. Table 7–3 highlights important theoretical views of relationships in nursing practice.

It is helpful for nurses to have a clear conceptualization of the difference between professional and social relationships. Social relationships are generally not specifically goal oriented; they exist for the mutual purposes of sharing, pleasure, and companionship. Professional relationships, in which roles are clearly defined, exist for a specific purpose. The structure of these relationships is generally time limited; professional relationships occur in specific places and focus on the needs of the client rather than the helping person. There is an instant intimacy between nurse and client based on the client's state of need and dependency, often involving bodily exposure.

TABLE 7–3 RELATIONSHIPS IN NURSING PRACTICE

Peplau[a]	"Nursing is a significant therapeutic interpersonal process."[b] It is a learning experience for both client and nurse. As the *relationship* evolves, roles are clarified and mutual collaboration and problem solving occur. Four relationship phases include: orientation, identification, exploitation, and resolution. These parallel the phases of all relationships as well as the nursing process.
Hall[c]	The "core" of nursing involves therapeutic use of self and reflective techniques. "To look at and listen to self is often too difficult without the help of a *significant figure (nurturer)* who has learned how to hold up a mirror and sounding board to invite the behaver to look and listen to himself."[d]
Orlando[e]	The nurse is defined by the *process of interaction* with the client rather than by the activities carried out. "Learning how to understand what is happening between herself and the patient is the central core of the nurse's practice and comprises the basic framework for the help she gives to patients."[f]
King[g]	*Interpersonal relationships* in nursing are based on perception, judgment, action, reaction, interaction, and transaction. Nurses use interpersonal relationships to assist clients to work toward health.
Levine[h]	Nursing is a *human interaction.* The patient's environment includes the nurse. People are dependent on their relationships with others.
Parse[i]	Relationships are central to the process of health maintenance. The nurse's willingness to participate in meaningful relationships with clients is crucial to effective nursing care.

[a]Peplau, H.E. (1952). *Interpersonal relations in nursing.* New York: Putnam.
[b]Peplau. *Interpersonal relations,* p. 16.
[c]Hall, L. (1959). *Nursing—what is it?* Virginia State Nurses' Association.
[d]Hall, L. (1965). Another view of nursing care and quality. Washington, DC: Catholic University Workshop.
[e]Orlando, I.J. (1961). *The dynamic nurse–patient relationship: Function, process and principles.* New York: Putnam.
[f]Orlando. *The dynamic nurse–patient relationship,* p. 4.
[g]King, I.M. (1971). *Toward a theory of nursing: General concepts of human behavior.* New York: John Wiley & Sons.
[h]Levine, M.E. (1973). *Introduction to clinical nursing* (2nd ed.) Philadelphia: F.A. Davis.
[i]Parse, R.R. (1981). *Man–living–health: A theory of nursing.* New York: John Wiley & Sons, pp. 54–55.

The intimacy felt by the client may not be experienced by the nurse in the same way (the client is concerned only with his or her own problem and caretakers; the nurse has many clients). The nurse may not realize his or her importance to a particular client and therefore, for example, may not say good-bye when leaving for vacation, being transferred, or working a different shift. It is a common occurrence for hospitalized clients to say, "Whatever happened to that night nurse who was so kind?"

On the other hand, nurses may be struck by the shared sense of intimacy with their clients and give "too much." For example, a nurse may work extra hours without extra pay. Although admirable at times, such giving, if it were frequent, could have adverse consequences for the nurse, such as fatigue, no time for personal life, and so on.

Giving too much to patients or one's chosen profession usually means that the individual is giving at his or her own personal expense. Only when people know how to take care of and give to themselves can they authentically give to others. Some nurses have an overdeveloped sense of responsibility for the welfare of others and suffer guilt when they fail to "fix" the patient's problems. Being preoccupied with someone else's needs protects nurses from acknowledging their own needs. Some people, particularly adult children of alcoholics, derive a sense of self-worth from taking care of someone who is unable to care for themselves. They look for opportunities to do what they are good at—rescuing and caretaking—to the exclusion of their own needs and wants.[52] Participation in Adult Children of Alcoholics, Alanon, and other types of support groups can help nurses find self-identity and a new belief system based on a sense of worth, choice, and trust.

Many nurses vacillate between being too detached from or too involved with their clients. Detachment is usually a process to protect themselves from over-involvement. Over-involvement occurs when nurses are unable to balance the natural compassion that they feel for their clients with their own personal needs. The dangers of "enabling," whereby nurses help (but often infantilize) clients and family members, to their own detriment, is becoming increasingly recognized by nurses. Only with experience and peer support can nurses easily develop a balanced attitude toward clients. Regular contacts with a nurse mentor (role model) who has mastered this balance is a tremendous help for nurses struggling with this issue. Siegal, in *Love, Medicine, and Miracles*, says,

> This so-called detached concern we've taught is an absurdity. Instead we need to be taught a *rational concern*, which allows the expression of feeling without impairing the ability to make decisions. It is our role to help the patients mobilize *their* mental powers against disease. We can help by touching, praying, or simply sharing on an emotional level.[53]

Nursing Diagnoses for Relationships

The North American Nursing Diagnosis Association (NANDA) defines *Relating* as a human response pattern involving establishing bonds.[54] There are four nursing diagnoses that can be used to assess the quality of relationships. They are social isolation; parenting, altered: actual and potential; sexual dysfunction; and family processes, altered.

Social isolation is a state of aloneness experienced by the individual and perceived as imposed by others and as a negative state. Defining characteristics include:

- lack of supportive significant others
- poor communication skills
- withdrawal
- feelings of difference from others
- inadequate or absent purpose in life.

Altered parenting is an inability in nurturing figures to create an environment that promotes optimum growth and development of another human being. Characteristics include:
- physical and psychological trauma
- inappropriate caretaking behavior
- frequent accidents
- statements of resentment toward the child

Sexual dysfunction is a state in which an individual experiences a change in sexual function that is viewed as unsatisfying, unrewarding, or inadequate. Defining characteristics include:

- alterations in perceived sexual role
- limitation imposed by disease or therapy
- inability to achieve desired satisfaction
- change of interest in self or others

Altered family processes is a state in which a family that normally functions effectively experiences a dysfunction. Assessment findings include:

- inability to meet needs of family members
- lack of respect for autonomy
- rigid role function
- unhealthy family decision-making process.

NURSES MODEL RELATIONSHIP SELF-CARE

Nurses have more contact with clients than do any other health care providers. These frequent contacts enable nurses to teach clients about the value of relationships in promoting health. Some of this teaching occurs in formal presentations. The way in which nurses model self-care in their personal and professional relationships, however, is usually even more powerful. Figures 7–1, 7–2, and 7–3 present assessment tools for this self-care area with the Clinical Application.

In their personal lives, nurses can practice relationship self-care by:

- Sending birthday and anniversary cards to friends and family.
- Planning lunch with a friend once a month.
- Volunteering at one community agency.
- Making a "special time" for each family member every week.
- Completing the self-care skills described in Tables 7–1 and 7–2.

Nurses also can model self-care by the ways in which they develop and maintain professional relationships. Examples include:

- Celebrating special occasions with co-workers; for example, giving baby showers or "toasting" promotions.
- Creating once a month "networking luncheons" with peers and mentors.
- Communicating assertively with supervisors and co-workers.
- Treating co-workers with trust and respect; for example, accepting absent days without interrogation.
- Recognizing phases of relationships in getting to know new staff members.
- Maintaining clarity as to the parameters of the nurse's role ("cannot be all things to all people").
- Forming support groups at work to deal with topics such as death, high staff turnover, and so on.

In addition to observing these examples, clients also learn about relationships from their interactions with nurses. Nurses promote relationship self-care during all clinical contacts. Examples include:

- Encouraging hospitalized nursing mothers to continue nursing, if possible, and providing breast pumps.
- Maintaining flexibility regarding visiting hours.
- Providing privacy for clients during visiting hours.
- Helping clients identify boundaries of nurse–client relationships.
- Helping clients prepare for separation from nurses and roommates.
- Properly separating from clients during shift or job changes.
- Involving family and friends in client care.
- Teaching clients about community support systems.
- Helping parents and friends participate in alternative birth centers or delivery rooms.
- Helping nonambulatory clients protect themselves from isolation and alienation.
- Touching clients with warmth and empathy.
- Recognizing that different clients need different levels of caring.

The relationship between the client and the nurse is a powerful representation of the value that each places on relationships. Treating clients with respect, empathy, and warmth promotes relationship self-care through modeling. Nurses frequently assume that time spent with clients must be filled with treatments and procedures; however, simply the *presence* of a caring individual is important. Therapeutic human contact and communication is an essential part of nursing care.

CLINICAL APPLICATION

Case Presentation

Bob is a 22-year-old college graduate who moved into his first apartment three months ago. His roommate travels in his job, so their contacts are infrequent. Bob contracted infectious hepatitis (hepatitis A) when he spent six weeks on active Army reserve duty and has been recuperating in a medical unit. He is three weeks into the icteric phase of the illness. He is afebrile, has lost 10 pounds, and his stools are becoming dark again. He also has an elevated alkaline phosphotase, SGOT, and SGPT. Bob's serum bilirubin is 7 mg per 100 ml, and he is still experiencing a fullness in the right upper quadrant of his abdomen. During the prodromal phase of his illness, Bob experienced acute bouts of nausea, vomiting, and diarrhea. With the onset of the jaundice these decreased in severity. During the last two days, however, the frequency and severity of the symptoms have increased. On a scale of 1 to 10, with 10 being the most nauseated, Bob identifies his nausea as a 9.

Nursing notes indicate that his symptoms seem to increase in the mid-afternoon and early evening, the usual visiting hours. During report nurses noted that, except for brief visits from his roommate, he has no outside contacts, spends no time on the phone, and has no cards or flowers at his bedside.

Further assessment by the nurse assigned to his care revealed that Bob had been working long hours and taking graduate classes at a local university. The financial requirements of being on his own and furthering his education left little time for other interests. He had enjoyed membership in a YMCA tennis club but had given that up. His parents had moved to another city, curtailing frequent visits. He had dropped his weekly phone conversations with a sister who lived nearby and had not called her in over a month.

Bob admitted that he felt lonely, overwhelmed, and withdrawn after the experiences of the past few months. His biggest priorities had been work and school. Since graduation he had not spent time with old friends. He had some difficulty making new friends and had always been a little unsure of how to initiate conversations. He was proud of his ability to handle the demands of his new life, however.

When the nurses assigned to the evening shift began spending a few extra minutes with Bob, his complaints of nausea decreased. He seemed eager to talk and was willing to explore his feelings as he became more physically comfortable. Bob's complaints of nausea during visiting hours seemed directly related to his unspoken need for human closeness. He was aware that seeing other clients greeting their visitors was emotionally painful and reminded him of the absence of relationships in his life. Interactions with the nurse at those times were comforting, and he stated that it was easier for him to complain than to admit that he needed companionship.

The nurse helped Bob evaluate the status of his *current relationships,*

```
┌─────────────────┐
│   Assessment    │
└─────────────────┘
```
• self-care demand
• assets
• limitations

which were upset by a change in work and school demands. He had overlooked his need for continued relationships. Uncertainties about *communication abilities* had further inhibited him from reaching out to make new social contacts. In high school Bob had acquired a circle of close friends who competed with him on the track team. Again, however, he had lost contact with them. He began dating in college but indicated that his financial burdens and lack of social skills had limited his experiences.

Bob remembered the close relationships he had with his family while growing up and the feelings he still shared with them. He also recalled that his parents had few friends outside the immediate family. His parents had prided themselves on being able to "make do," and he witnessed both of them working overtime with little time left for play or socializing.

The fact that Bob had been able to form good relationships early in life was a major asset. His relationship with his roommate was also important.

Bob's *total health care state* showed no serious problems. He drank only occasionally and did not smoke, but his dietary habits consisted of many "fast-food" meals. The hepatitis was resolving and no difficulties in recovery were anticipated. His ability to be physically active would be curtailed for several weeks, however. His drinking would be restricted for approximately six months.

Bob completed the Support System Exercise (Fig. 7–1). His support list included several old friends and his sister. Bob was surprised at the number of people he could list. He recognized that over time (and especially in the last six months) he had pulled away from most of them. He discussed his ideas and responses to the Intimacy Checklist (Fig. 7–2) with the nurse and also completed the Relationships Self-Assessment (Fig. 7–3). He discovered that much of his focus on work and school was a cover-up for his uneasy feeling about making social contacts.

He was anxious to reestablish contact with his sister and friends and expressed interest in talking further with the nurse about his feelings about relationships. Bob and his nurse decided to begin talking on a regular basis about relationship self-care. They began with the formulation of a self-care diagnosis.

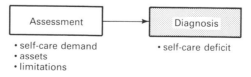

Bob concluded that he had two major self-care deficits in the area of relationships. They were:

Inability to initiate and maintain close relationships

and

Inability to communicate needs clearly to others due to lack of assertion skills

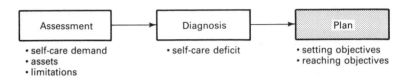

SUPPORT SYSTEM EXERCISE

This experience is designed to help you determine what is occurring in your own relationships with others and to help you to examine the strengths and weaknesses of your personal support system.

Materials needed: Three pieces of paper, a pencil or pen.

Procedure:

On the first piece of paper draw a circle in the center about the size of a 50¢ piece. Put your name inside the circle. Draw circles around the first one. The other circles represent the people in your individual support group. Think about your closest and strongest relationships. Think of the people you feel comfortable with and can turn to if you have a problem. Fill in the names rapidly in the circle just as they come to mind. Put the names of those who are supportive now as well as other significant persons who have provided such relationships for you throughout life.

Secondly, go through your memory of school mates, neighbors and friends at work or church. Thumb through your address book. On the second sheet list those peoples names who came up that you find yourself wishing to be in closer touch with. This list could include old friends or new friends you would like to get to know better.

As you write, you will probably find yourself becoming aware of a special affection for some of these persons, the ones you immediately feel like writing or talking to. These people have been important in your life, but that feeling may have gone unexpressed. On the third sheet of paper put the names of these people should you find that such feelings arise.

The last part of the exercise is to decide what to do with the lists and diagrams. Remember the kinds of relationships experienced with each person. Is there a person that you would like to contact right now? How do you feel about these people? How could you strenghten these bonds?

This simple activity is part of relationship self-care.

Figure 7–1. Support system exercise. (Reprinted with permission from Ferguson, T. Your support group. *Medical Self-Care. 7.* 9.).

Bob's reponses to Support System Exercise:

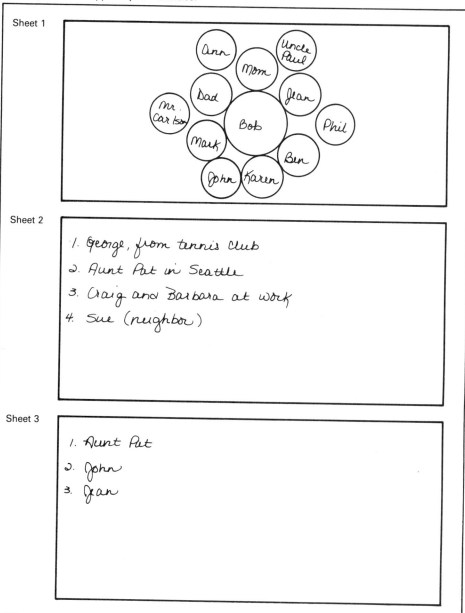

Sheet 1

Sheet 2

1. George, from tennis club
2. Aunt Pat in Seattle
3. Craig and Barbara at work
4. Sue (neighbor)

Sheet 3

1. Aunt Pat
2. John
3. Jean

Figure 7–1. (cont.)

Intimacy Checklist

Problems in relating are revealed by their own unique symptoms. In evaluating your own feelings about relating ask yourself if any of these 10 warning signs apply to you:

1. Do you consider yourself a closed person, controlled or up tight?
2. Are you frequently angry with the people close to you?
3. Do you use sarcasm, teasing and putdowns in relating with others?
4. Is your life so structured that the thought of doing something different, going someplace new or meeting new people makes you feel anxious?
5. Do you arrange your life so that you are always busy, involved with organizations or outside actvities? Are you seldom alone with yourself or with your family?
6. Do you find it hard to feel or show emotion?
7. Are other people often angry with you?
8. Do you need approval constantly?
9. In social situations, must you have a few drinks or use drugs before you feel comfortable?
10. Do you have vague feelings of anxiety most of the time?

If you answered "yes" to one or more of these questions you may have some difficulty in close relationships with others. Your "yes" response can be shared with a trusted friend or relative to help you gain an understanding of these feelings. With clients, the answers to the questions can be a part of the beginning of the assessement phase of treatment and a starting point for therapeutic interaction.

Figure 7–2. Intimacy checklist. (Reprinted with permission from Fast, B. (1978). *Getting close.* New York: Berkley Publishing Group, pp. 3–4.)

Setting Objectives

Bob and the nurse initially decided to concentrate on his reestablishing contact with one or two primary support persons. This would be a realistic, non-threatening start. Progress toward intimacy could begin after he had become more comfortable.

He decided he wanted to rejoin the tennis club, spend more time with friends, and get to know classmates and co-workers better. He realized that he had to do this slowly and to monitor carefully the amount of exercise he got during this recuperation period. At first he would exercise for only 15 minutes twice a week with planned rest periods for 30 to 45 minutes twice a day. He eventually wanted to begin dating again. The first step seemed to be spending structured time with friends. The nurse helped him write a self-care contract for this area (Fig. 7–4).

Reaching Objectives: Nursing and Client Actions

Bob set up appointments to talk with his nurse every other day. The specific actions that he took to meet his goals are presented in Figure 7–4 and Table 7–4. Specific nursing actions and roles are outlined in Table 7–4. They reviewed the Support System Exercise (Fig. 7–1) and discussed his feelings about the

RELATIONSHIPS SELF-ASSESSMENT

Complete the following self-assessment to help you look at the role of relationships in your life now. On the scale below circle the numbers which best indicate you and your life during the past year:

	Almost Never	Seldom	Often	Almost Always
1. There are people in my life upon whom I can rely . . .	1	2	(3)	4
2. My close relationships are satisfying . . .	1	2	(3)	4
3. Every week I plan time just for me . . .	(1)	2	3	4
4. I plan time together with others weekly . . .	1	(2)	3	4
5. I am comfortable meeting new people . . .	1	(2)	3	4
6. I am comfortable with the people I work/go to school with . . .	1	2	(3)	4
7. I can "be myself" when I am with friends . . .	1	2	(3)	4
8. My schedule includes time for socializing . . .	1	(2)	3	4
9. I make an effort to meet new people . . .	(1)	2	3	4
10. I maintain contact with old friends . . .	(1)	2	3	4

1. Connect all the circles down the length of the page. Look at the pattern that your connected line makes. You might also turn your page sideways to get an even more clear visual picture of relationships in your life right now. What does it seem to be saying to you?

2. Now add up your total score: _____ *21*

Circle which range it was in:
10–19   (20–29)   30–40

If your score was in the 10–19 range you might want to make some changes in your relationships. Which aspects do you think need the most work? How many "1's" did you mark on this assessment? __*3*__ These might serve as a clue to help you think about making changes in this area of your life.

3. How would you like this self-assessment to look six months from now? Are you interested in planning toward these improvements?

4. Remember to congratulate yourself for your efforts to improve this area of self-care.

Figure 7–3. Relationships self-assessment. (Adapted with permission from Baldi, S., et al. (1980). *For your health: A model for self-care.* South Laguna, CA: Nurses Model Health, p. iv.)

people on his lists. Bob began to contact these people. He remained in the hospital ten more days. His nurse provided a model of open and caring communication with Bob that encouraged him to share his feelings with others. They discussed Bob's time management, and the nurse helped him rearrange his schedule to accommodate time for his tennis games (when he was physically able) and other social activities. They also discussed contacts he could make while still confined at home.

SELF-CONTRACT

MY GOALS:

Short-term — by the end of six weeks I will . . . Spend an hour with John or Sue at least once a week

Long-term — by the end of six months I will . . . Have made one new friend. Spend an evening each week with friends or on a date.

ENVIRONMENTAL PLANNING: (all the steps I will take to reach my goal)

1. Phone my sister and parents.
2. Re-activate my membership in the tennis club.
3. Evaluate and change my schedule to allow time for myself each week.
4. Write or call the people in my primary support group.
5. Write or call those important people in my life whom I've lost contact with.
6. Read a book on assertion training — attend a class when I am recovered.
7. When I return to work have lunch at least twice a week with my co-workers in the company diningroom.

THOUGHTS AND ACTIONS

Helpful thoughts:	Helpful actions:
I enjoy being with friends. I will be more comfortable the more I get to know people.	Calling a friend. Setting up a tennis game. Reading an article about relationships.
Non-helpful thoughts:	Non-helpful actions:
I don't know what to say. I feel ackward with new people. What if they don't like me?	Cancelling a lunch date. Working on Sundays.

MY REWARD (if I meet my goal) Short-term — A new tennis racquet.

THE COST: (if I fail to meet my goal) Wax my roommate's car

REEVALUATION DATE: 10/1

I agree to help with this project:

_____Gale_____
(Support person)

I agree to strive toward this goal:

_____Bob_____ 8/15
(Your signature)   (date)

Figure 7–4. Self-contract. (Format adapted with permission from Baldi, S., et al. (1980). For your health: A model for self-care. South Laguna, CA: Nurses Model Health, p. 47.)

The nurse provided Bob with reading material about relationships that he could study during his recuperation. The nurse also talked to him about assertion skills and recommended an assertiveness training workshop at the local YMCA.

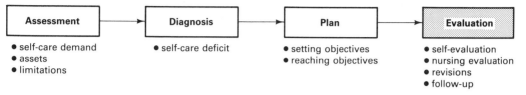

TABLE 7–4 NURSING CARE PLAN

Reason for consultation: Increase in nausea associated with loneliness   *Client:* Bob

Assessment	Plan	Evaluation

Self-care demand
  Need for development and maintenance of ongoing relationships
Assets
  Good family relationships
  Current discomfort is motivating
  Intelligence and verbal skills
  Previous positive experiences with tennis at YMCA
  Open relationship with nurse
  History of close friendships in past
  Intact relationship with roommate
  Good health prior to this illness
Limitations
  Long recuperation period
  Current illness and hospitalization
  Family theme of not sharing problems "with outsiders"
  Poor time management; over-scheduled with work and school; little time for self and/or relationships
  Financial stress
  New work and school status leading to numerous new relationships
 	
Diagnosis
 	
Self-care deficit:
  Inability to initiate and maintain close relationships
	Setting objectives
	  Six weeks: Spend one hour with John or Sue at least once a week.
	  Six months: Make one new friend; spend an evening each week with friends or a date.
	Reaching objectives
	  Client actions
	    Phone sister and parents.
	    Reactivate membership in tennis club.
	    Change schedule to allow time for one hour with John or Sue.
	    Read book on assertion training and attend class when I am recovered.
	    Plan to have lunch at least twice a week with co-workers.
	    Write or call important people in my life with whom I have lost contact.
	  Nursing actions
	    Teach value of relationships in health promotion; provide reading material for recuperation.
	    Describe and model assertion skills; refer to assertiveness workshop at YMCA. Refer to *Your Perfect Right* on assertive communication.
	    Model relationship self-care.
	    Consult during contracting process.
	    Provide guidelines re: recuperation period for hepatitis.
	Reevaluation date
	  At discharge from hospital in 10 days.
	  Phone contact in six weeks and six months.
		Met *Not met*
		X
		
		(not yet evaluated)
		
		X
		X
		
		X
		
		X (signed up for class)
		
		(have done for last 2 weeks)
		
		X (wrote three letters)
		
		X
		
		X
		
		X
		X
		
		X
		X
		
		X
		Needed revisions
		  Will need to monitor carefully his physical status; guard against additional fatigue.
		Client follow-up
		  Plan to call in six months. Goal is to teach self-care process and decrease dependence on nurse.

After several meetings, Bob reported that he had already spoken with his sister, and she was planning to visit him. His sister and his nurse became the first members of his reestablished primary support group. His sister had worked her way through graduate school and understood the demands on Bob's finances and time. She gave him moral support and encouragement.

Bob reported that he had felt quite lonely in his struggle with school and work and did not easily share his feelings with others. As he became comfortable in this, he initiated contacts with other support group members and planned to spend weekly time with friends.

Bob was able to interact readily with his primary support group; his isolation and loneliness decreased. It was unnecessary to revise his self-care plans. Bob began to understand that he had a tendency to withdraw into his work instead of reaching out toward others. He knew that he could return to the nurse for consultation if his difficulties returned. Table 7–4 presents a nursing care plan for this clinical situation.

SUMMARY

This chapter described the link between relationships and physical and emotional health. Correlations between poor interpersonal relationships and the presence of cardiovascular disease, cancer, increased mortality, and poor mental and physical health were explored.

The role of the nurse in modeling relationship self-care was a primary focus of this chapter. The way in which nursing theory emphasizes relationship issues was discussed. Differences between social and professional relationships were described. Specific self-care skills for nurturing relationships and managing relationship conflicts were presented. A clinical application illustrated how these concepts, combined with nursing process and self-contracting, can be used to help clients learn self-care behavior.

STUDY QUESTIONS

Personal Focus

1. Rate yourself as a model of relationship self-care.
2. What stage of life development are you in? Discuss the relationship tasks you are encountering.
3. Name some ways you maintain close relationships in your life.
4. Do you notice blocks in your ability to form relationships? Discuss these with a friend.
5. Set a relationship goal for yourself.
6. Discuss three differences in your professional and social relationships.

Client Focus

1. How is relationship self-care promoted with clients in your work setting? What are some ways it could be improved?
2. Evaluate the communication skills of one of your clients. Describe how those skills enhance or limit the formation and maintenance of the client's relationships.
3. Name some ways that relationship self-care may benefit total health. Practice describing the link between relationships and illness to a client.
4. Ask one client about his or her pets. How does the pet promote your client's health?
5. Complete a relationship self-care plan with a client.

REFERENCES

1. Mahler, M. (1975). *The psychological birth of the human infant.* New York: Basic Books.
2. Freud, S. (1953). Three essays on the theory of sexuality. In *Standard edition of the complete psychological works of Sigmund Freud.* London: Hogarth Press.
3. Erikson, E. H. (1950). *Childhood and society.* New York: W.W. Norton.
4. Erikson, E. H. (1959). Identity and the life cycle. Selected papers in *Psychological Issues, 1* (1). New York: International Universities Press.
5. Secord, P.F., & Backman, C.W. (1964). *Social psychology.* New York: McGraw-Hill.
6. Brown, M. Editors. (1979, October). Ingredients of friendship. *Psychology Today,* pp. 49–53.
7. Gaylin, W. (1976). *Caring.* New York: Alfred A. Knopf, p. 92.
8. Augsburger, D. (1982). *Caring enough to hear and be heard.* Venture, CA: Regal Books.
9. Muldary, T. (1983). *Interpersonal relations for health professionals: A social skills approach.* New York: Macmillan.
10. Stern, D.N. (1985). *The interpersonal world of the infant.* New York: Basic Books.
11. Greenwald, J. (1985). *Creative intimacy: How to break the patterns that poison your relationships.* New York: Jove Books.
12. Fromm, E. (1962). *The art of loving.* New York: Bantam Books.
13. Swinford, P. & Webster, J. (1989). *Promoting wellness: A Nurse's Handbook.* Rockville, MD: Aspen.
14. Wilson, H.S. & Kneisl, C.R. (1987). *Psychiatric nursing* (3rd ed.). Reading, MA: Addison-Wesley, pp. 118–120.
15. Scarf, M. (1987). *Intimate partners: Patterns in love and marriage.* New York: Ballantine Books.
16. Halpern, H. (1982). *How to break your addiction to a person.* New York: Bantam Books.
17. Woititz, J. (1985). *The struggle for intimacy.* Deerfield Beach, FL: Health Communication.
18. Norbeck, J. (1981). Social support: A model for clinical research and application. *Advances in Nursing Science, 3*(4), 45–59.

19. Johnson, J. & Klein, L. (1988). *I can cope: Staying healthy with cancer.* Minneapolis, MN: DCI Publishing, pp. 161–162.
20. Krier, B.A. (1988, June 26). Why so many singles? *Los Angeles Times,* Sec. VI, p. 1.
21. Bohan, K. (1989, Winter). As the pendulum swings. In *University Service News.* Irvine, CA: University of California.
22. Bowlby, J. (1969). *Attachment and loss* (Vols. I–II). New York: Basic Books.
23. Spitz, R.A. (1965). *The first year of life* (in collaboration with W. G. Cobliner). New York: International Universities Press.
24. Harlow, H. (1978). *The human model: Primate perspectives.* New York: John Wiley & Sons.
25. Berkman, I.F. & Syme, S. (1979). Social networks, host resistance, and mortality: A nine year follow-up study of Alameda County residents. *American Journal of Epidemiology, 1098*(2), 186–204.
26. Lillienfeld, A.M., Levin, M.S. & Kessler, I.I. (1972). *Cancer in the United States.* Cambridge, MA: Harvard University Press.
27. Brown, J. (1970). Nutritional and epidemiological factors related to heart disease. *World Review of Nutrition and Dietitian, 12,* 1–42.
28. Thomas, C.B., & Duszynski, C.B. (1974). Closeness to parents and the family constellation in a prospective study of five disease states: Suicide, mental illness, malignant tumors, hypertension, and coronary artery disease. *Johns Hopkins Medical Journal, 134,* 251.
29. Moriyama, I., Krueger, D.E., & Stamler, J. (1971). *Cardiovascular diseases in the United States.* American Public Health Association, Vital and Health Statistics Monograph Cambridge, MA: University Press, p. 2.
30. Wolf, S., & Goodell, H. (1976). *Behavioral science in clinical medicine.* Springfield, IL: Charles C. Thomas.
31. Young, M., Benjamin, B., & Wallis, C. (1963). Mortality of widowers. *Lancet, 2,* 454.
32. Nuckolls, K.B., Cassel, J., & Kaplan, B.H. (1972). Psychosocial assets, life crises and the prognosis of pregnancy. *American Journal of Epidemiology, 95*(5), 431–441.
33. Leshan, L. (1961). A basic psychological orientation apparently associated with malignant disease. *The Psychiatric Quarterly, 35*(2), 314–330.
34. Holmes, T.H., & Rahe, R.H. (1967). The social readjustment scale. *Journal of Psychosomatic Medicine, 2,* 214.
35. Gore, S. (1978). The effect of social support in moderating the health consequences of unemployment. *Journal of Health and Social Behavior, 19*(2), 157–165.
36. Maddison, D. (1968). The relevance of conjugal bereavement for preventive psychiatry. *British Journal of Medical Psychology, 41*(3), 223–233.
37. Marmot, M.G., & Syme, S.L. (1976). Acculturation and coronary heart disease in Japanese-Americans. *American Journal of Epidemiology, 104*(3), 225–247.
38. Carter, H., & Glick, P. (1970). *Marriage and divorce: A social and economic study.* American Public Health Association, Vital and Health Statistics Monograph Cambridge, MA: Harvard University Press.
39. Brown, G.W., Bhrolchain, M.N., & Harris, T. (1975). Social class and psychiatric disturbance among women in an urban population. *Sociology, 9*(2), 225–254.
40. Miller, P., & Ingham, J.G. (1976). Friends, confidants and symptoms. *Social Psychiatry, 11,* 51–58.
41. Body and soul. (1988, November 7). *Newsweek,* pp. 87–88.

42. Toufexis, A. (1987, March 30). Furry and feathery therapists. *Time*, p. 74.
43. Katcher, A.H., et al. (1983). Looking, talking, and blood pressure: The physiological consequences of interaction with the living environment. In A.H. Katcher & A.M. Beck (Eds.), *New perspectives on our lives with companion animals*. Philadelphia: University of Pennsylvania Press.
44. Thompson, D. (1989, January 8). A personable trio of pet therapists. *Los Angeles Times*, View Section.
45. Davis, J. (1988). Animal-facilitated therapy in stress mediation. *Holistic Nursing Practice, 2*(3), 75–83.
46. Francis, G., Turner, J., & Johnson, S. (1985). Domestic animal visitation as therapy with adult home residents. *International Journal of Nursing Studies, 22*(3), 201–206.
47. Muschel, I.J. (1984). Pet therapy with terminal cancer patients. *Social Casework: The Journal of Contemporary Social Work, 65* (8), 451–458.
48. Bolin, S.E. (1986). Effects of companion animals during conjugal bereavement. *People-Animals-Environment, 4*(2), 2021.
49. Brown, E. (1982, March). Are pets good for your health? *MS. Magazine*, p. 23.
50. Lynch, J.E., et al. (1982, October 3). A presentation on the television program *60 Minutes*. Columbia Broadcasting System.
51. Curtis, P. (1982, August). Our pets, ourselves. *Psychology Today*, pp. 66–67.
52. Beattie, M. (1987). *Codependent no more: How to stop controlling others and start caring for yourself*. New York: Harper/Hazelden.
53. Siegel, B.S. (1986). The privileged listener. In *Love, medicine, and miracles*. New York: Harper & Row, pp. 11–32.
54. North American Nursing Diagnosis Association. (1987). *Taxonomy I with Complete Diagnoses*. St. Louis: Author.
55. Alberti, R. & Emmons, M. (1982). *Your perfect right: A guide to assertive living*. California: Impact Publications.

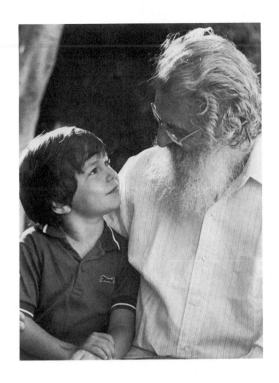

Planners make canals,
Archers shoot arrows,
Craftsmen fashion woodwork,
The wise man molds himself.

Buddha, as quoted in P. Lal, The Dhammapada
(New York: Farrar, Straus & Giroux,
1967), p. 85

8 Psychological Self-Care

LEARNING OBJECTIVES

Upon completion of this chapter, readers will be able to:

1. Define psychological self-care.
2. Identify three components of psychological health.
3. Describe six methods for nurturing psychological health.
4. Discuss the ways in which psychological self-care skills might be used during a crisis.
5. Discuss three criteria for referring clients or self for counseling or psychotherapy.

DEFINITIONS

Psychological Self-care   A constellation of activities practiced on a regular basis to promote psychological health; developing an integrated and balanced personality.

Crisis   A situation or event that a person perceives as stressful and that cannot be resolved in a reasonable period of time with ordinary coping skills.[1]

INTRODUCTION

Throughout history, many writings have contained references to psychological self-care. The Old Testament refers to a self-care tool still popular today—music. "And whenever the evil spirit from God was upon Saul, David took the lyre and played it with his hand; so Saul was refreshed, and was well, and the evil spirit departed from him."[2]

Over time, personal responsibility for health began to take a secondary role to dependence on physicians.[3] More recently, the emergence of the holistic health movement has re-emphasized individuals' responsibility for their own well-being. The philosophy and practice of holistic health is based on the mind–body–spirit connection. The treatment of one area should not be undertaken without respect for the totality.[4] True health reflects psychological and somatic harmony. Psychological self-care enhances physical and spiritual well-being.[5]

Discussion of psychological health engenders tremendous interest and acceptance today. Popular publications routinely feature current information about "how to" find happiness, recognize depression, know if therapy is indicated, assess self-esteem, and acquire a myriad of other skills.[6-8] *The Book of Tests* by Nash and Monchick is described as the "ultimate collection of quizzes to help a person discover what he or she is really like."[9]

Television presents a full gamut of activities and ideas for achieving psychological health. In recent years psychology has assumed an important status in radio programming. As millions from coast to coast listen, therapist and caller discuss problems in daily living. In newspapers, Ann Landers and Abby Van Buren provide their readers with tips for dealing with life's problems. All these media provide self-care information to the public.

Table 8–1 presents different theoretical views of psychological health. Common themes of balance and equilibrium in the individual's life are readily apparent in each perspective.

CHARACTERISTICS OF PSYCHOLOGICAL HEALTH

Jourard defines a healthy personality as a "way for a person to act, guided by intelligence and respect for life, so that as his needs are satisfied, he grows in awareness, competence, and the capacity for love."[10]

Psychological health encompasses many components; the most important being the following issues.

Self-Esteem

Self-esteem has two interrelated aspects: it entails a sense of personal efficacy and a sense of personal worth. It is the conviction that one is competent to live and worthy of living.[11] Self-worth exists when a person feels useful and valued.

Behavior is a good indicator of a person who has positive or negative self-esteem. People who are emotionally healthy are able to identify their assets and limitations and accept both aspects of themselves. They are not plagued by feelings of inferiority or inadequacy. These individuals adhere to a collection of *values* upon which their sense of self-esteem is based. They have a pretty definite idea of what is right and are able and willing to defend these views. At the same time they are flexible and willing to listen to other points of view without feeling

TABLE 8–1 THEORETICAL VIEWS OF PSYCHOLOGICAL HEALTH

Theorist	Date	Psychological Health is:
Plato[a]	400 B.C.	Harmony between mind and body: balance.
Aristotle[b]	300 B.C.	Practice of the Golden Rule: everything in moderation, nothing in extreme.
Freud[c]	1917	The ability to love and work.
Maslow[d]	1954	The ability to meet a hierarchy of human needs in an orderly progression.
Rogers[e]	1961	The continuous development of a realistic perception of self.
Erikson[f]	1963	Cohesiveness, maintenance of a stable identity in a variety of situations over time.
Glasser[g]	1965	Meeting personal needs without depriving others of the ability to meet their needs.
Ellis[h]	1973	Accepting personal responsibility for behavior.

Nursing theorists have also defined psychological health in discussing the general concept of health.

Peplau[i]	1952	Forward movement of the personality toward creative, constructive personal and community living.
Hall[j]	1966	The ability to achieve self-actualization and self-love.
King[k]	1971	The ability to adapt to internal and external stress and achieve maximum potential for daily living.

TABLE 8–1 (cont.)

Paterson and Zderad[l]	1976	An openness to and awareness of self; the ability to make responsible choices and become "more" as humanly possible in particular life situations.
Watson[m]	1979	Sensitivity to self and others, promotion and acceptance of positive and negative feelings in self and others.
Parse[n]	1981	Capacity for growth, the ability to change from what one is to what one wants to be.

[a]Taylor, A.E. (1956). *Plato: The man and his work* (6th ed.). New York: Meridian Books.

[b]Jaeger, W. (1934). *Aristotle: Fundamentals of the history of his development.* Oxford: Clarendon Press.

[c]Freud, S. (1917). Introductory lectures on psychoanalysis. In *Standard edition of the complete psychological works of Sigmund Freud.* London: Hogarth Press.

[d]Maslow, A. (1962). *Toward a psychology of being.* Princeton, NJ: D. Van Nostrand.

[e]Rogers, C. (1961). *On becoming a person.* Columbus, OH: Charles E. Merrill.

[f]Erikson, E. (1968). *Childhood and society.* New York: W.W. Norton.

[g]Glasser, W. (1965). *Reality therapy.* New York: Harper & Row.

[h]Ellis, A., & Harper, R.A. (1975). *A new guide to rational living.* Englewood Cliffs, NJ: Prentice-Hall.

[i]Peplau, H.E. (1952). *Relations in nursing.* New York: Putnam.

[j]Hall, L.E. (1964). Nursing: What is it? *Canadian Nurse, 60*(2), 150–154.

[k]King, I.M. (1971). *Toward a theory for nursing: General concepts of human behavior.* New York: John Wiley & Sons.

[l]Paterson, J.A., & Zderad, L.T. (1976). *Humanistic nursing.* New York: John Wiley & Sons.

[m]Watson, J. (1979). *The philosophy and science of caring.* Boston: Little, Brown.

[n]Parse, R.R. (1981). *Man–living–health: A theory of nursing.* New York: John Wiley & Sons.

threatened. People with high self-esteem enjoy new challenges, feel respected, and have patience when things do not turn out well immediately.[12]

Self-Awareness and Self-Knowledge

Self-awareness is considered a primary component of psychological health. Developing and maintaining self-awareness is a lifelong process. This difficult task is best approached with patience, humor, and a commitment to be honest but not excessively critical of oneself. Certain self-care activities can be very helpful with this process. (Refer to Chapter 10 for additional exercises.)

Satisfying Interpersonal Relationships

Psychologically healthy individuals are able to find commonalities between themselves and those who, on the surface, are quite different from them.[13] This includes the ability to establish close, loving, and collaborative relationships. An individual need not have many relationships, but a few intimate and rewarding ones are important. (See Chapter 7 for more about relationships and self-care.)

Environmental Mastery

Stress Management

The effects of life stress can be moderated through a variety of methods, including deleting unnecessary stressors, taking responsibility for and monitoring one's pace in life, establishing priorities, saying "no" to activities that will result in too much pressure, and anticipating stressful events. Psychologically healthy people take care of themselves in order to be in the best physical and emotional condition to cope with stress.[13]

Awareness of Thought and Action Patterns

People act in ways that are consistent with their thoughts and beliefs about themselves. The significance of cognitive models of learning in self-care nursing was discussed in Chapters 4 and 6.

Beliefs such as "I can't lose weight" or "people never recover from cancer" inhibit growth and health. When one perceives a situation from a completely different point of view, altered behavior is possible. A change in clients' perceptions of themselves or of the situation indicates a major shift in one of their belief systems. The ideas of "I should" or "ought to" behave in a certain way and "I am guilty if I do not live up to my own expectations" provide the clues for identifying basic attitudes and beliefs that are limiting.[14] Exploration of childhood beliefs and feelings may be necessary to link beliefs, attitudes, and behaviors with issues that relate to the past. Psychological self-care involves an on-going exploration of this link.

Self-love and self-acceptance are the cornerstones for the foundation of emotional and mental health.[15] The development of a healthy personality and psychological wellness is not a single task but a lifelong process involving a variety of areas. It is often difficult to differentiate psychological self-care issues from spiritual and relationship self-care issues. They overlap in many ways and some of the technical approaches for practicing self-care are similar. (Also see Chapters 7 and 10.) No matter what activity the client chooses to engage in, the central themes of self-love and acceptance will facilitate psychological development.

NURTURING PSYCHOLOGICAL HEALTH

There are a number of general skills related to psychological self-care. The following techniques and exercises are provided as broad guidelines for nurturing psychological health.

- Developing inner awareness
- Values clarification
- Expression of feelings
- Communicating effectively
- Assertiveness training
- Affirmations
- Time management

Developing Inner Awareness

Among other techniques for developing and maintaining self-awareness are imagery/visualization, transcendental meditation, relaxation, inner dialogue, dream analysis, and thoughtful, consistent contacts with nature, art, or music. These self-care skills are discussed in Chapters 9 and 10.

Journal Keeping. To promote self-development, journal keeping goes beyond the chronological account of day-to-day experiences. The journal is kept in a separate book, and entries are made several times per week. Ultimately, it will include a collection of subjective feelings, states of mind, and states of emotion.[16] These entries reflect real feelings and experiences that, soon after their occurrence, are likely to disappear from view even though they are present and exerting an important influence.

Journal keeping promotes psychological well-being by:

- Verbalizing and clarifying thoughts and feelings
- Stimulating *introspection*
- Categorizing life experiences to uncover *cycles* of behavior
- Accepting increased *responsibility* for personal choices
- Facilitating *change*
- Exploring a deeper *meaning* in life[17]

Figure 8–1 demonstrates a sample entry in an intensive journal. (Chapter 10 describes the use of journals to promote spiritual self-care.)

Values Clarification

Values are ideals and concepts that are important to people. People take care of themselves according to their beliefs and values. If they believe that exercise will keep them healthy, they will follow an exercise program. By the same token, if self-care activities are not believed to be valuable, they probably will not occur. *Values clarification* identifies a systematic method for teaching the process of valuing.[18,19]

One values clarification exercise that many have found particularly helpful is to list and then rank in order "The Ten Most Important Things in My Life" (see Fig. 8–2). It is important to note that there are no correct or incorrect answers. The purpose of the exercise is simply to stimulate thought and self-awareness.

Expression of Feelings

> All I wanted to do was to live in accord with the prompting which came from my deepest self. Why was that so very difficult?
>
> Herman Hesse[20]

People are often unaware of their feelings. Many people find it difficult to express feelings, to put intense internal experiences into words. Learning to acknowledge and express one's feelings is a lifelong process.

May 16th

I had worked with Mary for several years but wasn't really aware how special she was to me. I remember the feeling that came over me when I learned she had cancer. At first I couldn't accept it; neither could she ... But going through that experience with her changed my life. As I sat by her bed and held her hand, my throat felt choked and tight, with tears rolling down my cheeks. I always envisioned myself in that situation, and felt sure I wouldn't be able to handle it. But when it actually happened, I discovered resources I didn't know I had. I was able to talk to Mary, cry, and just be with her. Together, we walked down that lonely path ~ there were some beautiful spots along the path ~ but it was painful, too. When it was all over and Mary was gone, I began to realize just how much she had done for me. She had reawakened my sense of spirituality and had put my life in better perspective. Nearly every day that goes by I realize how much her death caused me to move to a new level of maturity. As I write this a tear trickles down my cheek again, but that's all right because, with Mary's help, I know that my feelings are just another natural part of my life.

B.

Figure 8–1. Sample entry, intensive journal.

The Ten Most Important Things in My Life

Directions: On a blank sheet of paper write down the ten most
important things in all of the aspects of your life.
Then, rate the entries in order of their importance.

Example:

1. Love and respect of my family	#1
2. Financial security	#3
3. Professional achievement	#8
4. Good health	#2
5. Being a good parent	#7
6. Concern for and service to others	#9
7. Development of hobby skills	#10
8. Reduction of stress	#5
9. Free time to play and recreate	#6
10. Friends	#4

Figure 8–2. The Ten Most Important Things in My Life. Format used with permission from Bolles, R. N. (1978). *Three boxes of life*. Berkeley, CA: Ten Speed Press, p. 112.

The problem begins in childhood if parents tell their children over and over again not to trust their own perceptions, but to rely upon the parents.[21] For example,

> Child: Mommy, I am hungry.
> Parent: You couldn't be hungry, you just finished eating.

or

> Child: That was a stupid birthday party.
> Parent: No it wasn't, everyone had a great time.

This continuous contradiction of feelings confuses children about their own feelings. As adults, people continue to deny their own and other people's perceptions by giving advice, defending the other person, or analyzing the situation. Empathic responses (tuning into the feelings of another) from others allow people to acknowledge and experience their own feelings.[22]

Learning to be empathic with self and others takes practice and patience. Some simple guidelines for identifying and expressing feelings are:

- Be still. Quietly pay attention to your inner feelings and bodily sensations.
- Let yourself *feel* all the different feelings present.
- One by one, give each feeling a name. "I feel irritable." Be as specific as you can. Try out different words until you find one that resonates with your emotion. Table 8–2 has a comprehensive list of feeling words.
- Share some of your feelings with another person, or write them in a journal. Begin with "I feel" not "I think."
- Ask another person to listen to you with full attention, and acknowledge your feelings with a "Mmm, I see."
- Practice telling another person how his or her behavior affects you by using "I feel" statements rather than "You make me" (e.g., "I feel worried and upset when you don't call to tell me you will be late coming home.").

Communication

Psychological self-care in the area of communication includes such aspects as:

- Regularly assessing one's communication patterns and style.
- Developing and maintaining an ability to give and receive accurate messages.
- Recognizing and limiting the expression of anxiety during communication.
- Regularly attending to nonverbal as well as verbal communication.
- Educating oneself regarding the role of culture and values in the communication process.
- Educating oneself about predictable communication skills of different age groups (toddlers, adolescents, etc.).
- Developing and maintaining assertion skills while limiting personal aggressiveness and passivity.

Assertiveness Training

Assertiveness training is a technique aimed at reducing anxiety and developing social skills. Assertive people are thought to be able to:

- Experience greater ease in establishing close relationships.
- Prevent situations in which others take advantage of them.
- Express, both verbally and nonverbally, a wide range of negative and positive thoughts and feelings.
- Recognize important interpersonal needs and acquire the skills necessary to meet them.[23]

TABLE 8–2. FEELING WORDS

Affectionate	Courageous	Happy	Resentful
Afraid	Deferential	Hopeful	Respectful
Aggressive	Defiant	Hopeless	Sad
Airy	Dependent	Horrified	Scared
Alarmed	Depressed	Humble	Seductive
Angry	Determined	Immobilized	Self-assured
Annoyed	Dishonest	Impatient	Sexy
Anxious	Disappointed	Inadequate	Silly
Appealing	Dominant	Independent	Spineless
Ashamed	Dull	Insecure	Stretched
Beaten	Ecstatic	Irritated	Strong
Belligerent	Edgy	Itchy	Submissive
Bewildered	Embarrassed	Jealous	Surprised
Bored	Empathetic	Joyful	Sympathetic
Breathless	Enraged	Light	Talkative
Burdened	Envious	Locked in	Taut
Bushed	Estranged	Lonely	Tender
Calm	Evasive	Loving	Tense
Carefree	Excited	Mixed-up	Terrified
Cautious	Fearful	Nauseated	Thankful
Choked up	Firm	Needy	Threatened
Close	Frisky	Open	Thrilled
Cold	Frustrated	Panicky	Timid
Comforted	Furious	Paralyzed	Tolerant
Compassionate	Giddy	Peaceful	Torn
Confident	Grateful	Pleased	Two-faced
Confused	Grief-stricken	Powerless	Uptight
Contemptuous	Grumpy	Proud	Vacant
Contented	Guilty	Quiet	Warm
Cooperative	Gutless	Relaxed	Weepy

(Adapted from Leg, M. (1978). *The six levels of a happy marriage.* Ligouri, MO: Ligouri Press.)

In assertiveness training, people are taught to differentiate between assertive, passive, and aggressive behaviors.[24] The ability to acknowledge and monitor anxiety is emphasized.[25]

Affirmations

An *affirmation* is a positive thought consciously chosen to be immersed into the consciousness to produce desired results.[26] The technique of affirmation is a method to replace undesirable beliefs with beliefs that contribute to one's well-being and happiness. See Table 8–3 for an example of how to implement this technique.

Affirmations help to identify and change limiting and negative beliefs that prevent an individual from expressing his or her true self. Emotional blocks within the personality keep one stuck in immature and distorted belief systems about self, other people, and the world. Activities designed to assist the person to make a change in the belief system allow for a release of repressed emotions, which frees the mind to re-evaluate the situation and make a new decision based on a clearer perception of the actual circumstances.

Manifestation of a changed belief is accomplished when one's desires, beliefs, and expectations are congruent. If a client is affirming for a particular result and it does not materialize, the nurse can help examine which of the factors was not present. For example, one may *desire* to be rich and work fervently toward this goal but not ever meet one's *expectations* of wealth. Upon closer examination the person discovers a deep conviction that "money is the root of all evil." This underlying *belief* from early childhood conditioning actually works against one's desire and actions. The sabotaging belief needs to be identified and re-evaluated before the three necessary factors (desire, belief, and expectation) are aligned and support each other.

The use of affirmations is an important self-care activity to move a client toward greater self-love and higher self-esteem. Sondra Ray's book, *I Desire Love*,[26] gives specific affirmations for several issues and presents an exercise for ferreting out sabotaging beliefs.

TABLE 8–3. SELF-LOVE AFFIRMATION

1. Consciously *know* that you can change any belief, no matter how deep-seated it may be.

   "I believe I am unlovable."

2. *Affirm* for the desired result by putting a positive thought that you choose to immerse into your consciousness.

   "I, (*your name*), am learning to love myself more everyday."

   Repeat the affirmation several times each day until it becomes totally intergrated in your consciousness.

3. *Visualize* the end result in your mind's eye, seeing in detail exactly how you want it to be. Feel the emotions of joy and satisfaction of achieving your goal.

   "I see myself appreciating my good qualities and others doing so also. I accept my limitations."

4. *Act* as if it is already true. Expect the results to happen and be the things you desire now.

   "I treat myself well now by acknowledging one positive quality each day."

   Know, act, and feel is the formula to manifestation of one's desires.

Time Management

Every area of personal and professional life requires time management. Psychological self-care involves developing and maintaining an ability to manage time effectively.

Extensive courses on time management are offered in community centers and employment agencies. Most of these courses focus on helping people learn to establish clear-cut goals and specific plans for reaching short-term and long-range life goals.

Assessing time usage and planning each day can be accomplished through a worksheet similar to that shown in Figure 11–2 (page 222). It can initially be used to assess the time now well utilized or wasted. It can then serve as a planning device and daily schedule for weekday and weekend time management. Many daily activities can be included in the plan together with more long-term goal-directed activities. This process calls attention to some of the easily forgotten ingredients of psychological health: relaxation, exercise, laughter, and meaningful socialization.

PREPARATION FOR CRISIS AND LOSS

Crisis is popularly used to describe anything from a bad day to a major life change. Technically, a crisis is a situation or event that a person perceives as stressful and that cannot be resolved in a reasonable period of time with a person's usual coping skills.[1] Any crisis must be evaluated through the eyes of the affected person; everyone experiences life situations in different ways and with varying thresholds of tolerance. Sudden inheritance, which is usually thought of as a positive occurrence, can also elicit as much stress as a family death or an automobile accident.

Crisis situations are either maturational or situational. *Maturational crises* take place in the process of normal growth and development, or maturation. These crises are transition points, when role changes required by new levels of development are difficult and cannot be achieved for some reason.[1] Once a person knows that certain stresses, such as graduation, marriage, retirement, or bereavement, will be experienced, self-care efforts can be directed toward learning new roles, and gathering needed support.

Situational crises are reactions to events that are likely to be sudden, unexpected, and often unfortunate. They may also be pleasant or have both happy and unhappy elements. Accidents, illness, changes in relationships, and economic changes are all experiences that could precipitate situational crises.

Crises often result when an event brings some *loss* to the person involved, such as the death of a relative or loss of a parenting role. That loss can take on exaggerated and unrealistic proportions in the person's life because of a distortion of the *meaning* of the situation (e.g., "My life will not go on" or "I will never feel better again"). As a result, daily *functioning* deteriorates. At this point, people often show poor judgment or simply forget, because of preoccupation and worry, to use resources and coping skills that they would have normally used. Within four to six weeks the crisis period ends, and some resolution occurs. Many people learn new, more effective coping skills; some return to past levels of functioning; unfortunately, a few deteriorate even further—often requiring hospitalization for physical or emotional illness.

Consider the situation of a 56-year-old widow and mother of five whose youngest child has just finished college and moved away from home. With this same set of circumstances, one woman might breathe a sigh of relief and exclaim "Free at last!" A second might experience insomnia, loss of weight, and episodes of crying for no apparent reason.

Why are these reactions to the same event so different? A number of balancing factors influence people's reactions to stressful events including:

1. Perception of the event.
2. Number and quality of support people and other resources.
3. Strength and number of coping skills, such as good health and self-care skills in many areas.[1]

In the example above, the first woman perhaps had strong support systems and may have taken self-care steps to prepare herself for this major life change, the second woman may have had few support people in her life, may have been unable to learn new roles (and skills) in society, and thus felt she had reached the "end of her importance in life."

Assessment of Coping Skills

Figure 8–3 presents one aid in the process of assessing the effectiveness of current coping methods. Self-awareness includes some understanding of how and why specific coping approaches were chosen.

Table 8–4 presents a self-care worksheet for nurses to use in learning, practicing, and teaching psychological preparedness for crises. Psychological self-care includes a commitment to building a repertoire of coping methods that promote wellness and help to deal effectively with stressful situations.

Nursing Diagnoses for Psychological Health

There are several nursing diagnoses that can be used to describe a client's psychological state of being.

Disturbance in self-concept: body-image occurs when there is a disruption in the way one perceives one's body. Chronic illness, surgery, loss of functioning or body part can change the way a person feels, thinks, or views himself or herself. A disruption in how one perceives one's self-esteem can be related to

Assessment of Coping Methods

Which of the following methods of coping with stress do you usually use? Do you consider them *"healthy"* for you or *"harmful"* for you?

Coping Method:	Healthy for me	Harmful for me	Coping Method:	Healthy for me	Harmful for me
Listening to music			Overworking		
Performing physical activity			Engaging in self-pity		
Having sex			Having a temper tantrum		
Smoking cigarettes			Going for a ride		
Overeating			Praying		
Drinking liquor			Chewing gum		
Knitting/sewing			Spending money		
Cooking			Writing poetry		
Taking drugs (street or prescribed)			Daydreaming		
Trying to ignore the problem			Biting your fingernails		
Pretending something doesn't bother you			Talking to yourself		
Thinking things over			Playing an instrument		
Going to a movie or watching TV			Watching TV		
Talking with friends			"Moping"–isolate yourself, do nothing		
Leaving town			Talking to a therapist		
Throwing things			Add your other ways here:		
Cleaning the house					

Figure 8–3. Assessment of coping methods. (Reprinted with permission from Baldi, S., et al. (1980). *For your health: A model for self-care.* South Laguna, CA: Nurses Model Health, p. 22.)

pathophysiological changes, required treatments, or situational or maturational crises (e.g., divorce, loss of a job, menopause).[27]

Ineffective coping is an impairment of adaptive behaviors and problem-solving abilities of a person in meeting life's demands and roles. The loss of usual coping mechanisms when someone is faced with a major life change, such as disruption of a relationship, illness, natural disasters, can result in a crisis situation.

TABLE 8–4. SELF-CARE WORKSHEET: PSYCHOLOGICAL PREPAREDNESS UNDERSTANDING AND MANAGING CRISIS EVENTS

Assessment

What event has happened (e.g., death, retirement, etc.)?

How does it make me feel (e.g., sad, angry, confused)?

How have I been coping since the event occurred?

   Which ways are positive for me?

   Which ways are negative for me?

Whom/what resources do I have available now?

   Which am I using?

   Why am I not using certain ones?

Are my communication skills impaired right now?

Is my normal daily functioning impaired?

How is my body reacting to this stress? Am I ill?

Clarification—diagnosis

Why does this event upset me so much?

What else does it mean to me? How is it a threat to my self-image?

In what way could I be misperceiving or distorting the meaning of this event?

What would I have done in the past to deal with this problem?

What advice would I give a friend regarding this problem?

Problem solving—self-care actions

I know that during this period I should:

   Manage my time carefully

   Mobilize and increase my self-care skills

     Plan for increased rest and sleep periods

     Choose the foods I eat carefully

     Attend to my physical and environmental needs

     Practice deep-breathing when I get anxious

     Take time out to review the problem carefully

     Plan personal time for spirituality, play, and relaxation

   Limit additional life changes (e.g., do not change jobs, buy a new house, etc.)

   Communicate effectively

     Speak to people whom I might have misunderstood

     Practice assertion skills

     Clarify my words, feelings, and thoughts

   Use support systems (friends, minister, family, etc.)

     Seek support from more than one person if necessary

     Utilize community support

   Structure my activities

     Set small goals

     Keep busy without making life too chaotic

   Educate myself about normal growth and development

     Stages of grief

     What to expect at crisis points

   Give myself time

     Do not try to "sweep the problem under the rug"

     Give myself permission to talk to others about my stress (final resolution may take months or years)

TABLE 8–4. (cont.)

Evaluation
What have I learned from this?
What will I do differently next time?
Will I feel more confident to handle a crisis in the future?
What long-term coping skills would I like to change?
Who or what was most helpful to me during this crisis? How can I maintain and nourish that support system?
What self-care deficits led to my reaction to this crisis?
Do I need to improve my wellness state?
Do I need to establish better support networks?
What type of self-contract can I make regarding these needs?

Grieving related to an actual, anticipated, or perceived loss can alter an individual's ability to implement self-care activities. Reduced self-esteem, anxiety, depression, and ineffective coping can occur with dysfunctional grieving.

Anxiety is always present to some degree. Severe anxiety, however, can interfere with a client's ability to learn, concentrate, and complete tasks of everyday living. Moderate levels of anxiety can interfere with using self-care techniques that promote healing and wellness.

Powerlessness is a perceived lack of personal control over certain events or situations.[28] Clients need to be assisted to re-establish a sense of control to prevent feelings of helplessness and hopelessness. Apathy, anger, and depression can result from feeling powerless. Decreased self-esteem and feelings of low self-worth are inherently present when individuals feel out of control in their environment.

Several nursing interventions for the above diagnoses are suggested in this chapter and other chapters on relationships, spirituality, relaxation, and sexuality. The case presentations in each chapter demonstrate how to interface self-care activities with nursing orders.

USE OF PSYCHOLOGICAL SELF-CARE IN CONJUNCTION WITH TRADITIONAL SYSTEMS

For some people, referrals to psychiatrists, mental health nurses, psychologists, or other qualified professionals may need to be employed along with self-care approaches. The nurse is often in an important position to help clients reach appropriate mental health specialists.

Most nurses are able to identify acutely psychotic or suicidal clients. These people require assistance from mental health specialists. Close supervision and medication may be necessary during an acute episode. This does not mean that self-care approaches are inappropriate with this type of client. *Self-Care approaches can be used with traditional medical approaches.* For example, medications are helpful for some types of depression; they may be readily used along with ongoing self-care practices of exercise, sleep, and nutrition, which are also helpful in alleviating depression.

The actual decision of whether or not to make a referral is often complicated. It is important for nurses to be able to describe client behavior and to know when it exceeds "normal limits." Figure 8–4 describes common behav-

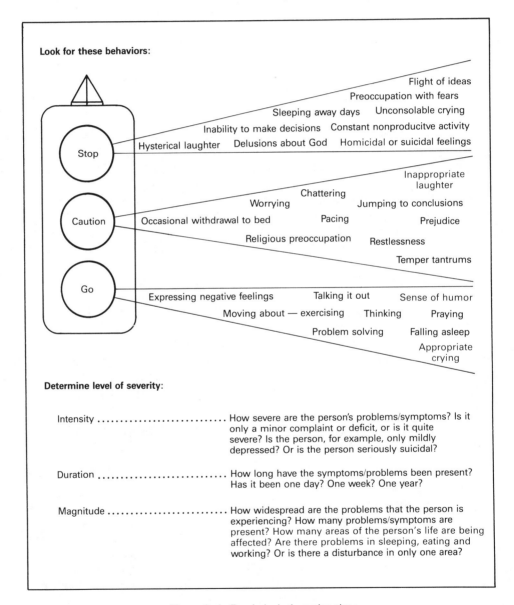

Look for these behaviors:

Stop
Flight of ideas
Preoccupation with fears
Sleeping away days   Unconsolable crying
Inability to make decisions   Constant nonproducitve activity
Hysterical laughter   Delusions about God   Homicidal or suicidal feelings

Caution
Inappropriate laughter
Chattering
Worrying   Jumping to conclusions
Occasional withdrawal to bed   Pacing   Prejudice
Religious preoccupation   Restlessness
Temper tantrums

Go
Expressing negative feelings   Talking it out   Sense of humor
Moving about — exercising   Thinking   Praying
Problem solving   Falling asleep
Appropriate crying

Determine level of severity:

Intensity . . . . How severe are the person's problems/symptoms? Is it only a minor complaint or deficit, or is it quite severe? Is the person, for example, only mildly depressed? Or is the person seriously suicidal?

Duration . . . . How long have the symptoms/problems been present? Has it been one day? One week? One year?

Magnitude . . . . How widespread are the problems that the person is experiencing? How many problems/symptoms are present? How many areas of the person's life are being affected? Are there problems in sleeping, eating and working? Or is there a disturbance in only one area?

Figure 8–4. Psychological warning signs.

iors in terms of those that are "normal," those that require observation, and those that require treatment. It provides a general guideline for nurses, clients, and family members to use when concerned about any problematic behavior pattern.

Here are several guidelines to use when deciding whether to make a referral:

1. Ask the client. If clients have been struggling with self-care approaches and continue to feel upset, they are often quite open about acknowledging their need for professional assistance.
2. Assess present psychological problems in terms of *magnitude, intensity,* and *duration.* Problems that are quite severe, affect many areas of the person's life, and have not improved over time, often call for professional intervention in addition to self-care practices. (Fig. 8–4 further describes these criteria.)
3. One of the most important assessment criteria as to whether or not psychotherapy is necessary is whether or not the client is *stuck* at any one stage of development. It is crucial to evaluate whether or not change and growth are occurring. If there are indications that the person is *not* continually repeating problematic behaviors, adequate self-care practices may solve the problem.
4. Use common sense. Nurses usually have an intuitive sense about the necessity for outside consultation from mental health specialists. This intuition and insight can be used in making good judgments.
5. When in doubt it is appropriate to refer the client for a consultative opinion. This safe route is often the most responsible and ethical action.

After the referral is discussed with the client, it is ideal to give the responsibility back to the client. By allowing the client to gather additional information and to make appointments, the nurse is encouraging self-care. The client's independence and collaboration are consistently encouraged. (See also Table 17–8, Locating Self-Care Resource.)

NURSES MODEL PSYCHOLOGICAL SELF-CARE

Nurses' psychological self-care skills are modeled in all of the ways that they manage home and work life. Many of these skills overlap with other self-care areas, such as sleep and exercise. Nurses who are rested and physically fit are likely to appear psychologically healthy.

In their personal lives nurses can model psychological self-care by:

- Practicing one self-awareness activity on a regular basis, for example, journal keeping or visualization.
- Planning for maturational crisis points.
- Maintaining at least two close support systems.
- Practicing assertive communication.

- Making "I" statements and practicing expression of feeling words.
- Obtaining counseling when needed.

In clinical interactions, nurses' psychological self-care skills are reflected in the ways nurses promote psychological health in clients. These actions include:

- Allowing clients to cry when sad or frightened; not closing off this type of communication.
- Demonstrating a sense of humor and balance.
- Teaching clients about psychological needs.
- Encouraging and facilitating expression of feelings such as anger, joy, and so on.
- Helping clients learn to use support systems.
- Acknowledging and respecting different cultural and social styles of emotional expression.
- Referring clients for counseling when indicated.

Clients observe nurses on a daily basis. Clients are aware of nurses who are anxious, angry, or withdrawn. They also notice nurses who are empathic, calm, and available to "be with" their clients.

CLINICAL APPLICATION

Case Presentation

Hester is a 59-year-old, middle-class, married, Protestant woman who owns her own accounting firm. She had married children and grandchildren. She has always been a very independent and active person. She manages her life with a high degree of organization and planning. She speaks softly but is a powerhouse of authority and leadership. Her health had generally been excellent except for moderate hypertension.

Nine months ago, during a monthly breast self-exam, she discovered a lump on the upper outer quadrant of her right breast. Surgery was performed, the lump was malignant, but there was no evidence that it had spread to the lymph nodes. The breast was removed in a simple mastectomy. She had adjusted well to the surgery and to the cancer diagnosis. Her family expressed surprise at how well she accepted and coped with the whole experience. Within a matter of weeks, she was back at work and involved in all of her previous activities.

Two weeks ago, as part of a routine checkup, a mass was discovered in her abdomen. After further diagnostic studies a hysterectomy was performed, and the mass was discovered to be a malignant tumor. Once again there was every reason to believe that the cancer had not spread from its primary site and that the two cancers were unrelated.

At this time her condition is stable; however, she no longer initiates conversations. When approached, she only offers superficial remarks. When her nurse noticed this, a discussion with Hester revealed her concerns about a second diagnosis of cancer. Hester stated that she felt depressed and anxious about the outcome of her illness. For the first time in her life she felt unable to cope.

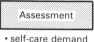

- self-care demand
- assets
- limitations

Hester gains most of her *self-esteem* from her achievements. She grew up in a working-class family; her family and close friends support her current work-oriented *values* and *life-style*.

Hester's *health care status* is very much in the forefront. Her husband, Edward, reports that Hester works very diligently to regain her physical integrity, but he has concerns about his wife's "stiff upper lip." She is uncommunicative about her feelings.

Hester has many *self-care assets*. She has a strong social support group. Until recently she did monthly breast self-examinations, monitored her own blood pressure twice weekly, adhered to a dietary regime of high complex carbohydrates and reduced fat and sodium, and tried to take a brisk one-mile walk daily. She is aware that she is a "workaholic" but has been trying to make changes in that area of her life.

Hester completed the psychological self-assessment tool Figure 8–5. Her husband also completed a peer assessment tool to provide his perception of her psychological self-care skills. Their responses were very similar. Hester volunteered that she prided herself in being self-sufficient and independent. She found it very difficult to admit that she was having a hard time coping with her illness.

It became apparent that Hester's inability to express her feelings was a detriment to her psychological health. She needed to deal with her loss of physical integrity and her fear of death. Hester was experiencing a situational crisis and needed to learn some new coping skills.

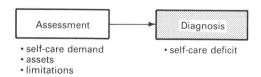

Hester and the nurse agreed that Hester had a psychological self-care deficit:

Inability to express inner feelings without intervention due to inadequate knowledge and skills

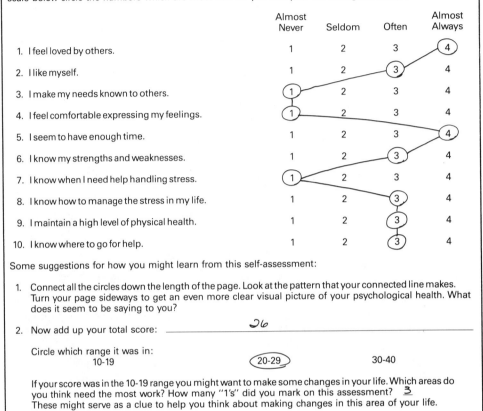

Figure 8–5. Psychological self-care assessment. (Adpated with permission from Baldi, S., et al. (1980). *For your health: A model for self-care.* South Laguna, CA: Nurses Model Health, p. v.)

Hester had always used denial as a style of coping and was unaware of many of her feelings. In Hester's family, feelings were to be contained and not expressed. She grew up with the motto, "If you can't say something nice, don't say anything at all." If the nurse initiated a discussion about feelings, Hester would initially respond with a puzzled look. As the nurse restated the comment, Hester would gradually begin to demonstrate a slight glimmer of understanding. She was motivated to become more self-aware but had to be carefully guided.

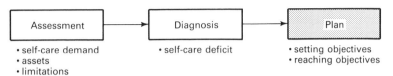

Assessment → Diagnosis → Plan

• self-care demand   • self-care deficit   • setting objectives
• assets   • reaching objectives
• limitations

Setting Objectives

Hester and the nurse clarified their respective roles in helping Hester increase her ability to express feelings. They then developed a self-contract (see Fig. 8–6). Hester said that she wanted to be able to express spontaneous feelings to others as the first step in the change process.

Reaching Objectives: Nursing and Client Actions

The nurse helped Hester increase her knowledge of the importance of feelings and "how to" express them. To facilitate this process, the nurse:

- Taught Hester how to tune in to her feelings.
- Taught Hester how to make "I feel" rather than "I think" statements.
- Provided a list of feeling words for Hester to use (see Table 8–2).
- Taught Hester the process and technique of journal writing as a method for expressing feelings.
- Encouraged the support and concern of Hester's husband by teaching him to give empathy.
- Described the program to the unit staff so that they could give Hester praise, feedback, and empathy.
- Modeled skills in this area by the expression of feelings and the use of role-play.

Figure 8–6 and Table 8–5 describe specific steps that Hester took to reach her goal. Hester completed a list of reasons for always keeping her feelings inside. Her ideas included:

- No one in my family expressed feelings, except my father when he lost his temper.
- I was always told to keep quiet and mind my own business; I was also told not to talk back.
- It always seemed easier to keep my feelings to myself and "keep the peace at any cost."
- I'm really uncomfortable with my negative feelings, and I don't want anyone to know that part of my personality.

Hester continued to work on her contract plans. The nurse met with Hester daily and with Hester and Edward together every few days. She was discharged

TABLE 8–5. NURSING CARE PLAN

Assessment	Plan	Evaluation	
		Met	Not met
Self-care demand	*Setting objectives*		
Need for improved ability to express feelings	Six weeks: "I will express at least three spontaneous feeling statements per week to another person."		X
Assets	*Reaching objectives*		
Bright, pleasant, agreeable	Client actions		
Self-sufficient	Make reason list.	X	
Highly motivated	Practice "I statements" four times a week.	X	
Practices self-care, does breast self-exam, monitors blood pressure	Use tape recorder, practice with mirror.	(only once)	
Limitations	Keep records of project.	X	
Past learning to "keep feelings inside"	Research assertion training.	X	
Denial of fear of death	Involve husband in plan.	X	
Temporarily not working	Keep appointments with nurse.	X	
Recent change in body image	Practice journal writing.	(tried it once)	
Recurrent hospitalization during last year			

Diagnosis	Nursing actions	
Self-care deficit Inability to express inner feelings without intervention due to inadequate knowledge and skills	Provide list of feelings words.	X
	Teach journal writing process.	X
	Teach use of "I statements."	X
	Model and role-play for client.	X
	Facilitate husband's involvement.	X
	Involve unit staff.	(most of staff are enthusiastic)
	Keep all appointments.	X
	Continually assess client's fear of death and readiness to talk about this issue.	X
		Needed revisions Plan to work on specific expression of angry feelings.
	Re-evaluation date	Client follow-up
	Every day with Hester during hospitalization.	Feels that self-care project was successful. Plans to meet with nurse in six weeks. Has given self the reward.
	Every three days with client and husband.	Follow-up re: fear of recurrent cancer and fear of death.
	Six week follow-up after discharge.	

SELF-CONTRACT

MY GOALS:

Short-term — by the end of six weeks I will . . . *Express at least three spontaneous feeling statements per week to another person.*

Long-term — by the end of six months I will . . . *Express negative or frightening feelings about my illness to at least one other person once a week.*

ENVIRONMENTAL PLANNING: (all the steps I will take to reach my goal)

1. Make a list of at least 4 reasons why I might keep my feelings locked inside of me.
2. Make at least ten practice "I-statements" using my list of feeling words four times per week. Record compliance or non-compliance.
3. Keep a graph to chart my progress in expressing my feelings.
4. Research an Assertion Training Class and establish a tentative future date for registering for the class.

THOUGHTS AND ACTIONS

Helpful thoughts:	Helpful actions:
It is healthy for me to express my feelings.	Ask Edward to comment on my expression of feelings and to compliment me!
Non-helpful thoughts:	**Non-helpful actions:**
I got along fine for 59 years without worrying about expressing feelings, why start now?	Whenever I feel the least bit uncomfortable I will bury myself in my work.

MY REWARD   (if I meet my goal) Short-term: Dinner-cruise with Edward on boat at Ports of Call Village. Long-term: Trip to Seattle to see son and daughter-in-law.

THE COST: (if I fail to meet my goal) Wash and dry all the crystal in the china cupboard.

REEVALUATION DATE: 2-15 for six week evaluation
6-1 for six month evaluation

I agree to help with this project:

_____Edward Enderle_____
(Support person)

I agree to strive toward this goal:

_____Nester Enderle_____
(Your signature)   (date)

Figure 8–6. Self-contract. (Adapted with permission from Baldi, S., et al. (1980). *For your health: A model for self-care.* South Laguna, CA: Nurses Model Health, p. 47.)

2½ weeks after she began her self-contract. The nurse agreed to call them at home every other week for the first three months.

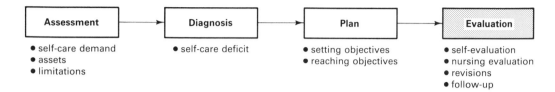

In addition to their frequent informal evaluation contacts throughout the first six-week period, Hester, Edward, and the nurse met six weeks after the initiation of the self-contract for a formal evaluation of progress. Hester was still awkward about saying what she felt. Her awareness of her negative feelings was increasing, however, and it was becoming more difficult for her to "sweep those feelings under the rug."

Hester reported that her husband's ability to empathize was improving and he helped her to meet her short-term goals. She indicated that occasionally her co-workers, who visited her often, gave her a second glance when she related a particularly emotionally-charged feeling, but all were accepting of her personal growth. Hester discovered that she had the most difficulty with her negative or angry feelings. She decided to rewrite the self-contract to reflect this new awareness.

The nurse was aware of Hester's initial inability to discuss concerns about her physical status, fear of cancer, and fear of death. At the evaluation session Hester indicated that she feared the cancer would recur. Although she was not able to express concerns about death per se, she did begin to talk about *loss* and reported three episodes in which she had cried after thinking about all she had been through.

Hester expressed great pride in all that she had accomplished. "I've always been good at doing tasks and being organized and dependable, but this is different . . . I'm learning to do something that I've never been able to do, and I feel so good about myself." She was also happy that she had given herself her "contract reward" of a dinner cruise with her husband.

Hester rewrote her self-contract to cover the next six-week period. Hester and Edward agreed to telephone the nurse if they experienced any problems or had questions. They made an appointment for the three of them to meet again in six weeks. Table 8–5 presents a sample nursing care plan for this clinical situation.

SUMMARY

In this chapter views of psychological health from different psychological and nursing theorists were discussed. Components of psychological health were explored. Included were self-esteem, self-knowledge, satisfying interpersonal relationships, environmental mastery, and stress management.

Techniques for nurturing psychological health were presented. Self-awareness, communication, time management, preparation for crisis and loss, development and maintenance of social support systems, and affirmations were areas in which specific techniques were delineated.

A clinical presentation illustrated the integration of psychological self-care in an acute care setting, emphasizing its use with traditional systems. The role of the nurse as a model of psychological self-care was also explored.

STUDY QUESTIONS

Personal Focus

1. How do you rate yourself as a model of psychological health for your family, friends, and clients?
2. Who are your personal models of psychological health?
3. What are your current psychological self-care goals?
4. Assess your current coping skills. How could you alter coping patterns that are maladaptive?
5. Practice completing one affirmation.

Client Focus

1. Role-play how you would explain to a client the meaning and technique of self-care.
2. Help a client assess his or her current time management skills. Help the client plan for more effective time management.
3. Help a client practice self-care during a crisis by using the worksheet in this chapter (Table 8–4).
4. Discuss the ways in which psychological self-care is facilitated or blocked in your clinical setting.

REFERENCES

1. Aguilera, D.C., & Messick, J. (1982). *Crisis intervention* (4th ed.). St. Louis: C.V. Mosby, pp. 67–71.
2. 1 Sam. 16:23.
3. Brett, G.S. (1962). *A history of psychology* (3 vols.). New York: Macmillan.
4. Ferguson, M. (1980). The aquarian conspiracy: Personal and social transformation in the 1980s. Los Angeles: J.P. Tarcher, p. 245.
5. Washkoviak, L. (1989). Psychological, spiritual, and social wellness. In *Promoting wellness: A nurse's handbook*. Rockville, Maryland: Aspen pp. 243–269.

6. Goleman, D. (1988, February 4). Talking to oneself is good therapy, doctors say. *The New York Times*, Health section. V, p. 21.

7. Houck, C. (1989, January). How To beat a bad mood. *Readers Digest*, pp. 93–95.

8. Stone, H. & Winkelman, S. (1989). *Embracing ourselves*. San Raphael, CA: New World Library.

9. Nash, B.M. & Monchick, R.M. (1980). *The book of tests*. New York: Doubleday/Dolphin Books.

10. Jourard, S.M. (1974). *The healthy personality*. New York: Macmillan, p. 29.

11. Brandon, N. (1984). *Honoring thyself*. New York: Bantam Books, p. 183.

12. Wegscheider-Cruse, S. (1987). *Learning to love yourself: Finding your self-worth.* Pampano Beach, FL: Health Communications, p. 16.

13. Wilson, H., & Kniesl, C. *Psychiatric nursing* (2nd ed.). Reading, MA: Addison-Wesley, pp. 248–249.

14. Davidhizar, R. & Marabaugh, N. (1988). Avoiding self-defeating feelings. *AORN Journal*, 48(1), 92–94.

15. Mesher, A. (1982). *Journey of love*. Austin, TX: Arnan Publishing, p. 92.

16. Progroff, I. (1975). *At a journal workshop*. New York: Dialogue House Library, p. 77.

17. Capacchione, L. (1979). *The creative journal*. Chicago: Swallow Press.

18. Arnold, E. & Boggs, K. (1989). *Interpersonal relationships: Professional communication: Skills for nurses*. Philadelphia: W.B. Saunders, pp. 308–338.

19. Taylor, C., Lillis, C., & LeMone, P. (1989). *Fundamentals of nursing: The art and science of nursing care*. Philadelphia: Lippincott, pp. 58–79.

20. Hesse, H. (1965). *Demian*. New York: Bantam Books, p. xii.

21. Faber, A., & Mazlish, E. (1980). *How to talk so kids will listen, and listen so kids will talk*. New York, Avon, pp. 2–3.

22. Seamands, D. (1986). *Healing for damaged emotions*. Wheaton, IL: Victor B.

23. Cotler, S.B., & Guerra, J. (1976). *Assertion training*. Champaign, IL: Research Press, p. 3.

24. Arnold & Boggs, *Interpersonal relationships*, pp. 340–372.

25. Cotler & Guerra. *Assertion training*, p. 5.

26. Ray, S. (1980). *I deserve love*. Millbrae, CA: Celestial Arts.

27. Carpenito, L. (1987). *Nursing diagnosis: Application to clinical practice* (2nd ed.). Philadelphia: Lippincott.

28. Miller, J. (1984). *Coping with chronic illness: Overcoming powerlessness*. Philadelphia: F.A. Davis, p. 13.

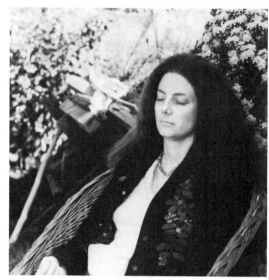

Blest, who can unconcernedly find
Hours, days, and years slide soft away
In health of body, peace of mind;
Quiet by day.

Sound sleep by night; study and ease
Together mixed, sweet recreation,
And innocence, which most does please
With meditation.

Edgar Allan Poe

9 Relaxation

LEARNING OBJECTIVES

Upon completion of this chapter, readers will be able to:

1. Define relaxation and differentiate relaxation from play or recreation.
2. List four characteristics of relaxation.
3. Describe three techniques through which relaxation can be achieved.
4. List the four essential components of all relaxation techniques.
5. List three benefits of regularly practiced relaxation.
6. Describe the major precautions to consider when beginning a relaxation program.
7. Practice one relaxation technique.

DEFINITIONS

Relaxation   "A natural and innate protective mechanism against 'overstress,' which allows us to turn off harmful bodily effects. This mechanism brings on bodily changes that decrease heart rate, lower metabolism, decrease the rate of breathing and bring the body back into what is probably a healthier balance."[1]

A neutral state. "Mental and physical freedom from tension or stress."[2]

INTRODUCTION

Relaxation includes a very specific set of behaviors. It involves the purposeful use of a set of techniques that focus attention in a nonanalytical way so as not to dwell on diversive, ruminating thought.[3,4] The first of these is the notion of *intention*. The individual chooses to focus attention on a particular object or field.

Second, these techniques are not dependent on any particular religious *beliefs* or practices. This does not imply that relaxation is not a part of any religious practice or that religion cannot be incorporated into the practice of relaxation. Quite the contrary, religion has played a significant role in the history of relaxation, but it is important to note that relaxation is distinct from religion or prayer.

Third, relaxation involves more or less *effort*, depending on individual skill level, to keep attention focused. The aim is to avoid sequential analytical thought.

Fourth, awareness of the *process* is more important than the content of the thoughts. Allowing distracting thoughts to come, to be noticed, and then to be released, is what is important. The specific focus of the relaxation exercise is not significant. An individual, for example, could choose to focus on a particular word, visualization, or sound and have equally satisfactory results.

Common examples of how people try to relax are not congruent with these characteristics. Frequently, play or recreation are given as examples or ways used to "relax." While playing Frisbee or watching television, however, it is not possible to focus attention and concentration on the process of relaxation. In these activities, new information and content must continually be processed or new problems solved. From moment to moment, one might need to decide to change the speed or spin of the Frisbee or to turn the television off.

Another frequent example of a means used to relax is sleep or naps. Sleep is physiologically very different from relaxation. During sleep, oxygen consumption decreases slowly over a period of hours to about 92 percent of normal. In relaxation, it decreases within the first three minutes to 80 to 90 percent of normal. In addition, alpha brain waves increase in intensity and frequency during relaxation, but not in sleep. Brain activity associated with the rapid eye movements (REM) of sleep does not occur in relaxation.[5]

HISTORICAL PERSPECTIVE

Throughout history, practices similar to relaxation have been described in religious and secular literature. Words used to describe the effect of these practices, such as peace, warmth, transcendence, ecstasy, and well-being, are the same as in descriptions found today.

The means used to achieve this relaxed state are also historically comparable. Essential elements in religious practices of all cultures remain constant. These elements are again very similar to the techniques used today to elicit relaxation.

As early as A.D. 354–430, St. Augustine described the need to "pass beyond this power of mind which is called memory" in order to quiet his thoughts. Christian mystical writings of the tenth century explained the need to eliminate all distractions and physical activity, including thoughts, in order to reach a higher level of consciousness. It was believed that this practice would help people in daily life by making them more efficient and tasks more enjoyable.[6]

In Judaism, the earliest form of mysticism dates back to the second century B.C. Merkabalism was a meditative practice involving chanting. In the thirteenth century A.D., the Jewish Kabbalistic tradition included meditative practices involving body posture, chanting, and breathing. The purpose of this meditation was to open up the soul's deeper regions and induce a state of ecstasy.[7,8]

These Judaic religious practices have been described as a Judaized version of the ancient Indian mystical practices of yoga. Indeed, several Eastern religions include meditative practices that extend the practice of relaxation into everyday life. Indian scriptures of the sixth century B.C., the Upanishads, describe the means of attaining a unified state. Zen and yoga employ specific techniques, including withdrawal from the senses, concentration, maintaining comfortable positions, repetition of phrases, and practicing specific breathing.

In Japan and China, Shintoism and Taoism include methods of prayer very similar to yoga. The objective is to concentrate on "nothingness" in order to achieve absolute tranquility.[9]

Cultures throughout the world employ meditative practices very similar to those of the Japanese and Chinese. Shamanism is a form of mysticism practiced in North and South America, Africa, and Indonesia.[10] Through the use of chants and trance-like states, feelings of ecstasy are achieved.

In addition to the religious and philosophical literature describing the practice of relaxation, writers of prose and poetry have descriptively portrayed a relaxed state. The works of Wordsworth, Tennyson, and Thoreau are explored by Spurgeon in her book, *Mysticism in English Literature*.[11] Entering a state of inner tranquility is described throughout the works of these authors. Practices of freeing the mind from distracting thoughts and spending time in a quiet environment were believed to be as helpful then as they are today.

Self-care through relaxation is not new but places new emphasis on an ancient self-care practice. Nurses today are involved in teaching prepared childbirth classes including the principles of breathing, body posture, and deep muscle relaxation. Preoperatively and postoperatively, clients are taught by nurses to breathe and relax as a means of controlling anxiety and pain. These same kinds of techniques are used to assist clients in going to sleep without medication or with decreased doses of medication. These are only a few examples of the use of some of the basic concepts of relaxation self-care.

THE RELAXATION RESPONSE

Physiology of Relaxation

Clinical relaxation has been described by Jacobson in specific physiological terms. It is reduced tension state in which skeletal and smooth muscle contractions are near zero, respiration diminishes in ratio and extent, the heart rate slows and force is decreased, and both systolic and diastolic blood pressure falls.[12]

Pelletier has describes psychophysiological changes that occur with deep relaxation.[13] In essence, these are exactly the opposite of the fight–flight response described by Selye.[14] In the *hypermetabolic* state of fight–flight, stimulation of the sympathetic branch of the autonomic nervous system leads to increased heart rate, respiratory rate, oxygen consumption, and perspiration. This group of responses involves neural, hormonal, and endocrine systems. What can be an adaptive response, in certain instances, is now believed to be connected to diseases of stress. In fact, the belief that sustained tension contributes to mental and physical illness is now a basic tenet of psychosomatic medicine.[15]

In relaxation, the physiological response is *hypometabolic*. This *parasympathetic* response results in a decrease in blood pressure, respiratory and heart rates, oxygen consumption, arterial blood lactates, and muscle tension. In addition, there is an increase in the production and amplitude of alpha brain waves and in skin resistance. These results vary in each person, but there is a tendency for them to occur together.

It is believed that a lowered arousal state of neurophysiological functioning "minimizes stress reactivity."[16] Individuals trained in relaxation are able to shift into a pattern of decreased sympathetic arousal when they are unable to avoid or overcome a stressor. This makes it possible to avoid the consequences of a prolonged stress reaction. As a result, there is an increased ability to cope with the strains and pressures of everyday life.

In addition to these clinical benefits, relaxation has been found to have a "carry-over" effect. That is, it has an effect on daily activities. Individuals who regularly practice relaxation are found to be more psychologically stable, less anxious, and to have a sense of greater personal effectiveness.[16]

TYPES OF RELAXATION TECHNIQUES

Many methods are used to elicit a relaxed state or response. These include deep breathing, autogenics, meditation, biofeedback, visualization or imagery and music.

Deep Breathing

Deep breathing originated as a Buddhist meditation technique. The meditator "watched" his or her breath flowing in and out of the nostrils. Counting the breaths further aided concentration.

Currently, deep breathing is used in a variety of clinical settings. Perhaps best known is in natural or prepared childbirth. Children and clients of any age are also taught this skill to aid in pain control and management of anxiety. An example of a deep-breathing exercise is found in Table 9–1.

The skill of deep breathing is prerequisite for success with other relaxation methods. Advantages of this technique include ease in learning, adaptability to a variety of settings, and value in integrating with other relaxation skills.

Autogenic Training

Autogenic training is highly structured and consists of six exercises practiced with a minimum of external stimuli. Attention is focused on particular body parts while specific phrases are mentally repeated. These exercises are listed in Table 9–2. They are intended to generate a particular physiological state and to teach passive concentration.

Meditation

Meditation is a set of techniques intended to enable an individual to focus attention. Although meditation had its historical origins in religion, it is in itself distinct from any specific religion or belief system. A specific form of concentration is the key to all types of meditation; attention is passively focused, nonanalytically and nonlogically.

There are two types of meditation. In one, attention is "opened up" so that the individual is receptive, in an undistracted way, to internal and external stimuli. In the other, attention is focused on a single object or a word (such as a candle or mantra), with all other objects excluded from awareness.

People who choose the latter approach may focus their attention on their breathing and on a phrase that they repeat over and over. This process achieves relaxation. It is an ancient technique that is simple to use and very effective. An example of one exercise is found in Table 9–3. This process takes only 15 to 20 minutes to teach, and it can help an individual in any stressful situation. In

TABLE 9–1. DEEP BREATHING EXERCISE

1. Although this exercise can be practiced in a variety of poses, the following is recommended. Lie down on your back on a blanket or rug on the floor. Bend your knees and move your feet about 8 inches apart, with your toes turned outward slightly. Make sure that your spine is straight.

2. Scan your body for tension.

3. Place one hand on your abdomen and one hand on your chest.

4. Inhale slowly and deeply through your nose into your abdomen to push up your hand as much as feels comfortable. Your chest should move only a little and only with your abdomen.

5. When you feel at ease with step 4, smile slightly, inhale through your nose and exhale through your mouth, making a quiet, relaxing, whooshing sound like the wind as you blow gently out. Your mouth, tongue, and jaw will be relaxed. Take long, slow, deep breaths that raise and lower your abdomen. Focus on the sound and feeling of breathing as you become more and more relaxed.

6. Continue deep-breathing for about 5 or 10 minutes at a time, once or twice a day, for a couple of weeks. Then, if you like, extend this period to 20 minutes.

7. At the end of each deep-breathing session, take a little time to scan your body for tension. Compare the tension you feel at the conclusion of the exercise with that which you experienced when you began.

8. When you become at ease with breathing into your abdomen, practice it whenever you feel like it during the day when you are sitting or standing. Concentrate on your abdomen moving up and down, the air moving in and out of your lungs, and the feeling of relaxation that deep-breathing gives you.

9. When you have learned to relax yourself using deep-breathing, practice it whenever you feel yourself getting tense.

(Reprinted with permission from Davis, M., Eshelman, E.R., & McKay, M. (1980). *The relaxation and stress reduction workbook.* Oakland, CA: New Harbinger Publications, pp. 31–32.)

TABLE 9–2. STANDARD AUTOGENIC TRAINING EXERCISES

Standard Exercise	Desired Physiological State	Phrase to be Repeated
1	Heaviness in the extremities	"My arms and legs are heavy"
2	Warmth in the extremities	"My arms and legs are warm"
3	Calm and regular function of the heart	"My heart is calm and regular"
4	Calm and regular respiration	"My breath is calm and regular" or "It breathes me"
5	Solar plexus warm	"My solar plexus is warm"
6	Forehead cool	"My forehead is cool"

(Reprinted with permission from Peper, E., & Williams, E.A. (1980). Autogenic therapy. In *Health for the whole person.* A.C. Hastings, et al. (Eds.), Boulder, CO: Westview Press, p. 133.)

TABLE 9–3. MEDITATION EXERCISE

Sit quietly in a comfortable position. Close your eyes. Deeply relax all your muscles, beginning at your feet and progressing up to your face. Keep them deeply relaxed.

Breathe through your nose. Become aware of your breathing. As you breathe out, say the word "one" silently to yourself. Continue for 20 minutes. You may open your eyes to check the time, but do not use an alarm. When you have finished sit quietly for several minutes, at first with closed eyes and later with open eyes.

Do not worry about whether you are successful in achieving a deep level of relaxation. Maintain a passive attitude and permit relaxation to occur at its own pace. Expect distracting thoughts. When these distracting thoughts occur, ignore them and continue repeating "one."

Practice the technique once or twice daily, but not within two hours after a meal, since the digestive processes seem to interfere with elicitation of anticipated changes.

(Reprinted with permission from Benson, H. (1977). Systematic hypertension and the relaxation response. *New England Journal of Medicine, 296,* 1152.)

hospitals, this technique is commonly used during labor and delivery and for pain control with medical–surgical clients.

Transcendental Meditation. Transcendental meditation (TM) focuses on the use of one phrase or *mantra* to achieve relaxation. The term *transcendental* means "going beyond" and indicates the goal of taking its practitioners beyond the familiar level of wakeful experience to a state of profound rest and increased alertness.[17]

The TM technique requires a course of special instruction. Once the instruction is completed, however, practice takes place independently and for maximal benefit should be practiced approximately 20 minutes twice a day.[18]

Through TM, people can achieve a profound relaxation response in which the heart rate slows, the metabolic rate decreases, and less oxygen is consumed. Problems that are seen as stress related (e.g., hypertension and insomnia) are within the client's control through TM. Meditators demonstrate significant decreases in anxiety and depression with increases in self-actualization. TM is also reported to help people decrease their consumption of food, alcohol, tobacco, and drugs.[19]

Biofeedback

Biofeedback is a mechanical method of providing physiological information to individuals leading to voluntary control of internal body activity. In biofeedback training, an assessment of physiological problems is made. As a result of continuous feedback, an individual is able to make physiological changes in body systems, such as warming the fingertips or lowering blood pressure.

Three conceptual principles are described by Pelletier as essential to biofeedback:

1. Any biological function that can be monitored electronically and fed back through the senses can be regulated by the individual.
2. Every physical change is accompanied by a mental change that can be conscious or unconscious, and conversely, mental–emotional changes are accompanied by changes in physiological state.
3. Deep relaxation facilitates the establishment of voluntary control.[20]

Biofeedback has been used with a variety of physiological measures. Clinically, the most commonly used are hand temperature, muscle tension, palmar skin conductance, brain electrical activity, heart rate, and blood pressure.

Training methods in biofeedback vary tremendously from one health care provider to another. Outcomes also vary and are dependent on several factors, including client motivation and ability to learn new skills, client expectations regarding outcome, and the skill of the trainer.[21]

Some clients and health care providers work together to incorporate principles of relaxation into the biofeedback training; others do not. Regardless of the technique used, relaxation is the goal. A benefit of biofeedback is that the client can know, by way of mechanical feedback, whether or not relaxation has been achieved.

Visualization/Imagery

Visualization or imagery is another relaxation technique. Some people use this method daily, but it has also been used on a temporary basis in acute clinical settings. This technique involves closing one's eyes and seeing with the "mind's eye." The person visualizes calm and pleasant scenes for the purpose of relaxation. For example, an individual might envision a sunset at the beach and think about it quietly for 20 minutes to achieve relaxation.

Imagery and visualization have been used in the treatment of physical illnesses such as headaches, hypertension, and cancer. The Simontons have used these techniques in working with cancer clients.[22] Clients envision a positive outcome for their illnesses and practice the technique three times a day for 10 to 15 minutes. A sample of their exercise is found in Table 9–4. This exercise can be adapted for many illnesses and conditions.

Imagery is also helpful in states of wellness. Visualizing successful marketing calls on customers, dynamic public speaking presentations, or a calm, relaxed, and peaceful state can increase a person's sense of well-being. Table 9–5 gives an example of a visualization exercise to help children wind down after school or following any fast-paced or emotionally charged activity.

These relaxation techniques can all be adapted to home practice with minimal teaching and cost. They do require extensive patience and effort, however, to become integrated into an individual's daily activities.

Music

Certain sounds can produce healing and relaxation. Some people consider music to be the most effective path to relaxation and recuperation.[23] Music with a

TABLE 9–4. VISUALIZATION EXERCISE

1. Sit in a comfortable position. Close your eyes and begin taking deep breaths. Concentrate on breathing, relaxing, and experiencing your lungs filling and emptying completely.
2. While relaxing and breathing deeply, visualize the diseased area. Picture the area and see the disease process within the area.
3. Visualize your white corpuscles attacking the disease process. The white corpuscles may be imagined in any form, such as an army, a lion, or a bulldozer. See the white corpuscles surround and penetrate the diseased area, overcoming and clearing the disease.
4. Imagine yourself well. See the formerly diseased area as healthy, vibrant, and fully functioning. Extend this visualization to see each organ system as happily fulfilling its function in harmony with all other functions. See and feel your entire body as healthy and vibrant.
5. Return your awareness to your breathing and slowly open your eyes.

(Reprinted with permission from Jasmin, S., & Trygstad, L.N. (1979). *Behavioral concepts and the nursing process.* St. Louis: C.V. Mosby, pp. 71–72. Modified from Simonton, S.M. (1977). Group process and imagery with cancer patients. In M.C. Brotman (Ed.), *Mind as healer, mind as slayer: A workbook.* Pacific Palisades, CA: The Center for Integral Medicine, pp. 7–1, 7–2.)

tempo of about 60 beats per minute, with an even rhythm, tends to slow the body processes down and has a sedating, calming effect.[24] This helps clients cope with a variety of psychophysiologic dysfunctions.

Nurses use music to help clients relax and to aid in pain reduction. Intensive care clients who listened to certain "healing tapes" have shown significant reductions in heart rate, depression, anxiety, and pain. Operating room clients have reported that listening to healing tapes through ear phones made their experience less stressful.[25]

Certain types of calming music will obviously be more effective with certain types of clients than others. For example, there is some evidence that

TABLE 9–5. VISUALIZATION EXERCISE: KITTY

"You're a kitty who's played all day; scaled the walls and leaped away." (If you're sitting, act it out with your arms; if standing, with your whole body.) "Meow . . . meow. Now it's time to slowly creep, to find a place where you can sleep. Curl up snug and I'll stroke your fur. Resting calmly, as you purr."

You can add: "I will reach out and stroke each resting kitten's furry back (or head), and you make a purring sound when I do."

(Reprinted with permission from Hirsch, H. (1980). *Relaxation techniques for young children: A guide for teachers and parents.* Boulder, CO: New Beginnings Publications, p. 50.)

clients who are experienced in listening to music are able to reach a deep relaxation state with the use of music more quickly than clients who do not usually listen to music. Nuses and clients must work together to develop a sound program that will be most effective for each person's particular preferences and needs. Bonny has produced a set of tapes called *Music RX* that are designed for hospital use.[25] Nurse authors have also provided extensive descriptions of the use of this relaxation modality with clients.[24,27]

Effectiveness of Specific Methods

The variety of methods and techniques present an array of choices for the client and the nurse. The selection of a particular method is influenced by knowledge, experience, and consideration of the client's illness, personality, and response to treatment.

In an extensive review of the literature, Shapiro does not find any significant differences in the outcomes of specific relaxation methods. He points out that further research is necessary and that the distinction must be made between beginning practitioners of relaxation and those with advanced skills. Limitations in research design and methodology may be responsible for the failure to demonstrate the clear advantages of certain techniques.[28]

There is some evidence that a somatic treatment (e.g., progressive relaxation or biofeedback) may be particularly effective with muscular problems such as tension headaches. Cognitive approaches (i.e., autogenic training or meditation) may be a better choice for disorders with a cognitive aspect such as test anxiety, insomnia, or depression. Combinations of techniques appear to produce more cumulative effects than a single technique for treating psychosomatic disorders.[29] Thus, nurses may want to suggest that clients try a number of different approaches to relaxation until they find the particular "fit" that is best for their needs and skills.

Uses in Clinical Settings

An increased understanding of the neurophysiology of relaxation has contributed to its current application in the treatment of many health disorders. These include muscle contraction headache, migraine headache, essential hypertension, Reynaud's disease, anxiety, asthma, and drug and alcohol dependence.[21] Specifically, in both prospective and retrospective studies, the ability of individuals to improve their health in very dramatic ways has been demonstrated.

In an extensive review of clinical literature, Titlebaum points out that nurses can and *do* use relaxation techniques to reduce tension, anticipatory anxiety, blood pressure, and pain.[30] Relaxation skills are used in clinical settings to increase concentration, sense of control, ability to block inner dialogue, and suggestibility. They are also used clinically to promote sleep, slow the heart rate, and warm or cool parts of the body.

Examples of research in this area include:

- Nurses found a reduction of anxiety, crying, stalling, and other distress behavior in children receiving repeated lumbar punctures following a program of desensitization, guided imagery, suggestion, and relaxation training.[31]
- Cholecystectomy patients who were taught relaxation as a method of postoperative pain management reported a decrease in anxiety and an increase in perceived control of their pain.[32]
- Cancer clients practicing guided relaxation/imagery reported less emotional distress, nausea, and physiological arousal following chemotherapy infusions than control subjects.[33]
- Improved T-cell activity, increase in natural killer cell activity, and changes in B-cell measures have been shown in cancer patients who practiced relaxation with guided imagery.[34]
- Guided imagery has been shown to have a significant impact on the self-esteem, anxiety, and drinking behavior of alcoholics.[35]
- Imagery has been used to facilitate grief work in families with dying relatives.[36]

Nursing Diagnosis and Relaxation Self-Care

No one nursing diagnosis is more relevant to relaxation self-care than any other. Teaching relaxation skills is clearly a major nursing intervention in diagnostic areas such as anxiety, sleep pattern disturbance, fear, and certain types of sexual dysfunction. Since this skill is so central to *all* stress management, it should probably be considered as an intervention for most clients regardless of their health problem or nursing diagnosis.

PRECAUTIONS RELATED TO RELAXATION

Regardless of the method used, relaxation, when practiced regularly, will allow an individual to achieve a physiological state characterized by *hypometabolic activity*. Serious attention must, therefore, be given to those conditions in which an individual's health and safety can be affected.[37]

These conditions include (1) mental disorders in which an individual is in a psychotic state and (2) clinical disorders that can be affected by a change in metabolic rate. Diabetes, hypertension, chronic respiratory disease, epilepsy, and hyperthyroidism or hypothyroidism are but a few examples.

Physical symptoms need to be medically evaluated prior to the initiation of relaxation self-care practices. It is absolutely necessary to rule out any organic pathology underlying a client's symptoms and complaints. It would be highly unprofessional to assume, for example, that a client's headache is caused solely by tension. Any physical disorder must have concurrent medical attention throughout the course of relaxation training and practice.

Perfectionistic clients may feel pressure to "perform" by relaxing "well." This undermines the benefits of the activity and increases client anxiety unless the nurse is tolerant of this behavior and able to provide new options.

DEVELOPING AND MAINTAINING RELAXATION SELF-CARE SKILLS

There are a variety of factors that facilitate the practice of relaxation. These are particularly helpful in initial phases of learning relaxation techniques.

Fundamental to *all methods* used to achieve relaxation are:

1. A quiet environment
2. Focused attention
3. A passive attitude
4. A comfortable position[38]

The specifics of how these are utilized may vary, but the basic components remain constant. It is necessary to decrease logical thinking and problem solving. To achieve this state, one needs to develop a passive, nonjudgmental attitude in which distracting thoughts are observed and simply allowed to occur.

It is necessary, at least initially, to practice this nonjudgmental passive concentration in a quiet, comfortable environment. This allows fewer distractions and frees the individual to focus attention. Adequate support for the back and extremities is important so that large muscle groups and bones are truly supported and not held in position by tension and effort.

Other considerations in developing relaxation self-care skills include:

- *Deep breathing:* This skill is applicable in a variety of settings. Many times, it is helpful just to take two or three deep breaths while sitting in traffic on the freeway, taking off in a plane, getting ready to give a talk, or in the midst of some tedious task.
- *Privacy:* Providing for privacy is essential to learning relaxation skills. The individual must be free from interruptions to allow total concentration on the technique. Considerations include taking the telephone off the hook, providing for child care, hanging a "Do Not Disturb" sign on the home or office door, and securing commitment from others not to interrupt during this time.
- *Music:* Soothing music can lower pulse and blood pressure. This might be played in the car while on the freeway, at home during the hectic late afternoon rush (instead of television), while getting ready for work in the morning, or for an hour before bedtime.
- *Comfort:* Physical and emotional comfort are essential to the practice of relaxation. Considerations include loose, comfortable clothing, a warm place, a comfortable chair, time to practice, giving oneself permission to have this time alone, and allowing one's mind to wander and then return to the practice of relaxation.

There are so many ways to achieve relaxation that it is important to remember several points. First, what works for one individual may not work for another. As with other self-care practices, each person must find his or her own way. Visualization may work better for one person, while someone else may find chanting or music more helpful.

Second, it is important to begin slowly. Again, as with other self-care practices, the individual cannot expect to be able to achieve immediate results. Individuals need to begin with a few minutes each day and gradually increase time. Practicing for 15 to 20 minutes once or twice a day will be sufficient to achieve psychophysiological benefits. It is possible to spend too much time in relaxation, but, as Benson points out, several hours daily would be necessary to produce any negative side effects.[39]

Over time, with practice and patience, the individual will be able to find his or her own way to relax. The relaxation skill can then be integrated into daily self-care programs.

NURSES MODEL RELAXATION SELF-CARE

Nurses often confuse relaxation with play or recreation. They think of it in the colloquial sense (e.g., reading or watching television). Even nurses who use relaxation techniques with their clients, such as breathing techniques to assist with labor or controlling postoperative pain, frequently identify these techniques only with clinical situations. They are rarely used in the nurse's personal life.

Nursing is highly stressful. Burnout and high attrition levels are discussed at length in both lay and professional literature as resulting from too much stress over too long a period of time. Relaxation has been shown to reduce the harmful effects of ongoing stress and to increase coping skills.

Specific self-care actions that promote relaxation in the work setting may include:

- Practicing relaxation skills instead of drinking coffee at break.
- Taking time out for relaxation after a particularly stressful event, such as a cardiac arrest.
- Offering relaxation music tapes to clients.
- Providing privacy for clients to practice relaxation skills.
- Teaching clients relaxation skills as an adjunct to pain or sleeping medication.
- Trying alternative methods such as visualization or deep breathing to reduce a client's pain *before* administering medications.
- Asking for classes in relaxation skills for nurses.
- Using a relaxation self-assessment tool with clients and colleagues.

The nurse is also a model of this self-care skill for family and friends. There are many situations in which knowledge of relaxation and a willingness to share the technique can benefit others. Uses of this self-care activity in the nurse's personal life include:

- Using relaxation skills when children return from school "wired up."
- Providing for private "quiet time" two to three times during the day and right before bed.
- Teaching children to practice relaxation as they approach such stressful situations as tests at school or visits to the doctor or dentist.
- Being an advocate and model of relaxation skills for family and friends.
- Actively lending tapes and written materials on relaxation to friends.
- Spending a few minutes with one's spouse for assisting with relaxation before he or she takes medication for a headache.

Anyone (client, family, or friend) can be stressed by many situations. By spending a few minutes to teach a simple relaxation technique such as deep breathing, the nurse becomes a model for a healthier life-style.

CLINICAL APPLICATION

Case Presentation

Mary is an 18-year-old Caucasian, Lutheran, middle-class nursing student. In a visit to the hospital's employee health department, she complained of fatigue, headache, and irritability that had lasted for two weeks. A health history and physical examination revealed no abnormal findings.

```
┌─────────────────────────┐
│      Assessment         │
└─────────────────────────┘
• self-care demand
• assets
• limitations
```

The occupational health nurse gathered data regarding Mary's *assets* and *limitations* in the areas of self-care practices, life-style, developmental level, family background, sociocultural orientation, and health care state. The nurse found that Mary's *life-style* left her with little time for herself. She had taken a part-time job every other weekend in the intensive care unit at the local medical center to gain experience and to earn tuition and spending money. She also spent 10 hours a week in class and an average of 30 to 40 hours studying. While excited about her role as a student, Mary found it necessary to be continuously "on top" of all cases. She felt a need to read and study constantly.

Many was feeling torn as a result of the new demands at school and work. Many of her friends had eight-hour-a-day jobs with plenty of time for socializing and dating. Her high school boyfriend was attending college across the country, and they had not seen each other for a year due to *financial* restrictions.

When not at work or school, Many spent her time studying. She was not involved in any *social* or community groups. Although she did attend student meetings once a month, Mary encountered difficulty just finding time to have her hair cut. She had two close female friends who were also nursing students and had similar life-styles. She found them supportive.

Mary's family held beliefs and values consistent with their *sociocultural background*. Family members were expected to work hard, not ask for help, and delay gratification. Vacations were rare, and recreation was allowed only after "all the work was done."

Mary's *physical examination* revealed no physical cause for her symptoms, but she suffered from fatigue, headaches, and irritability, which had been increasing for the past two weeks. At the interview she reported feeling "too tired to get out of bed." She explained that she had been having difficulty falling asleep and on several occasions slept only four or five hours. This was markedly different from two weeks before when she regularly slept for eight uninterrupted hours. As a result, she believed that just when she needed to be "on top of things," she was finding it more difficult to concentrate. She was "so worried" that she found herself "snapping" at her friends and hospital staff for things "I would ordinarily laugh at."

Mary knew the effect of life-style on health, particularly for her clients in intensive care. Somehow, she had never considered that this also applied to her. A summary of her *self-care skills* revealed:

- Three well-balanced meals daily.
- No regular exercise; no knowledge of target heart rate.
- No knowledge that recreation and play were important to health.
- No knowledge of relaxation.

Mary completed the relaxation self-assessment tool. Her responses are shown in Figure 9–1.

Her symptoms began just after taking on her part-time job. She was feeling tense and anxious about her work expectations. Since that change she had been unable to sleep and, as a result, her school, work, and relationships with friends were affected. In addition to these demands, Mary did not take time for herself to exercise, play, or relax. Mary and the nurse worked together to arrive at her self-care demand:

Need for improved relaxation skills

After this demand was identified, they assessed Mary's

- Knowledge of relaxation as a hypometabolic process.
- Knowledge of specific relaxation techniques.
- Previous experiences with relaxation.
- Coping style.
- Preference regarding specific relaxation techniques.

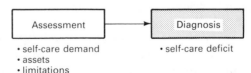

RELAXATION SELF-ASSESSMENT

Complete the following self-assessment to help you look at the role of relaxation in your life. On the scale below circle the numbers which are most true for you and your life during the last year:

		Almost Never	Seldom	Often	Almost Always
1.	It is easy for me to find a place to be alone in my house.	1	2	3	4
2.	My feet are warm when I go to bed at night.	1	2	3	4
3.	My neck and shoulders are relaxed.	1	2	3	4
4.	I fall asleep within ten minutes of going to bed.	1	2	3	4
5.	When I shake hands with people my palms are dry.	1	2	3	4
6.	I practice deep breathing when I am tense.	1	2	3	4
7.	When I put my hands to my face they are warm.	1	2	3	4
8.	I am able to function in an emergency situation.	1	2	3	4
9.	When I notice that I am tense I am able to calm down.	1	2	3	4
10.	It's easy for me to focus my attention and block out distracting noises.	1	2	3	4

1. Connect all the circles down the length of the page. Look at the pattern that your connected line makes. Turn your page sideways to get an even more clear visual picture of relaxation in your life right now. What does it seem to be saying to you?

2. Now add up your total score: _____ 20

   Circle which range it was in:
   10-19   20-29   30-40

   If your score was in the 10-19 range you might want to make some changes in how and when you relax. Which aspects do you think need the most work? How many "1's" did you mark on this assessment? 3 These might serve as a clue to help you think about making changes in this area of your life.

3. How would you like this self-assessment to look six months from now? Are you interested in working toward those improvements?

4. Remember to congratulate yourself for your efforts to learn to relax.

Figure 9–1. Relaxation self-assessment. (Reprinted with permission from Baldi, S., et al. (1980). *For your health: A model for self-care.* South Laguna, CA: Nurses Model Health, p. 132.)

After gathering the data, the self-care deficit was collaboratively defined as:

Inability to relax regularly due to lack of knowledge and skill

The diagnosis was based on the physical symptoms she was experiencing (with no physical basis) as well as the number of stressful areas in her life.

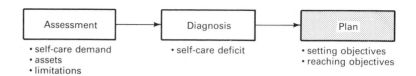

Setting Objectives

There were several considerations in formulating Mary's goal:

- Fitting practice time into her daily schedule.
- Finding time to learn a relaxation technique.
- Finding a quiet, uninterrupted place to practice.
- Providing for comfortable clothing and chair.
- Providing for relaxation tapes.
- Gaining support from her roommate to allow her privacy and to assist in giving rewards.

Mary and the occupational health nurse wrote a self-contract (Fig. 9–2). Their mutually agreed upon goals were:

Short-term (six weeks):	To do abdominal deep breathing for 5 minutes, four times a week.
Long-term (six months):	To do abdominal deep breathing for 10 minutes, twice a day, four times a week.

Reaching Objectives: Nursing and Client Actions

Mary and the nurse identified several actions that Mary would carry out to reach her goal. These included:

- Learning about hypometabolic states and why they are important.
- Attending relaxation classes at the hospital community forum.
- Learning abdominal deep breathing from the occupational health nurse.
- Talking with her roommate, Marilyn, to gain support.
- Identifying five effects that practicing relaxation might have on her lifestyle and symptoms.
- Bringing a comfortable chair from home to her dorm room.
- Finding a quiet spot in the hospital where she could be uninterrupted for 10 minutes.
- Providing a weekly reward.

The nurse's responsibilities in the self-care plan were:

- Instructing Mary in abdominal deep breathing with a return demonstration.
- Providing her with written materials about relaxation.
- Calling her weekly to see how her practice was going.
- Explaining relaxation precautions to her.

SELF-CONTRACT

MY GOALS:

Short-term — by the end of six weeks I will . . . *be doing abd. deep breath. 5 min 4x week*

Long-term — by the end of six months I will . . . *be doing abd. deep breath. 10 min/*
ENVIRONMENTAL PLANNING: (all the steps I will take to reach my goal) *2x day 4x week*

1. Set aside time after school.
2. Arrange with Marilyn to not interrupt me.
3. Bring a livingroom chair from home.
4. Weekly rewards of one new music tape.
5. Learn about hypometabolic states.
6. Attend relaxation class.

THOUGHTS AND ACTIONS

Helpful thoughts:	Helpful actions:
I'll feel better.	Scheduling activities to keep time free after school.
Non-helpful thoughts:	Non-helpful actions:
It really won't work.	Leave the T.V. on during practice.

MY REWARD   (if I meet my goal) *Short-term - Concert c̄ "Plasmatics" June 20*
Long-term - A weekend camping trip

THE COST: (if I fail to meet my goal) *Do Marilyn's laundry x 4 weeks*

REEVALUATION DATE: *June 12*

I agree to help with this project:

___*Marilyn*___
(Support person)

I agree to strive toward this goal:

___*Mary*___
(Your signature)   (date)

Figure 9–2. Self-contract. (Adapted with permission from Baldi, S., et al. (1980). *For your health: A model for self-care.* South Laguna, CA: Nurses Model Health, p. 47.)

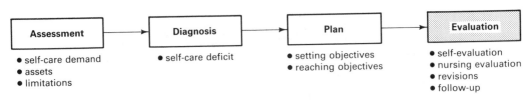

In the joint six-week evaluation appointment, Mary reviewed her self-contract. The nurse helped her look at the following:

- Were there changes in her symptoms?
  Was she sleeping better?
  Had her headaches and irritability decreased?
- Did she meet her goal?
- What was most difficult for her?
  Time
  Place
  Giving herself permission
- Did she get her rewards? If not, why not?
- What were effects of nurse's weekly calls?
- Were instructions and materials sufficient?
- Had she brought the chair from home?
- Had she attended the classes at the hospital forum?

Mary accomplished her goal of doing abdominal deep breathing for five minutes, four times a week. There were many times, however, when that was difficult for her to do. After a busy day, Mary found it extremely difficult to concentrate on the deep breathing. Her mind kept wandering back to her schoolwork or her clients. Remembering what the nurse had told her, she gave herself permission to be distracted and then to try the exercise again.

During the six-week period, Mary had not brought a chair from home. She had decided that this required too much effort to transport and decided instead that she would get one from the school's maintenance department.

There were a few days during the six weeks that Mary did not want to do the exercises. Her roommate was instrumental in helping her find the motivation to do them. Marilyn would call her on the unit to remind her about how much better she would feel if she did the relaxation exercise instead of drinking a soda on her coffee break. Initially, Marilyn got into the role of being critical of her when she had not practiced at the exact time she said she would. This issue was discussed during the first weekly telephone call with the nurse, and the process of positive reinforcement was reviewed. Marilyn gave Mary her weekly rewards of music tapes and had purchased concert tickets as the reward for accomplishing her six-week goal.

Mary's physical symptoms decreased. She found herself being much less irritable and fatigued. She was still having difficulty falling asleep some nights but described this as being about "half as often as before." She found that if she practiced the deep breathing immediately before going to bed, it was easier for her to fall asleep.

This accomplishment stimulated a new sense of caring for herself and resulted in her wanting to work on an exercise program with a new self-contract. In addition, Mary became interested in trying relaxation skills with her clients before automatically administering analgesics to them. Table 9–6 presents a nursing care plan for this clinical situation.

SUMMARY

Beginning with an historical perspective, this chapter presented relaxation as a self-care skill. In addition, clinical uses and effects of relaxation were explored.

Types of relaxation techniques were discussed. These included deep breathing, autogenics, meditation, biofeedback, visualization/imagery, and music. Examples of each were given. Also included were precautions for practicing relaxation and methods of developing and maintaining relaxation skills.

The nurse's role as a model of relaxation self-care skills was explored. Specific actions to promote this in the nurse's professional as well as personal life were given. A clinical application section explored the use of relaxation self-care with one client.

STUDY QUESTIONS

Personal Focus

1. How is relaxation integrated in your life-style? Rate yourself as a model of relaxation self-care.
2. Is relaxation clearly differentiated from play in your life? From spirituality?
3. How do you feel physically after practicing relaxation? How do you feel emotionally?
4. In what ways might you develop and maintain relaxation self-care in your life?
5. Listen to one relaxation music tape. Share your reactions with your friends.

Client Focus

1. Describe one client with whom relaxation might be utilized.
2. What changes, either symptomatic or behavioral, would you anticipate?
3. What precautions might it be necessary to consider in working with this client?
4. Discuss the ways in which nurses could model relaxation self-care skills in your clinical setting.

TABLE 9–6. NURSING CARE PLAN

Reason for consultation: Fatigue, headache, and irritability lasting for two weeks   *Client:* Mary

Assessment	Plan	Evaluation
		Met — *Not met*

Self-care demand
  Need for improved relaxation skills
Assets
  Nurse, understanding of anatomy, physiology
  Motivation to learn
  Place to practice
  Supportive roommate
Limitations
  Lack of knowledge about relaxation
  History of "work ethic"
  Lack of time
	Setting objectives
	Six weeks: "will be doing abdominal deep-breathing 5 minutes four times a week."
	Reaching objectives
	<u>Client actions</u>
	  Learn about hypometabolic state.
	  Attend relaxation class.
	  Learn abdominal deep-breathing from nurse.
	  Gain Marilyn's support.
	  Get chair from home.
	  Find quiet spot in hospital to practice.
	  Provide weekly reward.
	<u>Nursing actions</u>
	  Instruct in abdominal deep-breathing.
	  Provide written materials.
	  Phone weekly.
	  Explain precautions.
		X (Met)
		
		X (Met)
		X (Met)
		X (Met)
		X (Met)
		X (Not met)
		X (Met)
		X (Met)
		X (Met)
		X (Met)
		X (Met)
		X (Met)
		X (Met)

		Needed revision Needs more information re: sleep self-care
Diagnosis	Re-evaluation date	Client Follow-up
Self-care deficit Inability to relax regularly due to lack of knowledge and skill	Joint appointment with nurse in 6 weeks.	Encourage attendance at self-care class series. Establish another self-contract. Encourage clinical application.

REFERENCES

1. Benson, H. (1975). *The relaxation response.* New York: Avon Books, pp. 25–26.
2. McCaffrey, M. (1979). *Nursing management of the patient with pain* (2nd ed.). Philadelphia: J.B. Lippincott, p. 137.
3. Shapiro, D.H. (1982). Overview: Clinical and physiological comparison of medication with other self-control strategies. *American Journal of Psychiatry, 139*(3), 268.
4. Benson. *Relaxation response,* p. 97.
5. Benson. *Relaxation response,* p. 90.
6. Benson. *Relaxation response,* p. 112.
7. Benson, H. (1974, July–August). Your innate asset for combating stress. *Harvard Business Review,* pp. 98–99.
8. Scholem, G. (1967). *Major trends in Jewish mysticism.* New York: Schocken Books, p. 139.
9. Fujisawa, C. (1959). *Zen and Shinto.* New York: Philosophical Library.
10. Benson. *Relaxation response,* p. 135.
11. Spurgeon, C. (1970). *Mysticism in English literature.* Port Washington, NY: Kennikat Press.
12. Jacobson, E. (Ed.). (1967). *Tension in medicine.* Springfield, IL: Charles C. Thomas, p. 24.
13. Pelletier, K.R. (1977). *Mind as healer, mind as slayer.* New York: Dell, pp. 197–208.
14. Selye, H. (1956). *The stress of life.* New York: McGraw-Hill, pp. 47–124.
15. Titlebaum, H.M. (1988). Relaxation. *Holistic Nursing Practice, 2*(3), 17–25.
16. Pelletier. *Mind as Healer,* p. 200.
17. Bloomfield, H.H. Cain, M.P. Jaffe, D., & Kory, R. (1975). *TM.* New York: Dell, p. 96.
18. Bloomfield et al. *TM,* p. 36.
19. Bloomfield et al. *TM,* p. 56.
20. Pelletier. *Mind as Healer,* p. 265.
21. Hastings, A.C., Fadiman, J., & Gordon, J.S. (Eds.). (1980). *The complete guide to holistic medicine: Health for the whole person.* Boulder, CO: Westview Press.
22. Simonton, S.M. (1977). Group process and imagery with cancer patients. In M.C. Brotman (Ed.), *Mind as healer, mind as slayer: A workbook.* Pacific Palisades, CA: The Center for Integral Medicine.
23. Hill, A. (1988, September–October). Healing Tapes. *Medical Self-Care, 48,* p. 73.
24. Swinford, P., & Webster, J. (1989). *Promoting wellness: A nurse's handbook.* Rockville, MD: Aspen.
25. Bonny, H., & McCarron, N. (1984). Music as an adjunct to anesthesia. *Journal of the American Association of Nurse Anesthetists, 52,* 55–57.
26. Halpern, S., & Savary, L. (1985). *Sound health.* San Francisco: Harper & Row.
27. Dossey, B., Keegan, L., Guzzetta, C., & Kolkmeier, L. (1988). *Holistic nursing: A handbook for practice.* Rockville, MD: Aspen.
28. Shapiro. Overview: Clinical and physiological, p. 269.
29. Lehrer, P.M., & Woolfolk, R.L. (1984). Are stress reduction techniques interchangeable, or do they have specific effects?: A review of the comparative empirical literature. In R.L. Woolfolk & P.M. Lehrer (Eds.), *Principles and practice of stress management.* New York: Guilford Press.
30. Titlebaum. Relaxation.

31. McGrath, P.A., & DeVeber, L.L. (1986). "Helping children cope with painful procedures. *American Journal of Nursing, 11,* 1278–79.
32. Wells, N. (1982). The effect of relaxation on postoperative muscle tension and pain. *Nursing Research 31*(4), 236–238.
33. Burish, T., & Lyles, J. (1981). Effectiveness of relaxation training in reducing adverse reactions to cancer chemotherapy. *Journal of Behavioral Medicine, 4,* 65–79.
34. Squires, S. (1987). Visions to boost immunity. *American Health, 6*(6), 54–61.
35. Hughes, W. (1982) Guided imagery training as treatment for alcoholism. (From *Dissertation Abstracts International, 43B,* Abstract No. 8302246)
36. Collison, C., & Miller, S. (1987). Using images of the future in grief work. *Image, 19*(1), 9–11.
37. Vines, S. (1988). The therapeutics of guided imagery. *Holistic Nursing Practice, 2*(3), 34–44.
38. Benson. *Relaxation response,* pp. 159–161.
39. Benson. *Relaxation response,* p. 172.

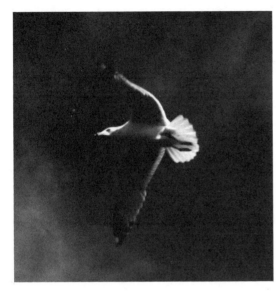

A spiritual man is one who listens to the dictates of his soul.

Victor Frankl, *The Doctor and the Soul*
(New York: Bantam Books, 1965), p. xvi

10 Spirituality

LEARNING OBJECTIVES

Upon completion of this chapter, readers will be able to:

1. State a personal definition of spirituality.
2. List and describe 12 characteristics of spirituality.
3. Describe the relationship between spirituality and each of the following: philosophy of life, religion, intuition, and hope.
4. Describe the significance of spirituality for health.
5. Discuss the development of spirituality throughout the life span.
6. Identify common methods for the development of spirituality.
7. Discuss the nurse's role in helping clients practice spiritual self-care.

DEFINITIONS

Spirituality   A component of health related to the essence of life; the vital principle in human beings that gives life to the physical organism in contrast to its purely material aspects; relating to the soul as opposed to the body; "the breath of life."

Religion   Belief in a power such as a being or eternal principle, greater than the human being, that has created or affects the world. This belief frequently involves practices in relation to this power such as prayer, proper conduct, or ritual observance of faith.

Philosophy of life   The belief system that a person forms for the conduct of life.

Spiritual self-care   Activities that help one relate positively and consistently to his or her deepest inner self in ways that help the person become "spirited"—vital, alive, aware, conscious, and loving. These practices include attention to the nonmaterial parts of the self.

INTRODUCTION

Spirituality is the ability to express qualities of one's *spirit*, or essence, through the human personality. An assessment of spirituality can be based on the degree of joy, love, freedom, clarity, spontaneity, and responsibility that the individual demonstrates. It is rarely fixed and may change radically during a lifetime. No path to spiritual development can be judged as being better or worse simply because it is different. One path may demand an ascetic life limited to the barest essentials. Another method may accommodate abundant material goods and an active social and family life.

Spirituality is highly variable and is a very private issue. People experience their spirituality in different ways at different times. A religious service or a sunset may be experienced as an integrating spiritual event. Both may have quite an opposite affect on some other occasion if mood or circumstance change.

The goal of spiritual self-care is to become "spirited": vital, alive, aware, conscious, and loving. Relating positively and consistently to one's deepest inner self is a major part of spiritual self-care.

People who regularly practice spiritual activities are healthier in body as well as mind.[1] People who integrate spirituality into their lives often report that they feel better, peaceful, or comfortable. Spiritual resources are a source of calm and strength during crises. Even surviving and healing from serious illness have been related to one's degree of hope and faith in a higher being.

Frankl,[2] May,[3] and others have written in depth about the role that spirituality played in helping people survive concentration camp internment during World War II. People who found value and meaning in their lives and a place in humanity were better able to tolerate those devastating experiences. They were less suicidal and were even able to risk their own lives in altruistic service to others.

Timerman has emphasized this effect in his moving account of Argentinian injustice, *Prisoner without a Name, Cell without a Number*.[4] The comfort and support of his values, attitudes, and life philosophy helped Timerman endure torture and the isolation of imprisonment.

Holistic approaches to health and self-care all emphasize the importance of spiritual health. In contemporary clinical situations, however, the spiritual components of health care are often ignored.[5] In one study less than one-third of clients' spiritual problems were recognized as such by 74 percent of a sample (N=35) of oncology nurses.[6] Nurses and clients often place their spiritual development after exercise, nutrition, and other more "concrete" and quantifiable "physical" self-care practices. This is unfortunate.

Spiritual self-care can provide a vital, deepening, and unifying force within each person and can integrate physical, mental, and social dimensions. Banks has identified four major aspects of spirituality:

- A unifying force within individuals
- A meaning in life
- A common bond between people
- An individual perception of faith[7]

HISTORICAL PERSPECTIVE

In many ancient societies it was believed that spiritual forces ruled human destiny. Physical and mental illnesses were considered to be vengeful afflictions sent by the gods or other supernatural forces. Sometimes the sufferers had transgressed taboos. Treatment was administered by the tribal shaman or medicine man. In later years sufferers were treated in temples by priests. Although some physical means of treatment (herbs, splints, fasting) may have been used, the primary healing forces were nonmaterial.

With the development of scientific medicine, starting as early as 500 B.C. in ancient Greece, India, and China, the distinction between body and spirit (soul) and later body, mind, and spirit came to be recognized.[8] As scientific knowledge progressed, treatment of the body became primary. Patients went to hospitals and asylums to be treated by scientifically trained physicians and surgeons. Although spiritual needs were still recognized (for example, many hospitals were maintained by religious orders and chaplains were available), these needs became more and more de-emphasized. This has especially been true during the past 100 years of Western culture. Today, physicians and nurses are increasingly specialized and sophisticated machinery is considered essential. Modern medicine in the United States has become highly technical and complex. The spiritual dimension has been considered last; the client has become increasingly dehumanized.

As a reaction to this dehumanization there has been an increase of interest in the spiritual aspects of health and illness. This resurgence includes self-care and holistic health, and seeks an integration of body, mind, and spirit. Mainstream members of the American Medical Association have even begun to call for research studies regarding the impact of prayers by family members on the health of intensive care patients. The long-term influence of this movement on health care in the United States is as yet unclear.

SIGNIFICANCE OF SPIRITUALITY IN NURSING

The nurse is in a strategic position to help promote the client's spiritual dimension. Nurturing the spirit helps people mobilize and reaffirm their internal strengths and resources. It helps them find meaning in health, illness, and suffering.[9]

Nurses may find it difficult to provide spiritual care even when the need is quite apparent. They may be unsure of their own spirituality, uncomfortable about sharing it, and may even fear ridicule from peers. A conflict in spiritual values between nurse and client may complicate this problem.

Nursing practice involving spiritual care often focuses on the "religious component" of spirituality. In hospitals with specific religious affiliations, nurses often baptize ill babies, call ministers to perform last rites, and provide for the religious needs of clients in a variety of ways. Nursing literature has focused on the referral process (for example, when and how to call a member of the clergy) and presented basic information about the ways in which the needs of specific religious groups can be met in the hospital. Taylor, Lillis, and Lemone have presented an excellent review of world religions, including guidelines for nurses and other clinicians for helping clients meet their religious needs while hospitalized.[10] Potter and Perry describe application of the nursing process to meet the spiritual needs of clients.[11]

The Concept of Spirituality in Nursing Literature

Nurse theorists have recognized the importance of the spiritual development of clients. Abdellah et al. describe one important nursing activity as facilitating client progress toward achievement of personal spiritual goals.[12] Henderson defines the ability to worship according to one's faith as a primary client need.[13] Watson presents the installation of faith–hope as a major, carative factor in nursing.[14]

Dickinson presents a practical way of integrating spiritual care into everyday nursing but also suggests that spiritual care involves a broader search for meaning.[15] Colliton believes that spiritual care should be based on a universal concept of "inspiriting" rather than centering around specific religious concepts. She believes that the role of the nurse should be to inspire and "inspirit" hope with loving care: "For nurses to respond with compassion to a client's spiritual needs, they must be willing to meet the client spirit to spirit and help in his or her experience of illness as a spiritual journey."[16]

Fish and Shelly have developed a text and workbook for a Christian approach to spiritual care. They stress prayer, Bible reading, and "therapeutic use of the nurse" to intervene during spiritual distress.[17] Stoll has developed a spiritual history guide that is divided into four areas: (1) concept of God or deity, (2) source of strength and hope, (3) perception of the significance of religious practices, and (4) perceived relationship between spiritual beliefs and states of health.[18] Forbis encourages clients to examine the relationship between their belief systems and their health behavior.[19]

CHARACTERISTICS OF SPIRITUALITY

It is difficult for many nurses to differentiate between spirituality and similar concepts. The following summaries show how spirituality and self-care relate to other ideas.

Philosophy of Life—A Link to Spirituality

Spirituality and life philosophy are intimately connected. Everyone has a conscious or unconscious philosophy of life, a system of rules, beliefs, and values. A person's philosophy of life is the way in which basic spiritual faith is expressed. That philosophy may be connected to serving others or to following a specific moral or ethical code. It may or may not be linked to a specific religious orientation.

The specifics of an individual's belief system are not as important as the process of learning to develop harmony between the internal and external worlds. Frankl states, "the moment we realize the Universal Spirit we can be in perfect harmony with all different beliefs."[20]

Spirituality underlies a person's philosophy of life. It may be highly developed or extremely rudimentary. If one's spirituality is underdeveloped or shortsighted, his or her behavior and philosophy of life may be more inconsistent and vulnerable to poor functioning (physically or mentally) under stress.

There may be gaps between what people say they *believe* and how they actually *behave*. Some people go to church every week but do not practice their spiritual and philosophical values (e.g., love, forgiveness, hope). In assessing spiritual concerns it is important to explore how an individual's beliefs and values are integrated into daily life. Spiritual self-care encourages this exploration on a regular basis.

God as a Spiritual Concept

The concept of an infinite and powerful force permeating all nature is basic to many people's spirituality. The name commonly given this ultimate source and power is *God*. The concept may also be referred to as the Supreme Being, the

Creator, Cosmic Force, Higher Intelligence, Universal Energy, Infinite Love, Divine Energy, or the Source. These terms have held a variety of religious and philosophical meanings in human history.

Belief or disbelief in a higher power is based on each person's psychological makeup, experience, and upbringing. One's God is frequently symbolic of one's conscience or unconsciousness. Sometimes people will project onto this concept their unresolved conflicts with authority figures. They may fear the judgment and punishment of a God who is really their internalized "critical parent" or become angry at a God who has not performed according to their expectations.[21]

Spirituality Is Not Necessarily the Same as Religion

Religion involves belief in a specific doctrine, faith in a higher power, and some form of public or private religious practice. Many people derive great benefit from religion and practice their spiritual self-care in this way. The sense of peace and communion with others that can be found in religious services often provides a crucial link for spiritual development. For others, participation in organized religion may be an empty action that does not fulfill their spiritual self-care needs.

Personal and Transcendent Dimensions of Spirituality

The *personal dimension* of spirituality refers to questions of individual existence, such as: Who am I? What is meaningful in my life? The task of personal growth is to develop a well-integrated, effective personality that helps the individual lead a rewarding and productive life. It may include "worldly" goals such as wealth and status. Pursuit of meaning and goals leads to personal growth and the development of a balanced, rhythmic personality. This is intimately linked to the ability to experience and express one's spirituality.

The *transcendent dimension* of growth relates to the meaning of life itself. Spirituality often involves transcending the reality of this universe to come into contact with a dimension of higher awareness and consciousness. It is an inner state in which the individual can contact and share in a larger universal energy. Meditation, prayer, chanting, and fasting are usually directed toward the transcendent dimension of spirituality.[22]

Many people have a tendency to favor either the personal or the transcendent dimension of spirituality. The goal of spiritual self-care is to balance each of these necessary dimensions. Nurses play an important role in helping clients with this balance and integration.

Peak Experiences

Maslow described *peak experiences* as moments of great awe, intense happiness, profound insight, rapture, bliss, or ecstasy.[23] These experiences can be stimulated by many things, including music, athletic achievements, sexual union, beauty, or a religious service. Sometimes these experiences are sudden and unexplainable. "Ordinary" events can be experienced in an extraordinary spiritual manner. These more commonplace peak experiences are similar to the transcendent religious experiences that are encountered in nearly all faiths.

Paterson and Zderad see nursing as a struggle with others through "peak experiences related to health suffering."[24] They believe that through these interactions both nurse and client "become more in accordance with their human potential."[24] Parse also discusses nursing as an activity in which clients are helped to "reach beyond" and to "live several modes of experience all at once."[25] She sees health as being linked to this ability to transcend ordinary living situations in order to develop all aspects of the self.[25]

Intuition and Spirituality

Jung divides the personality into four distinct, interlocking quadrants—intuition, feeling, thinking, and sensation.[26] Since the personality operates as a unit, the entire structure suffers from malfunctioning of any one of its components. Self-care is necessary in every quadrant. A physically healthy body cannot sustain itself without emotional, intellectual, and spiritual development. Use of intuition is a major spiritual self-care practice. Relating to one's inner world on a consistent basis can lead to an inner knowing that goes beyond intellectual knowledge. Something that "feels right" can reflect a deep wisdom from one's inner core or a transcendent level of consciousness. Openness to one's intuition is made difficult by energy-consuming anxiety, low self-esteem, chronic depression, or physical illness. This highlights the importance of a balance of good physical and psychological self-care practices.

People can learn to recognize, trust, and use their intuition in many different ways. Dream analysis, guided imagery, journal writing, and artistic processes are self-care techniques that help develop spirituality and intuition. Spirituality and intuition can also be developed through gardening, running, swimming, or during any activity in which the person is able to focus inward, daydream, and pay attention to inner experience.

Spirituality Often Includes Rituals

> Your spiritual practice must be a daily ritual. To truly develop your ability to contact and channel divine energy you should be regular and persistent in your practice.
>
> I Ching[27]

Rituals and religious practices are stabilizing forces. Kneeling, fasting, Bible reading, wearing shawls, meditating, and chanting are outward and visible expressions of faith. Prayer, common to all religions, brings one into the presence of a higher power and allows for the expression of dependence, appreciation, and faith. Besides traditional religious rituals, art, music, theater, and walks can be considered spiritual activities. Rituals provide a sense of continuity, a sense of belonging to a community, and a feeling of closeness with God or a higher force.

Many cultural rituals also provide a safe and protected setting in which strong emotions can be expressed and contained. Wedding ceremonies, graduations, and funerals represent important life passages. Ritualistic practices unite and link the inner and outer worlds by expressing deep spiritual and psychological truths in physical form.

To be effective in long-term health promotion, spiritual self-care must be practiced *regularly*. Spiritual rituals such as watching a sunset or saying a rosary provide this needed structure and consistency.

Love—the Core of Spirituality

"Our health and vitality can be limited only by our ability to love."[28] One element of spirituality is the expression of spontaneous love in all facets of life. Compassion, the ability to love and accept other people and situations, is possible only to the extent that the individual can accept and love himself or herself. One must care enough about oneself to resolve problems of low self-esteem and blocks to self-love.

Healing—Spirituality—Love. Throughout the ages every sage and healer has agreed that the essential healing agent is love. It is inexhaustible and all powerful. From the laying on of hands to biofeedback, it is the divine spark that underlies all healing techniques. True healing is an affirmation of wholeness and holiness.[29] Mother Teresa has given the message: "Go out and give love to all you meet. Do not be afraid to love."[30]

Unconditional Love. Unconditional love means loving people as they are and as they are not.[31] It is not conditional love—the selfish, businesslike love of "I love you if you please me." Unconditional love is a spiritual force that is related to healing and can be tapped into by practice. A preacher who heals by the "laying on of hands" does so through God's unconditional love. Perhaps only a saint is fully prepared to love other human beings unconditionally.

Unconditional love of oneself is also an ideal. The degree to which one can accept or love oneself as a worthwhile, though fallible, being will determine how loving one can be to others. Self-love leads to health; self-hate leads to illness and death.

Radiation of Spirituality

No one differs in the amount of spirituality he or she possesses; people differ only in the amount of spirituality that they realize and use. Twitchell describes a spiritual person as a distributor of universal love and energy.[32] Sanford uses the example of Christ to describe the same phenomenon.

You are a channel and through you Christ can reach others and lighten their darkness. Wherever you go light and love will radiate forth about you, creating peace and unity. Everyone will be better and happier by reason of your appearance in their lives.[33]

Spirituality may be manifested in a variety of ways. Beautiful surroundings, worthwhile activities, enjoyable friends, and optimum health can all be living examples of the powerful channeling of spiritual energy. A person's relationship with the outer world will reflect his or her inner psychological and spiritual nature. Spiritual development with depth, calmness, and self-acceptance will be manifested by an individual's positive relationships. Inner chaos will be reflected by poor relationships.

To Be Spiritual Is to Create

True creativity flows from one's deepest self. Art, music, and literature are examples of the translation of internal energy into physical form. Conventional artistic forms are not the only mode of creation, however; a person may create (call forth) a balanced life, a loving home, or healing forces from others. This is expressed in the Zen Buddhist concept of becoming an *artist in life*. Creativity is enhanced when spiritual self-care is practiced regularly.

Spirituality Expresses Itself as Joy

Spirituality includes an inherent joyousness. Inner joy is becoming who one really is and finding one's unique place in the universe.[34] It increases the ability to love and comes from a deep inner trust in the meaningfulness of life. The joy associated with play, humor, laughter, and sexuality are also spiritual experiences.

Spirituality Requires Responsibility and Choice

Being the most that one can be includes a conscious awareness of the daily choices that constitute life. It includes good health care decisions as well as the ability to live in accordance with one's professed morality. Spiritual development requires the embracing of responsibility and choices. "I know that I am capable of actualizing my possibilities, my self. So I am my choices not only in terms of my past but also in regard to my future, my possibilities."[35]

Centeredness Allows Expression of the Spirit

Centeredness is a fine tuning of sensitivity to life's inner patterns and processes.[36] Centering quietly within allows the person to recognize a state of balance and intuitive knowing. Looking within, acknowledging one's deepest needs, and tapping into a profound source of strength are part of the centering process.

To be centered means that the person experiences a true "present"; a focus on the process and activity going on in the moment rather than on the outcome.

The person is not behaving mechanically but is acting with purposeful intention. Centeredness results in a heightened sense of well-being. Spiritual self-care activities and religious practices can facilitate the ability to turn inward for peace and equanimity.

Spirituality Provides Faith and Hope

Faith is the belief in the trustworthiness of a person or idea that is not based on logical proof (e.g., a belief in God). Spirituality is the essence of life and allows for a belief in a power greater than ourselves. Faith has a powerful effect in helping people recover a sense of balance, tranquility, and hope. It offers three valuable gifts by: (1) diminishing fear, (2) redefining values, and (3) permitting acceptance of the outcomes of life's predicaments.[37]

Hope is the effect that accompanies faith and is characterized by the desire to accomplish a goal with some expectation that what is desired is attainable.[38] Hope includes confidence, faith, inspiration and determination. It requires a dependence upon others, choice, trust, perserverance, and courage.[39] Hope for a better future can be a powerful incentive for people to tolerate difficult situations and maintain motivation.

Hopelessness results when people believe that no help can be obtained, and the situation will remain the same or get worse. Loss of hope and confidence leads to a deep despair. Giving up seems to be the only viable option when the person is convinced that what is wanted is beyond reach and impossible. Hopelessness affects the client's response to treatment and can hasten death. In time of illness and tragedy, a sense of hope is essential for facing crisis and surviving adversity.

DEVELOPMENT OF SPIRITUALITY

The spiritual quest is a search for a way of life that brings knowledge, freedom, and joy. Spiritual self-care is directed toward the goal of higher consciousness, enlightenment, self-realization, and connection with a greater creative force. It is also an inner search into deeper levels of the self. It may include facing undesirable truths about oneself as well as discovering and developing talents and skills. Spiritual self-care constitutes a "way of life" requiring conscious commitment and persistent practice.[40]

There are many roads leading to the same goal of spiritual development. They include "the path to wholeness,"[41] "the process of individuation,"[42] and "finding the kingdom within."[43] All methods of spiritual growth include the same underlying message: "Look within, spiritual growth is within and not anywhere outside ourselves."[44]

Nurturing Spirituality

Particular activities that may help clients meet their spiritual objectives include ways to develop a relationship with one's inner world through:

- Prayer
- Meditation or "quiet listening to one's essence"
- Readings or poetry (religious or otherwise)
- Songs or chants, done alone or in groups
- Church or religious group activities, such as services, celebrations of holy days, feasts, and fasts
- Communion with nature through walks in the woods, running on the beach, walks in a park, and so on
- Inner dialogues with oneself or with a higher being (see Tables 10–1 and 10–2)
- Artistic processes such as music, drama, art, and dance
- Dream analysis to communicate with the unconscious by deciphering symbols, hidden wishes, and feelings
- Journal writing (see Table 10–3)
- Affirmations (positive thoughts that are repeated consciously to "program" the unconscious to produce desired results)
- Visual imagery

Ways to manifest spiritual energy in one's outer world include:

- Loving relationships with others
- Self-care of body
- Laughter, joyous expressions

TABLE 10–1. CONTACTING YOUR INNER HEALER

Purpose: To contact that part of you that heals, that part that has accumulated all the wisdom and knowledge of your body and psyche.

1. Enter a state of deep relaxation.
2. Imagine yourself in a peaceful place and experience its pleasure.
3. Wait calmly with the expectation that something will join you. It might be a person, an animal, or a plant.
4. Wait in a quiet and receptive state. Something will eventually enter your consciousness.
5. When you finally encounter your advisor, greet him or her warmly. Ask the healer's name, get acquainted.
6. Eventually your inner healer will respond to your questions about your illness.
7. Keep your dialogue simple, clear, direct, and explicit.
8. Ask the inner healer what needs to be done to remove the symptoms.

Jaffe, D. (1980). *Healing from within.* New York: Alfred A. Knopf, pp. 261–266. © 1980 by Dennis Jaffe, reprinted by permission of Alfred A. Knopf, Inc.)

TABLE 10.2. DIALOGUING WITH ILLNESS

Purpose: To explore the psychological and unconscious messages and meanings within a symptom, pain, or illness.

Task: To establish a dialogue with your inner self.

1. Choose a physical symptom or illness that is bothering you.
2. While in a deep relaxed state, imagine it taking a human form, or having a separate distinct voice.
3. In your mind, begin to create a dialogue between the afflicted area and your conscious self.
4. Ask your symptom why it exists.
5. Converse with your symptom, gathering information about its origin.

Resolution: Discover feelings you have not faced, or a source of anxiety or conflict in your life that made you susceptible to a particular ailment. Own and integrate parts of yourself that have been desired, forgotten, ignored, rejected, or despised. Plan a change and implement it.

Jaffe, D. (1980). *Healing from within*. New York: Alfred A. Knopf, pp. 257–261. © 1980 by Dennis Jaffe, reprinted by permission of Alfred A. Knopf, Inc.

- Service to others in need
- Sense of selflessness and feeling for others
- Commitment to higher consciousness
- Beautiful surroundings
- Forgiveness of others
- Empathy, compassion, and hope
- Self-love and unconditional love of others
- Group chants, meditation, and prayer
- Church services and activities
- Social gatherings
- Prayer and healing groups

No matter what activity the client chooses, the themes of centeredness, inner peace, and unconditional love will facilitate spiritual development. If nurses can realize that there are no boundaries to the definition of what can constitute a spiritual experience, they can be creative resources to help clients identify meaningful ways to practice spiritual self-care.

Consideration needs to be given to the *means* and *support* that clients have for their chosen activities. They will need quiet and compassion. The sharing of deep personal thoughts and beliefs can be enriching if accepted and devastating

TABLE 10-3. JOURNAL WRITING

Purpose: Tool for personal growth designed to help you find and love your inner self.

Task: To express innermost feelings and thoughts and make more conscious choices. To define and implement changes. To get a clearer sense of creative potential. To enrich relationships with others. To find deeper meaning in life. To deal with creative blocks and develop awareness and courage.

Forms of Expression: Drawing, doodles, and scribbles. Prose and poetry, dramatic dialogue and letters. Graphs and charts. Colors, abstract designs, images.

Setting: Quiet, private place, comfortable and conducive to self-reflection. Reserve block of uninterrupted time of 15 minutes or more.

Confidentiality: Arrange for a secure, private place in which to keep your journal. Be sure that it will not be casually picked up by someone else. This will enhance your ability to be open with yourself.

When and How Often: When you have something to express. When you want to work on specific exercises. When you simply want to be alone with yourself. During a major crisis or major transition. On a regular basis (daily, weekly).

Materials: Notebook with plain white paper (6 × 9 or larger). Pens, felt-tip pens of various colors.

Preparation: Gather materials and go to your private space. Use any relaxation technique you like. Take several deep breaths. Date the page in your journal. Begin.
  —How do I feel right now?
  —What do my inner and outer selves look and feel like at this time in my life?
  —What have been the key events and experiences in my life?
  —Where am I in my life right now?
  —Are there aspects of life I want to change?

(Adapted with permission from Capacchione, L. (1979). *The creative journal: The art of finding yourself.* Athens, OH: Ohio University/Swallow Press, pp. 5–27.)

if ridiculed or rejected. The nurse may play a key role in helping the client predict responses from friends and family. Friends and family may need assistance to provide trust and understanding.

Nurses must be capable of moving beyond their personal concepts of spirituality to allow others to express their needs in the language most appropriate for them. Fish and Shelly stress that "while it is important for a nurse to respect and recognize the difference in the way a person expresses his or her faith, it is significantly more important that a nurse comprehend *how similar are everyone's basic spiritual needs.*"[45]

The Spiritual Crisis

The spiritual crisis is a state of acute discomfort characterized by the loss of a sense of meaning or purpose in life. It can accompany psychological or physical stress, such as bereavement or physical injury and illness. During this crisis, a person's view of life fails to explain the meaning or value of suffering.

Expansion of the self, which includes finding new meaning for what has been done or a new direction with meaning, often necessitates letting go of old concepts and values. Crises often arise when people refuse to do this difficult letting go. A void then exists in which nothing new emerges while old concepts and values gradually cease to have meaning. A spiritual dilemma occurs when the person has no answers about life and a desperate need for meaning. Some people attempt to avoid this problem by working too hard, using intoxicants, or withdrawing in other ways. These solutions are usually only temporary, and a deep sense of despair frequently results.[46]

Often a crisis in spirituality is stimulated by crises with children, career changes, or the loss of a spouse. Sometimes individuals attempt to resolve this questioning by means of a divorce or other major life change. The real issue is to find one's own reckoning. It is not possible to run from this challenge without some symptomatic expression. Alcohol and drug use, compulsive sexuality, and overt neurotic symptoms may be seen as an individual attempts to push away feelings of emptiness and dread. Apathy, fear, and despair are frequently experienced.

A spiritual crisis can be *either* an opportunity for growth, through a search for new ways of thinking and being, *or* it can result in a regression to a lower level of functioning. The cycle of meaninglessness and despair is broken when a person finds new meaning in life. This may result from spiritual self-care practices. However the resolution takes place, a sense of new meaning and hope must come from within.

Nursing Diagnoses for Spiritual Concerns

Initially, the North American Nursing Diagnosis Association (NANDA) differentiated between spiritual concerns, distress, and despair. More recently, the diagnosis of *Spiritual Distress* is used for all spiritual concerns and the diagnosis *Hopelessness* for feelings of despair.

Spiritual Distress is defined as, "Disruption in the life principle which pervades a person's entire being and which integrates and transcends one's biological and psychosocial nature."[47] Major defining characteristics include concern with and questions about:

- The meaning of life and death or belief system
- Anger toward God

- The meaning of suffering
- Beliefs or the meaning of own existence
- Relationship with deity
- Moral or ethical implications of therapeutic regimen.

Hopelessness is defined as, "A state in which an individual sees limited or no alternatives or personal choices available and is unable to mobilize energy on own behalf."[48] Major defining characteristics are:

- Passivity, decreased verbalizations
- Decreased affect
- Profound, overwhelming, sustained apathy in response to a situation perceived as impossible and with no solutions
- Despondent verbal cues (e.g., "I might as well give up because there's no cure.")

SPIRITUALITY THROUGHOUT THE LIFE CYCLE

Childhood

The development and integration of spirituality is a life-long process. It begins when the infant first learns to trust that the environment is a safe and secure place. Consistent and predictable love from a parenting figure contributes significantly to the development of self-esteem and self-love. Spiritual and religious values are conveyed nonverbally during the child's early years and are the basis for the individual's beliefs.

Adolescence

Adolescence is a critical time in the formation of individual identity. The major task of this stage is to resolve *identity* versus *role diffusion*.[49] One of the most significant changes that occurs during this period is a new and often intense attention paid to spirituality and life philosophy. The normal adolescent reevaluates parental values, seeks and tests new philosophies, and eventually develops a personal life philosophy.[50] Like a snake shedding its skin, the adolescent sheds the values, beliefs, and conditioning given as protective guidance during earlier years. He or she must answer the question: "Who am I and how do I want to express myself?"

Adulthood

Transition into middle life is as critical as adolescence and in some ways more difficult. It is a time of reexamination and reevaluation. Questions such as "Why am I doing all this?" and "What do I really believe in?" are common.

The ability to understand and communicate with the inner world provides answers and constructive inner guidelines based on reflection and choice. Dass states, "There is nowhere you have to go to work on yourself other than where you are at this moment; everything that is happening to you is part of your work on yourself."[51]

Old Age

As people age they often have more time for spiritual self-care. An old Chinese adage explains that the first quarter of life is for growth, the second for work, the third for play, and the fourth for spirituality.

Many of the spiritual considerations of old age center on preparing for death. Accepting or fearing death depends on how one has lived. The courage to die is a result of having the courage to live. Acceptance comes with a sense of fulfilled potential. Fear, resentment, despair may occur when the individual has neglected to become all that was possible.[52] Although it is too late to live another life, the presence of faith and a life philosophy will help the individual develop a positive attitude toward death. Faith often provides humility and the ability to forgive oneself.

NURSES MODEL SPIRITUAL SELF-CARE

To be models of spiritual self-care, nurses need an inner strength and a commitment to a way of life that will be reflected in their nursing care.[53,54] Nursing students with a higher level of "spiritual well-being" have been found to have more positive attitudes toward providing spiritual care.[55]

Nurses face birth, death, severe loss, and other potential spiritual crises on a daily basis. In one recent study, 90 percent (of a sample of 230 nurses) affirmed that spiritual care is a responsibility of health care professionals. Sadly, 87 percent of the sample agreed that they were uncomfortable discussing spiritual matters with clients.[56]

> Clarity about one's life philosophy and spiritual beliefs often adds a sturdiness or reserve energy to one's mental and emotional states. This reserve energy provides more stamina and less vulnerability to intense or prolonged stressors.[57]

In their personal lives nurses model spiritual self-care by:

- Setting aside time and space for spiritual practices on a regular basis.
- Developing and enhancing inner awareness.
- Discussing life philosophy and spirituality with family and friends.
- Developing a spiritual support system or group.

Figure 10–1 in the Clinical Application Section and Table 10–4 present assessment tools to help the nurse explore personal assets and limitations in this self-care area.

TABLE 10–4. ASSESSING MY SPIRITUALITY

1. What is my own definition of spirituality? 2. Describe a spiritual experience I have had. 3. When do I feel most peaceful? 4. How do I express joy in my life? 5. What do I celebrate? 6. What gives me fulfillment? Why? 7. Do I have a purpose in life? If so, what is it? 8. Am I living my purpose now? How? 9. Do I have a process of relating to my inner world? If so, what is it? 10. Do I love myself? How do I show it?

(Adapted with permission from *Picture of health: A guide to assessing your well being.* (1979). Berkeley, CA: Health Education Unit, University of California at Berkeley, pp. 99–104.)

In professional interactions nurses model spiritual self-care in a variety of overt and covert ways. These include:

- Expressing joy, creativity, and peace in interactions with clients.
- Enhancing knowledge of different religious and spiritual rituals.
- Respecting clients' spiritual needs even when they are quite different from the nurse's belief system.
- Promoting time and privacy for clients' spiritual practices.
- Facilitating client access to ministers, family, friends, and other spiritual support systems.
- Referring clients to a different nurse, minister, or other person when client–nurse value conflicts limit the nurse's ability to be helpful (e.g., issues of abortion or discontinuing life support systems).
- Making time to talk with clients about fear of death, pain, meaning of illness, and other philosophical or spiritual concerns.

As nurses practice spiritual self-care, they will gain and maintain the reserves that are needed to help clients face spiritual crises. When nurses model spiritual self-care, clients will be more likely to value and practice this area of self-care in their own lives.

CLINICAL APPLICATION

Case Presentation

Chuck is a 47-year-old, middle-class Caucasian male recently admitted to the AIDS unit at the Veterans Administration hospital. He was hospitalized for further diagnostic tests after an MRI revealed an atypical lesion on his brain.

Chuck first noticed the diminished functioning of his right hand while writing Christmas cards in mid-December. Any unusual symptom was cause for alarm since Chuck had tested positive for the HIV virus. He had been a very sexually active gay man since his early twenties and knew that it was only a matter of time before he contracted the disease. Several of his friends and former lovers had already died from AIDS.

By the end of January, Chuck's right hand and foot exhibited signs of neuropathy. He was unable to write, eat, or hold anything with his right hand and was dragging his right foot as he walked. At the urging of his closest friend, Jim, Chuck finally went to a neurologist who confirmed his worst fear.

The physician believed that the lesion might be toxoplasmosis and started IV antibiotic therapy. This treatment was discontinued after 12 hours when Chuck broke out with a body rash and a high fever. Other diagnostic tests (e.g., CAT scan, lumbar puncture, and extensive blood studies) indicated that Chuck's immune system was completely intact. The physician concluded that he had an unusual form of AIDS whereby the virus bypasses the immune system and directly attacks the central nervous system.

Chuck was an only child whose parents had passed away within the last five years. He had no close relatives but had two very close friends and several casual friends. Five years ago when his father died, Chuck gave up his painting and wallpaper business, rented his house, and moved in with his 73-year-old ailing mother. His father's estate provided an adequate income from rental properties. Although he enjoyed the freedom of not working, the social contacts a work life provides were lacking in his life. Chuck had not initiated any new activities or met new friends since his father's death. He spent all his time working around the house and yard. He loved to garden and had a vegetable garden, several fruits trees, and an abundance of flowers.

Chuck's mother was not aware of his gay life-style. After moving in with her, he significantly curtailed his social activities and had been celibate since testing positive for the virus. He missed having sexual partners and hanging out at the gay bars. He had daily telephone contact with his friend of fifteen years, Jim, who also was gay and lived with his sick mother. At least once a week they got together for breakfast or lunch. Chuck also spent time with his childhood friend, Martha, going to dinner, plays, and movies. The holidays were spent with these friends, who Chuck considered his family after his mother's death one year before.

After a week of tests and consultation, the physician told Chuck that there was no treatment available, and no hope of recovery or remission. There would be no physical pain, no opportunistic infections, just slow gradual paralysis until he had lost all functioning. Chuck would be discharged as soon as arrangements could be made for home care.

Chuck reacted with fear and panic when told of his prognosis. There was intense crying with emotional outbursts about who would take care of his beloved dog, Mandy. He began to talk of suicide almost immediately. Since he had no insurance, he would have to pay for home care ($1800 a week) by selling one of his rental homes. He was very adamant that it was a waste of money.

| Assessment |

- self-care demand
- assets
- limitations

When the discharge nurse came to visit Chuck to evaluate his needs for home care, he was in a state of depression, turned toward the wall, with the window shades tightly closed. The nurse was aware of Chuck's suicidal threats and began the conversation with, "This situation seems so hopeless, it must feel like the only way out is to kill yourself." Chuck began to cry softly and asked, "Why is this happening to me? Why did I have to be a gay man in the 1980s?" After 30 minutes of talking about his feelings of despair, fear, and sadness, he told the nurse about his plan to take an overdose of pills once he was home. He stated emphatically, "I can not be a burden to my friends. It is a waste of money to have home care, just so I can waste away to nothing. I can't bear the prospect of being so helpless and dependent. I have a choice. I can kill myself."

The nurse realized that Chuck wanted to die before he lost control. His ability to cope stemmed from his hope and belief that he could decide when to die and not have to face the horror of the next few months. Chuck had been very frightened of getting AIDS and refused to read or listen to anything about the disease. His coping style was avoidance of the facts. Since his suicidal ideation was an immediate reaction to the bad news, the nurse wanted to prevent Chuck from acting impulsively out of panic. The idea was to explore his spiritual beliefs in order to help him cope with his impending death. The nurse asked Chuck if they could work together to explore the situation before he made any final decisions. Chuck expressed relief that someone seemed to comprehend his predicament with compassion and agreed that they would meet again after he had completed the spiritual self-assessment tool (Fig. 10–1).

The discharge nurse gathered data regarding Chuck's assets and limitations in the areas of self-care practices (see Table 10–5). Since learning of his positive HIV test, he had been listening regularly to a guided imagery audiotape about staying healthy given to him by his friend, Martha. This helped him deal with his anxiety about being in a high risk group for developing AIDS. He worked out at a gym three times a week, taking pride in looking slim and trim and younger than his 47 years. He ate a well-balanced diet and enjoyed cooking and entertaining his mother and few friends. He lead a laid-back life with minimal external stressors. Chuck, however, felt unfulfilled in his life and fearful of taking risks. He dealt with this emptiness by excessive drinking of alcohol. He still grieved deeply over his mother's death the year before.

After finishing the self-assessment activity, Chuck talked with the nurse about his religious beliefs. He stated that even though he called himself Catholic, he only went to church on Easter and Christmas and no longer derived

---

SPIRITUALITY SELF-ASSESSMENT

Complete the following self-assessment to help you look at the role of "spirituality" in your life now. On the scale below circle the numbers which best indicate you and your life during the past year:

	Almost Never	Seldom	Often	Almost Always
1. I feel comfortable with my own spirituality	1	②	3	4
2. I have a sustaining philosophy of life	1	②	3	4
3. My family and friends support my spirituality	1	2	③	4
4. I feel able to incorporate my spirituality in my home and work	1	②	3	4
5. I have a place for attending to my spiritual needs	1	2	③	4
6. I have a time for spirituality each day	1	②	3	4
7. I have a sense of peace with myself	1	②	3	4
8. I find meaning in my life and the world around me	1	2	3	④
9. I can define my philosophy of life	1	②	3	4
10. I have a purpose for living	1	2	3	④

Some suggestions for how you might learn from this self-assessment:

1. Connect all the circles down the length of the page. Look at the pattern that your connect line makes. You might also turn your page sideways to get an even more clear visual picture of spirituality in your life right now. What does it seem to be saying to you?

2. Now add up your total score: _24_

   Circle which range it was in

   10–19   (20–29)   30–40

   If your score was in the 10–19 range you might want to make some changes in your spiritual life. Which aspects do you think need the most work? How many "1's" did you mark on this assessment?_____0_____These might serve as a clue to help you think about making changes in this area of your life.

3. How would you like this self-assessment to look six months from now? Are you interested in planning toward these improvements?

4. Remember to congratulate yourself for the ways in which you are providing spirituality for yourself. Give yourself a pat on the back.

Figure 10–1. Spirituality Self-Assessment. (Adapted with permission from Baldi, S., et al. (1980). *For your health: A model for self-care.* South Laguna, CA: Nurses Model Health.)

many personal benefits from his religious upbringing. He stopped going to church when he "came out of the closet." Chuck had not ever explored nor engaged in any specific spiritual practices other than praying. He never felt the need for more than occasional prayer during times of crisis. He saw himself as a loving and giving man, living his life according to his personal code of ethics wherein people were to be treated fairly and honestly.

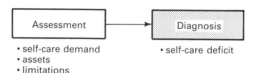

When the nurse asked about how suicide was viewed by the Catholic church, Chuck said it was a sin and unacceptable. After a few moments reflection, he asked, "Can I go to heaven if I kill myself? Will God understand and forgive me?" Chuck and the nurse agreed that he had a spiritual self-care deficit:

> Inability to cope with debilatating illness and impending death related to lack of strong inner resources and spiritual beliefs.

Chuck's deficit could also be identified as a spiritual crisis. His beliefs about God were not helping him face his illness. He had a conflict between his desire to avoid the emotional and mental suffering by taking his life and the fear of punishment from God for committing suicide. Chuck felt ill-equipped to face his prognosis because he lacked a belief system that gave meaning to his suffering. His religious beliefs, rather than being a source of strength during this time, were a source of fear and guilt for wanting to end his life while he was still in control and had a choice.

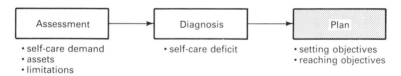

Setting Objectives

Chuck and the nurse clarified their respective roles in helping Chuck improve his spiritual self-care skills. Chuck said he wanted to die in a state of peace, and he was willing to work toward this resolution. Together they wrote a self-contract for Chuck (see Fig. 10–2). Although Chuck felt hopeless about not recovering, he no longer felt hopeless about not having any choices. He did not really know what it meant to die in peace, but the idea was appealing to him. He trusted the nurse enough to be guided in setting objectives that would help him use the resources available to work toward this goal. Since relating to his inner world was foreign to Chuck, the nurse did not suggest these activities but rather chose other techniques and discussion of issues as a way to foster spiritual awareness.

TABLE 10–5. NURSING CARE PLAN

Reason for consultation: Request to talk to nurse about terminal illness. *Client:* Chuck Taylor

Assessment	Plan	Evaluation		
			Met	Not Met
Self-care demand	Setting Objectives			
Need to develop spiritual beliefs to face illness	Two weeks: "I will spend at least 30 minutes a day talking to my friend, Jim, and the priest to explore and clarify my religious beliefs."		✕	
Need for spiritual support system during current crisis				
Assets	Reaching Objectives			
Catholic by upbringing	Client actions			
Supportive friendships with Jim, Martha	Explore my feelings about the Catholic Church, being gay, and my illness.		✕	
Enjoys gardening				
Prayer as a ritual				
Motivated during time of crisis	Meet with priest as soon as possible.		✕	
History of exercising at gym	Read inspirational literature daily.			
Limitations	Pray with my friends, Jim and Martha, daily.			
Terminal illness				Did 3 x/wk
Few past experiences with inner awareness	Spend time with my friends, share my loving feelings toward them.		✕	
No strong purpose in life	Pray for forgiveness, clarity and peace.		✕	Almost daily
Progressive physical debilatation				
Feelings of guilt and confusion				

Diagnosis	Nursing actions		Re-evaluation data	Client follow-up
Suicidal ideation	Review all the good things I have done in my life.	×		
Use of alcohol to numb anxiety	Nursing actions			
Recent death of mother	Discuss the importance of daily rituals such as meditation and journal writing.			
	Initiate conversations about the meaning of life and what gives meaning.	×		
Diagnosis	Clarify client's source of hope and strength.	×		
	Assist with life review.	×		
Self-care deficit	Teach how to do affirmations.			
Inability to find meaning in his present circumstances without spiritual intervention.	Arrange for follow-up system with staff.		Pt. Resistant	
	Teach self-contracting process and provide follow-up.	×		
	Arrange for tape recorder and guided imagery tapes on self-worth and love.	×		
	Re-evaluation data			**Client follow-up**
	Will discuss progress everyday with nurse.			Identified priest to meet with
	Will talk with nurse via telephone once a week after discharge for one month.			Has two friends who are comfortable with their own spirituality; meets with them daily.

SELF-CONTRACT

MY GOALS:

Short-term — by the end of six weeks I will . . . Spend 30 minutes/day talking to Jim, a priest, or the nurse to explore and clarify my Religious and Spiritual beliefs.

Long-term — by the end of six months I will . . . Come to a decision (about suicide, euthanasia, or living until my natural death) that is congruent with my beliefs.

ENVIRONMENTAL PLANNING: (all the steps I will take to reach my goal)

1. Meet with the hospital priest as soon as possible; go to confession.
2. Examine my feelings about the Catholic church, being gay, being ill.
3. Read inspirational literature for @ least 15 minutes daily.
4. Pray with my friend, Jim daily.
5. Spend time with my friends; share my loving feelings for them.
6. Pray for forgiveness.
7. Review all the good things I've done in my life.

THOUGHTS AND ACTIONS

Helpful thoughts:	Helpful actions:
I can find piece of mind before I die.	Calling a friend when I feel desparate
Non-helpful thoughts:	Non-helpful actions:
Killing myself is the only answer.	Withdrawing and being Non-communicative when I get scared.

MY REWARD (if I meet my goal) Jim and Martha will bring my favorite videotape. We'll have a "special evening."

THE COST: (if I fail to meet my goal) N/A

REEVALUATION DATE: 3/15

I agree to help with this project:

Jim Smith
(Support person)

I agree to strive toward this goal:

Chuck Taylor   2/15
(Your signature)   (date)

Figure 10–2. Self Contract. (Adapted with permission from Baldi, S., et al. (1980). *For your health: A model for self-care.* South Laguna, CA: Nurses Model Health, p. 47.)

Reaching Objectives: Nursing and Client Actions

The specific actions that Chuck decided to take are in his self-contract (Fig. 10–2). Since Catholic doctrine was the only one Chuck knew, he wanted to reconnect with this belief system and discuss his situation with a priest. He also realized that his friends, Jim and Martha, were very strong in their faiths and could be a source of support.

To help Chuck establish spiritual self-care practices the nurse:

- Offered to spend time praying with Chuck that he would find the right answer *for him.*
- Arranged for a tape recorder and more guided imagery tapes on self-love and self-worth for Chuck to listen to while in the hospital and at home.
- Discussed the importance of daily rituals in the development of spirituality; explored other rituals that Chuck might incorporate into his schedule.
- Initiatied conversations about "What gives meaning to your life?"
- Taught Chuck how to do affirmations to develop inner strength to cope with his situation.
- Assisted him in doing a life review of meaningful events, people, goals met, and achievements he could be proud of.
- Helped Chuck to clarify his past and current sources of strength and hope.

For Chuck to meet his goal of finding peace before he died required him to finish many areas of unfinished business in his life. It was not simply a question of, "Do I kill myself or not?" The bigger questions were, "What happens to my soul or spirit if I kill myself?" and "Is there a God that punishes suicide?"

Once Chuck understood the immensity of the task that lay before him, he became more depressed and felt overwhelmed with feelings of confusion. His philosophy and approach to life did not prepare him with the necessary skills to face these existential questions alone. He felt too sick and weak to develop new religious beliefs. It was easier to find hope and faith in the religion of his childhood. Visits with the priest helped him to begin to trust in God as an all-merciful being who does forgive and love all His children. Chuck began to remember how much comfort his religion gave him as a child.

Chuck never told his parents about his homosexuality and never fully accepted the moral rightness of being gay. He realized how he never wanted to admit the pain of having to live an alternative life-style. There seemed to be no other choice but to be himself.

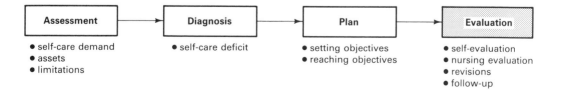

In his daily conversations with nurse, priest, and friends, Chuck started to openly acknowledge his conflicts about the meaning of his life and his illness. He saw how he had let his world shrink after his father's death and was unable to expand it again once he was free from taking care of his mother. His whole purpose for living had become his mother. Once she was gone, he had no other meaningful pursuits. Although it was too late to change the course of events, understanding what happened to him might ease the way to self-forgiveness.

Chuck had home care attendants from 7 A.M. to 7 P.M. as long as he could get around. Once he lost the ability to walk, attendants were there around the clock. The discharge nurse called once a week to discuss his spiritual self-care practices. He reported that he was unable to do much for himself anymore and was slowly losing the ability to form words. He feared the loss of speech and found it difficult to talk for long, especially over the telephone. Chuck had developed a relationship with his day nurse, who was instructed on how to help him with his spiritual ojectives. His closest friends worked out a system whereby someone would stop by each morning and evening to visit and pray with Chuck. Other friends were encouraged to call and come by as often as possible. Since so many of his friends had experienced the death of loved ones by AIDS in recent months, the friends formed a support group to help themselves cope with the grief and loss. Each friend's death reminded them of their own precarious status and uncertain future. Chuck refused to participate in any groups. He was a very private person and had always shunned groups.

Once Chuck began to feel some sense of control over his ability to find peace before he died, he gradually talked less of suicide and more about completing things before he died. Eventually all talk of suicide stopped. He started to believe that he could endure what life presented to him. He felt secure in his belief that when he died his parents would be waiting for him on the other side. This belief in an afterlife and the reuniting with his parents gave comfort to Chuck and helped him look forward to his passing rather than dreading it.

He continued to have fears about dependency and being a burden but was amazed by the amount of support he received on a regular basis. It was hard for him to allow in so much love and caring when he felt guilty and worthless. As Chuck continued to work on his spiritual practice of praying daily with a friend, reading inspirational materials, listening to tapes, and discussing his feelings and philosophy of life, he developed a stronger sense of self-love. He felt he deserved loving care until the very end.

As Chuck lost more functioning he became quieter and more depressed. Once his speech was gone it was difficult to know exactly how he was feeling. He seemed to enjoy having company and knowing someone was there. The attendants began to read to him and continued to play his tapes. Chuck died peacefully two months later in the presence of his closest friends, who talked to him about making the transition to the other side where his parents awaited him.

SUMMARY

This chapter explored the concept of spirituality as a component of health. Although no specific religious orientation was discussed, the ways in which spirituality is different from and similar to religion and philosophy of life were presented. Characteristics of spirituality such as love, joy, choice, and creativity were also explored.

Specific spiritual self-care activities that help people develop along both personal and transcendent levels of spirituality were presented. The way in which inner awareness and a sense of the meaning of life promote personal resources needed to meet crises was described. The role of the nurse as a model of spiritual self-care was emphasized. A clinical presentation described the use of nursing process and self-contracting in the integration of these concepts.

STUDY QUESTIONS

Personal Focus

1. State your personal definition of spirituality. What specific self-care activities help you feel most spiritual?
2. Rate yourself as a model of spiritual self-care.
3. Who are the models of spirituality in your life? Do you have adequate contact with these people?
4. Complete a self-contract for developing one area of spirituality in your life.

Client Focus

1. Describe the relationship between spirituality and philosophy of life as you would to a client.
2. How would you explain the relationship between spirituality and religion? Practice this with other students.
3. Make a list of four activities that would help a client develop a deeper relationship with his or her inner world. Practice describing these activities and teaching a client how to do them.
4. List the most typical spiritual concerns of your clients. Which concerns are of a personal dimension, and which are transcendent?
5. Describe the signs and symptoms that a client might experience during a spiritual crisis.
6. Help a client complete a self-contract in the self-care area of spirituality.

REFERENCES

1. Schnert, K. (1981). *Family doctor's health tips*. Deephaven, MN: Meadowbrook Press, pp. 56–61.
2. Frankl, V. (1963). *Man's search for meaning*. New York: Washington Square Press.
3. May, R. (1969). *Love and will*. New York: W.W. Norton.
4. Timerman, J. (1981). *Prisoner without a name, cell without a number*. New York: Vintage.
5. Dettmore, D. (1984). Spiritual care: Remembering your patients' forgotten needs. *Nursing 84, 15*, 46.
6. Highland, M. F., & Carson, C. (1983). Spiritual needs of patients: Are they recognized? *Cancer Nursing, 6*(3), 187.
7. Banks, R. (1980). Health and the spiritual dimension: Relationships and implications for professional preparation programs. *The Journal of School Health, 50*, 199–200.
8. Mora, G. (1975). Historical and theoretical trends in psychiatry. In A.M. Freedman, I. Kaplan, B.J. Sadock (Eds.), *Comprehensive textbook of psychiatry* (Vol. 1) (2nd ed.). Baltimore: Williams & Wilkins, pp. 1–75.
9. Stoll, R. (1979). Guideline for spiritual assessment. *American Journal of Nursing*, 1574.
10. Taylor, C., Lillis, C., & Lemone, P. (1989). *Fundamentals of nursing practice: The art and science of caring*. Philadelphia: Lippincott.
11. Potter, P., & Perry, A. (1989). *Fundamentals of nursing: Concepts, process, and practice* (2nd ed.). St. Louis: C. V. Mosby.
12. Abdellah, F.G., & Powers, S. (1960). *Patient centered approaches to nursing*. New York: Macmillan.
13. Henderson, V. (1966). *The nature of nursing*. New York: Macmillan.
14. Watson, J. (1979). *The philosophy and science of caring*. Boston: Little, Brown.
15. Dickinson, C. (1975). The search for spiritual meaning. *American Journal of Nursing, 10*, 1789.
16. Colliton, M. (1981). The spiritual dimension of nursing. In I. Beland & J. Passos (Eds.), *Clinical nursing patho-physiological approaches* (4th ed.). New York: Macmillan, p. 496.
17. Fish, S. & Shelly, J. (1978). *Spiritual care: The nurse's role*. Downers Grove, IL: Inter-Varsity Press.
18. Stoll. Guideline for spiritual assessment, pp. 1574–1577.
19. Forbis, P.A. (1988). Meeting patients' spiritual needs: Helping patients to fulfill spiritual needs is part of the nursing process. *Geriatric Nursing. 9*, (3) 158–159.
20. Frankl. *Man's search for meaning*, p. 96.
21. Phillips, J. B. (1961). *Your God is too small*. New York: Macmillan, pp. 19–21.
22. Brown, M. (1983). *The unfolding self*. Los Angeles: Psychosynthesis, pp. 20–24.
23. Maslow, A. (1968). *Toward a psychology of being*. New York: Van Nostrand Reinhold, p. 112.
24. Paterson, J.G., & Zderad, L.T. (1976). *Humanistic nursing*. New York: John Wiley & Sons, p. 7.
25. Parse, R.R. (1981). *Man-living health: A theory of nursing*. New York: John Wiley & Sons, p. 56.
26. Jung, C.G. (1923). *Psychological types of the psychological individuation* (H. G. Bagnes, Trans.). London: Kegan Paul, p. 547.

27. Reifler, S. (1974). *I Ching: A new interpretation for modern times.* New York: Bantam, p. 70.

28. Peck, D. (1978). Compassion and healing. *Holistic health handbook.* Berkeley, CA: And/Or Press, p. 267.

29. Dossey, L. (1984). *Beyond Illinois.* Boston: Shambhala, p. 176.

30. Beyette, B. (1982, June 9). *Los Angeles Times,* Sec. V, p. 2.

31. Green, W. (1976). *EST—4 days to make your life work.* New York: Pocket Books, p. 12.

32. Twitchell, P. (1970). *The flute of God.* Menlo Park, CA: IWP, p. 94.

33. Sanford, J. (1970). *The kingdom within.* Philadelphia: J.B. Lippincott, p. 44.

34. Siegel, B.S. (1989). *Peace, Love, and Healing.* New York: Harper & Row.

35. Paterson & Zderad. *Humanistic nursing,* p. 16.

36. Dossey, B.M. (1988). L. Keegan, C.E. Guzetta, L.G. Kolkmeier (Eds.) *Holistic nursing: A handbook for practice.* Rockville, MD: Aspen, p. 40.

37. Veninga, R. (1985). *A gift of hope.* New York: Ballantine, p. 232.

38. Miller, J. (1983). *Coping with chronic illness: Overcoming powerlessness.* Philadelphia: F.A. Davis, p. 287.

39. Beck, C., et al. (1984). *Mental health–psychiatric nursing.* St. Louis: Mosby, pp. 501–502.

40. Peck, M.S. (1978). *The road less traveled.* New York: Simon & Schuster.

41. Hart, D. (1972). The path to wholeness. *Psychological Perspective, 3*(2), 150.

42. Jung, C.G. (1964). *Man and his symbols.* London: Aldus, pp. 158–229.

43. Sanford. *The kingdom within,* p. 219.

44. Rajineish, B.S. (1973). *The psychology of the esoteric: The new evolution of man.* New York: Harper & Row/Perennial Library, p. 75.

45. Fish & Shelly. *Spiritual Care,* p. 37.

46. Heckler, R. (1983). Entering the place of conflict. In J. Welwood (Ed.), *Awakening the heart.* Boston: Shambhala, pp. 176–182.

47. North American Nursing Diagnosis Association. (1987). Taxonomy I with complete diagnoses. St. Louis: Author, p. 70.

48. NANDA. Taxonomy I, p. 99.

49. Erikson, E.H. (1950). *Childhood and society.* London: Penguin, pp. 259–61.

50. Sheehy, G. (1974). *Passages: Predictable crises of adult life.* New York: E.P. Dutton, p. 286.

51. Dass, R. (1976). *Grist for the mill.* Santa Cruz, CA: Unity Press, p. 12.

52. Kavanaugh, R. (1972). *Facing death.* New York: Penguin, p. 16.

53. DeYoung, S. (1986). Spiritual care and the unprepared nurse. *Journal of Christian Nursing, 3,* 32.

54. Swinford, P. & Webster, J. (1989). *Promoting wellness: A nurse's handbook.* Rockville, MD: Aspen.

55. Stoken, K.L., & Carson, V.J. (1986). Study measures nurses' attitudes about providing spiritual care. *Health Programs, 67*(3), 52.

56. Yancey, V. (1987). Spiritual care, attitudes and practices of intensive care unit nurses. Unpublished Master's thesis, St. Louis University, St. Louis, MO.

57. Kreiger, D. (1981). *Foundations for holistic health practices: The renaissance nurse.* Philadelphia: J.B. Lippincott, p. 186.

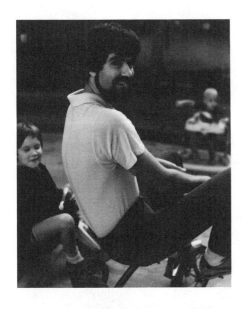

He who laughs, lasts.

Norman Cousins

11 Humor and Play

LEARNING OBJECTIVES

Upon completion of this chapter, readers will be able to:

1. Differentiate play from relaxation.
2. List eight characteristics of play.
3. Describe the role of play in healthy personality development.
4. Describe the relationship between laughter and emotional and physical health.
5. Describe and demonstrate a deep laughter response.
6. Complete a plan for behavior change in the self-care area of play.

DEFINITIONS

Play   A self-care activity engaged in simply because the person wants to.[1] At its best it is an activity free of constraint by others. Play can be free, spontaneous, joyful. It is not motivated primarily by competition. The positive effects of healthy play are not cumulative; play must occur on a regular basis.

Playfulness   An attitude and way of behaving in life that incorporates physical, social, and cognitive spontaneity. It included traits of manifest joy and a sense of humor.[2]

Humor   "That quality which appeals to a sense of the ludicrous or absurdly incongruous."[3] Humor implies an ability to perceive the nonserious component of situations and often leads to a feeling of relief. *Humor* and *laughter* are often used interchangeably.

Laughter   A spontaneous reaction in stressful or humorous situations. It is accompanied by behavioral responses that are indicative of amusement and pleasure, such as smiling, a change in facial expression, and twinkling eyes. Deep belly laughter leaves a person feeling free and renewed. It provides exercise for the lungs and entire cardiovascular system.

INTRODUCTION

Play is a term most commonly associated with children. Children have *play* time and *play*grounds. Primary education systems place a high value on play as a mechanism for both social and cognitive learning. Evidence of the significance of children's play in our society is seen in the fact that toy industries are multimillion-dollar enterprises.

Until recently, however, *play* was rarely associated with adults. It is now seen as a specific area of self-care for both children *and* adults throughout life. Play is clearly related to higher levels of creativity and mental and physical health. It is imperative that nurses begin to understand and integrate this concept into their own lives as well as into clinical practice.

Henderson, an early nursing theorist, recognized the importance of play and wrote about it as early as 1922. She defined play as activities that "have no serious motive; are carried on for the pleasure they give the participants; and from which there is no material gain."[4] She saw that diversion and playful activity must be provided to recuperating children and adults to facilitate the healing process.

Play is an activity engaged in simply because a person wants to.[1] Play is different for all people but it *always* provides diversion from daily responsibility and concerns. It is a time not constrained by others.[5] Some words commonly associated with play are *spontaneity, joy, humor,* and *restoration.* The activity of play can be understood and differentiated from other closely related and often overlapping activities.

CHARACTERISTICS OF PLAY: DIFFERENTIATING PLAY FROM OTHER ACTIVITIES

Play Is Not Relaxation

Play is quite different from relaxation (see Chapter 9). *Relaxation* implies a physiological, hypometabolic state, in which a person's total body system slows down with a decrease in heart rate and blood pressure. Relaxation is an integrated central and autonomic nervous system response in which one reduces both mental and physical activity to a minimum.[6] *Play*, on the other hand, is spontaneous, joyful, expressive, and often very active. Blood pressure and heart rate actually increase (and subsequently decrease) with joyful laughter and play. Improved circulation and cardiac efficiency related to increased oxygenation during play is similar to that provided by aerobic exercise.

Play May Be Exercise but Need Not Be

Exercise and play are often confused. One may exercise in a playful way, such as when a humorous attitude is adopted while playing tennis. Play may also involve an exercise activity such as playing a game of Frisbee with a group of friends. All exercise is not play, however, and all play is not exercise. Clients often have difficulty in differentiating these two activities. One client, for example, reported to the nurse that he jogged 15 minutes that day and thought that jogging was also his play activity. With further questioning, though, he stated that he perceived jogging as a "boring struggle," which he practiced because he knew it was good for his heart. Jogging was clearly not a playful activity for this client. Each person's *attitude* toward an activity has a major role in differentiating play from other activities.

Competition Is Not a Major Component of Play

Competition is not a *primary* motive of good play. While a person may *enjoy* winning a tennis game with a friend in healthy play, winning is not a prerequisite for having fun. Friedman has written about the difficulties faced by competitive, time-driven people when they begin sports or play activities.[7] The concept of doing something "just for fun" is foreign to most of these people. A constant need to win (for example, to have the *best* running time or the *best* score at racquetball) is often in conflict with their intellectual knowledge of the value of playing just for fun. Healthy play can provide situations in which everyone wins and no one loses.

Play May Be Passive or Active

Good play leaves one feeling refreshed, happy, and alive. It is frequently a spontaneous activity that provides release, exhilaration, and refreshment. This is quite different from the passive experience of watching television. People seldom feel good, happy, or alive after watching four hours of television. Although play is often active, it can be passive and still leave the person feeling exhilarated and refreshed. Murphy writes that fun stops when one *has* to play. She describes a common occurrence when school children are encouraged to go outside and "play" (for example, soccer or jump rope). In Murphy's example, 10-year-old Colin said, "No, I want to sit here on the windowsill and write a poem." Murphy points out that this, too, would leave Colin feeling refreshed, happy, and alive; this is true play.[8]

Work for One Person May Be Play for Another Person

It is important for nurses to pay attention to the fact that *perception of an activity as playful* is unique to the individual. Some people hate doing yardwork. For others this is an extremely playful activity, eagerly anticipated. Appreciation of these unique perceptions is vital. If the nurse considers something playful, he or she must understand that the client may have a very different perception of that activity.

Play Is a Preoccupied State

When engaging in true, healthy play a person becomes preoccupied and totally immersed in the pleasurable experience. Most adults are aware of children's inability to hear Dad calling them to dinner while they are engrossed in play. For adults it is more difficult and unusual for this state to be reached, although sexual play provides one example. Adults also occasionally become preoccupied during social play (playing cards, watching a stage play) and are able to "lose themselves" in the pleasurable experience.

Play Is Noncumulative

A common misconception is that fun time or playful times are only for weekends or yearly vacations. Some clients will intellectually understand that these types of playful time are vital for health but will participate in them only for brief, isolated periods. To be most effective in maintaining health and preventing or managing illness, play, like all other self-care activities, *must be practiced regularly*. People cannot "save up" all of their play activities for a yearly vacation and expect to obtain effective, long-term benefits.

Play Usually Involves Humor and Spontaneous Laughter

Play is *always* the opposite of seriousness, even though it may occur during serious times. A sense of freedom and stimulation is associated with the experience of a good laugh. The ability to laugh at oneself places stressful problems in a new perspective.

Play Involves Freedom of Choice

The experience of not being constrained by others or circumstances is a major component of play.[5] This, again, is a difficult and confusing area for many people. A client reported that she went bicycling with her children. The major motive in this activity, however, was to allay the guilt that she felt in having so little time for play with them. In this circumstance, the client was probably constrained by others (children) and was not experiencing the bicycling simply for her own pleasure.

HISTORY OF PLAY

Throughout history, the activity of play in the lives of both children and adults has been closely related to economics and religion. In earliest recorded history, play was for the rich. It was provided or supported by the poor (that is, slaves). Hedonism, or the pursuit of pleasure, was a very early philosophy that espoused pleasure, particularly of the senses, as having the highest value. Images of early Romans gorging themselves with large meals while they watched exotic dancers are associated with this philosophy. Early opponents of this way of life were known as ascetics. They proposed that all pleasure of the senses was sinful and should be avoided at any cost.

Traces of these opposing philosophies have been apparent throughout history. School discipline employed in Germany at the beginning of the eighteenth century readily displayed a common attitude of that period. According to Franke:

> Play must be forbidden in any and all of its forms. The children shall be instructed in this matter in such a way as to show them, through the presentation of religious principles, the wastefulness and folly of all play. They shall be led to see that play will distract their hearts and minds from God, the eternal God, and will work nothing but harm to their spiritual lives.[9]

In America, this type of religious conviction was also prevalent. The educational system of the Methodist Church in 1792 conveyed a typical attitude of the day about play:

> We prohibit play in the strongest terms . . . the students shall rise at five o'clock . . . summer and winter. . . . The students shall be indulged with nothing which the world calls play. Let this rule be observed with the strictest

nicety; for those who play when they are young, will play when they are old. (Discipline of the M.E. Church, 1792)[10]

Although such repressive attitudes sometimes still exist, play is now seen as a more central part of human development, not just of child development. Progress from the point when play was only for the leisure class has occurred. Child-labor laws have provided more play time, as well as more educational time, for children of all classes. Parks and recreation centers are now a common part of the landscape. Most are available to the public for free or at minimal cost. Remarkably, private industry is beginning to provide play time and recreation centers for adult workers. These practices have been directly tied to higher job performance and a decrease in employee turnover.[11,12]

Increasingly, people live to be 80 years old and beyond. Coupled with the incidence of earlier retirement, it is possible for a person to experience twenty to thirty years of retirement! This presents a challenge for older persons to learn to use their leisure time in pleasurable, fun ways. Often they have no prior history of play beyond the traditional family vacation time and must learn how to play. Senior citizen centers, community colleges, and other resources now help older people learn this skill.

THE VALUE OF PLAY

> Man alone suffers so excruciatingly in the world that he was compelled to invent laughter.
>
> Nietsche

Many different physiological and psychological theories of why people play have been proposed. There are overlapping components in many of these theories. Some focus only on the theoretical aspects of children's play and provide no discussion of this part of life for adolescents and adults. Theories about adult play center around the idea that people need these activities in order to relax, get rid of surplus energy, or practice life skills (including emotional and physical growth).

Freud has described the value of humor in helping people decrease anxiety. He wrote about the cathartic value of stage drama for adults. In his view, as adults watch play characters experience and master life stresses, they become better able to master their own.[13]

The value of play for healthy and ill children is rarely disputed. "Play therapy" for children has gained wide acceptance and respect. Most pediatric nurses are adept at the skill of helping children prepare for and master anxiety about illness, surgery, and even death through play. Play also creates situations in which children can reenact stressful events such as a tonsillectomy.

Psychodrama provides a similar type of play therapy for both children and adults. In this treatment model clients act out stressful situations and play many different roles in interactions until they, too, feel that they have mastered specific anxiety and gained new confidence.

Play as a part of the educational process for children has been solidly integrated. As early as 1921, Dewey facilitated this integration through his emphasis on the folly and uselessness of trying to suppress play in the lives of both children and adults.

> Education has no more serious responsibility than making adequate provision for enjoyment of recreative leisure, not only for the sake of immediate health, but still more if possible for the lasting effects upon habits of the mind.[14]

Play and Healthy Development

Play has been studied extensively in the social life of monkeys. Harlow has repeatedly documented the short-term and long-range value of play in the monkey world. Monkeys who play as young infants are more likely to play throughout their lives. When compared to monkeys deprived of play as infants, playing monkeys generally demonstrate higher levels of security and confidence, more normal sexual lives, and more healthy social interactions with peers.[15] Harlow translates these findings as having marked significance for studies about play in human beings.

Play is one of the earliest activities of children. Play provides a basis for many interactions between parents and children. Peek-a-boo provides an excellent example of the vital role of play in children's lives. At a very early age children begin to master anxiety through this game as they see that their parents do not disappear forever but quickly return.

Play often provides physical movement that is very different from motion at work or in other activities. Self-motion play, such as rocking or swinging, forms the basis from which other types of play evolve. The pleasure associated with *motion* is an important part of many play activities. Running, chasing, and jumping accompany "rough and tumble" play, which is beneficial in helping children and adults divert aggression in acceptable ways. Spontaneous laughter is frequently a powerful indication of the pure enjoyment experienced in this type of play.

A continuity of playfulness from childhood through adult life is positively related to emotional health.[11,12] Freud initially introduced the idea that to be emotionally healthy, a person must be able to work and love. A current perception is that to be truly healthy, persons must be able to love, work, *and play.*[18,19]

Gardner[20] and Lieberman[21] both emphasize humor and playfulness as helpful coping methods for adults. The ability to allow free time for oneself is an implicit part of a playful attitude toward life. The following quotation of Joseph

Welch captures the essence of what is meant by *free time* or *play time:*

> I would hope that I passed along to my sons a certain legacy of laziness, for without laziness no one can expect to be a whole man. You must, if you are to be happy, have the time to take an occasional look at life as it rushes past you. You must decorate it with a little humor or generosity or whatever pleases or delights you. Else you risk spending all your years on a treadmill racing to earn more money, attain more security, win more prestige, only to find at the end of the day that you've had no real target anyway, except death. You miss a lot if you run too fast, and you never reach your goals either, they always recede over the horizon.[22]

The importance of balancing one's "play life" with one's "work life" has been addressed by Jourard. He points out that it is important to train people to use leisure time in rewarding ways and as a meaningful balance to work. When people are unable to do this, free time is frequently seen as oppressive and related to anxiety rather than to freedom, spontaneity, and joy.[17] "The healthy personality calls for hobbies, interests, and leisure-time activities that provide enjoyment and sustain a 'joie de vivre.' "[23] This is a crucial concept for elderly people as well. Activities that are fun and pleasure giving increase their satisfaction with their lives and sustain their desire to keep active and involved with the world.

The therapeutic value of play in adult life has also been emphasized by Winnicott, a noted English psychoanalyst. He repeatedly states that the first priority in helping emotionally upset clients should be to help them to play. He believes that play is a major self-healing device. He later emphasizes that efforts to help people play are cost-effective since they decrease the need for traditional health care.[24] He sees play as universal and "belonging to health." It facilitates growth and health, and leads to an increase in creativity, communication, and group relationships.[25]

Furthermore, Winnicott believes that for professionals to help clients in this area they must be able to play themselves:

> If the therapist cannot play then he is not suitable for work. If the patient cannot play he needs to be helped to learn how to play before therapy can begin. Play is essential and is the only process towards creativity.[26]

He sees it as logical that people who have had a playful break from work routines usually return to work rested, more creative, and more productive.

Play, then, is clearly valuable. It provides both children and adults with a mechanism of catharsis and an opportunity to master anxiety. It provides rest and recreation so that individuals can return to work and other activities with new energy and creativity. As a self-healing, self-care device, it is cost-effective for clients. To be healthy, people must be able to love, work, *and play.*

Value of Humor and Laughter

> Laughter is the shortest distance between two people.
>
> Victor Borge, Humorist

To be healthy, people must have a sense of humor and be able to laugh with others and at themselves. Humor and laughter are components of good play. The value of laughter for physical and emotional health has been widely publicized; this area of self-care is thus not quite so foreign to clients as in the past.

Cousins[27] and Simonton and Matthews-Simonton[28] see laughter and humor as integral parts of holistic health. They believe that repeated occurrences of joyful and self-expressive states may be associated with physical and emotional wellness and with prolongation of life. Studies on humor have upheld this positive relationship. Humor gives very ill people one means of maintaining mastery and control over their environment.[29]

Cousins describes his use of comical movies to cure himself of a collagen disease, which had been diagnosed as terminal. He refused to accept pessimistic prognostic statements from his physicians and instead began to watch humorous films and practice regular, deep belly laughs for his self-prescription.[27] This procedure is now being used in clinical settings with ill clients. Many hospitals provide "living rooms" or "lively rooms" where clients are encouraged to watch funny movies and tell jokes to each other.[30,31]

Humorous play has been advocated for the treatment of grieving clients.[32–34] Nurses must consider the timing, setting, content of the humor, and receptiveness of the client in decisions to use humor in health care settings.[35] In the past, use of humor has been seen as dangerous.[36,37] Clients must sense that nurses are laughing *with them* and not *at them*. When timing is appropriate, however (and sensitivity and empathy are present), the use of laughter can move the therapeutic relationship to a more intimate and productive level. Laughter and humor bring a sense of perspective to the grieving person's overwhelming feelings of loss.

A person is physiologically incapable of smiling and frowning at the same time. Deep, spontaneous laughter is incompatible with the severe gloom of depression. Mindess points out that laughter enables a person to be momentarily free of inhibition and control.[38] This brief interlude usually leaves the person with a new appreciation of other parts of his or her personality. The ability to cope is thus strengthened.

Laughter, as a valuable preventive medicine, is also becoming widely accepted. Laughter is invigorating and stimulating and provides exercise for the cardiovascular system. There is some evidence that deep laughter stimulates the release of endorphins, which play a role in pain reduction.[39] It has been described as "stationary jogging." These changes during laughter are summarized in Table 11–1.

TABLE 11–1. PHYSIOLOGICAL EFFECTS ASSOCIATED WITH LAUGHTER

During deep laughter:
Increase in heart rate
Increased oxygenation to lungs
Stimulation of the adrenal glands
Increase in blood pressure
Release of endorphins
Immediately following deep laughter:
Subjective experience of relief
Decrease in heart rate
Decrease in blood pressure

(From Fry, W.F. (1977). The respiratory components of mirthful laughter. *The Journal of Biological Psychology, 19* (2), 39-50; Bushnell, D.D., & Scheff, T.J. (1979). The effect of laughter on mood, heart rate, and skin temperature. Second International Conference on Humor, Los Angeles; and Fry, W.F. & Salameth, W. (1987). *Handbook of humor and psychotherapy.* Sarasota, FL: Professional Resources Exchange.)

Infants smile and laugh spontaneously and with great joy. They have amazing power to make adults around them smile and coo. Unfortunately people laugh out loud less and less as they mature. Many children lose their sense of humor as they get older and enter the school world and the work world. Many adults find it difficult to laugh and play.

Robinson has written of the need for assessment of each client's sense of humor as part of the routine health assessment. She believes nurses need to pay more attention to this valuable coping skill in themselves.[40] Laughter and play can contribute to improved team work, decreased burnout and improved staff relationships. Nurses can learn to say, as quoted from Weinstein, "I take my job seriously, but myself lightly."[41] Techniques for helping people learn laughter and play skills are presented in Tables 11–2, 11–3, and 11–4. Samples of hospital humor are presented in Table 11–5.

Nursing Diagnosis and Play Self-Care

The nursing diagnosis of *Diversional activity deficit* is clearly related to the self-care area of play and humor. This deficit is an inability to occupy oneself in activities that pass time, entertain, distract, or gratify, because of internal or external factors that may or may not be beyond the individual's control. Hospitalization often leads to boredom as clients are unable to participate in their usual diversional activities. Some clients are unable or unwilling to play whether at home or in the hospital. The material presented in this chapter provides a structure for nursing interventions in this area.

TABLE 11–2. TECHNIQUES TO FACILITATE PLAY BEHAVIOR

Note: It is recommended that the nurse complete each of these activities before assisting clients to complete them. Nurses are also encouraged to add new activities to this list as they gather feedback from clients.

1. List three times or periods in your life during each week when you are free from responsibility.
2. Go back to your own childhood and think about the kind of play you enjoyed at that time.
3. Pay attention to your dreams and daydreams about play. For one month keep a journal record of your dreams. Pay attention to the ones that are particularly free, spontaneous, and joyful.
4. Plan to spend at least two hours each week watching children play. Do this for one month. Do you find yourself smiling inside as you watch them? What kinds of activities are they experiencing?
5. Plan to play with children during the week. If you have your own children, make a special effort to play with them "just for the fun of it" Did you laugh out loud during your play with them?
6. List three friends who are most playful and fun to be with. Think about how you could plan to spend more time with these people.
7. Think about the kind of environment or setting that you need for play. Do you need to be outside your home? Do you need to be wearing special "play" clothes? Is there a special room in your home where you feel most free and spontaneous?
8. Lock the bathroom door and look at yourself in the mirror. Try to think serious and then humorous thoughts. Smile at yourself in the mirror for two minutes.
9. Practice laughing with a friend. If necessary, have that friend tickle you. Tell each other jokes, go to a silly movie. Make a tape of yourself laughing and plan to play it back in privacy when you are feeling most depressed.

TABLE 11–3. ACTIVITIES TO USE TO DEVELOP A SENSE OF HUMOR

Directions:

Using the seven components of humor (flexibility, spontaneity, unconventionality, shrewdness, playfulness, humility, and irony) practice ways of enhancing your sense of humor, and of seeing your problems in a humorous way.

Flexibility

1. Look at the situation from many different points of view. For example, from a child's, parent's, spouse's, boss', religious person's, doctor's, nurse's, or alien-visitor-from-another-planet's point of view.

2. Be your problem, and ask, "What kind of clothes would my problem wear?" "What language would it talk?" "What songs would it sing?" "What mottos would it have?"

3. Make a list of dreams, hunches, fantasies, wild ideas, or wishes you have had. Review the list and see how it bears on your level of wellness.

Spontaneity

1. Decide how to solve a problem using intellectual or logical processes. Then solve the same problem using your intuitive or feeling reactions. Next, solve the same problem using a spiritual or cosmic approach.

2. Demonstrate different feelings through using facial expression, body posture, and any other mode but words. Some feelings to use are: anger, love, sadness, fear.

Unconventionality

1. Plan a day in your life as if you were living in a kibbutz in Israel, an Indian reservation, an Eskimo village, a spaceship circling the moon, or Krypton (Superman's birthplace).

2. Live one day as if you were Louis Pasteur, Florence Nightingale, Madame Curie, Wonder Woman, Albert Einstein, a favorite animal or bird.

Shrewdness

1. Give examples of how you are not who you seem to be.

2. Think about your friends, family, and other significant people. Draw up a list of people, and then write down at least one example of how each person is not who he or she seems to be.

Playfulness

1. Pretend your current predicament is a game. Write down the rules and chance factors that are operating, draw up game cards, a score sheet, and rules for who wins and loses.

2. Visualize your total life as a game. Chart "wins," "losses," and "rained out" events. List times of enjoyment, fun, sadness, and fear. Give a name to your life game.

Humility

1. State the meaning of life for you. Consider what would happen if that were *not* the meaning of life.

2. Pretend you are an ant or a mosquito. Try to expand on what your life would be like.

Irony

1. Think about how ironic life is, and to try to remember how happy events or relationships have included suffering, and difficult situations have brought happiness.

2. List your greatest desires or fears at the moment. Then look at the list and ask for each entry, "What difference does this make in terms of my total life or of the larger scheme of eternity?"

(Reprinted with permission from Clark, C.C. (1981). *Enhancing Wellness.* New York: Springer, pp. 187-188.)

TABLE 11–4. LEARNING DEEP BELLY LAUGHTER

The following exercise will help you practice deep belly laughter. These steps then can also be taught to clients.

1. Sit in a quiet room alone. Plan to stay there for about 10 minutes.
2. Loosen your belt, take off your shoes. Loosen any other tight clothing so that you will not feel restrained. Be sure to take off your tie.
3. Think of a funny joke or a ridiculous event in your life.
4. Begin to laugh out loud; laugh for at least 30 seconds.
5. If this is difficult for you, plan to do it with a friend. This approach is usually effective because both people give permission to each other to be silly.
6. If you are embarrassed when you first start, you may want to close your eyes. This will make everyone else disappear so that you can be more spontaneous.
7. For more assistance you may want to play a tape of people laughing or watch comedy movies for your planned laughter times. You may also find it easy to laugh if you look at yourself for a long time in a mirror.

NURSES MODEL PLAY SELF-CARE

Nurses cannot help their clients learn to play unless they are able to play themselves.[24] Figure 11–1 presents self-assessment questions to help nurses judge their own success in this area.

In their personal lives nurses model play self-care by:

- Playing on a regular basis, not only during vacation periods.
- Managing personal schedules to allow for daily periods free of responsibility.
- Expressing joy, enthusiasm, and humor with family and friends.
- Maintaining a humorous perspective during periods of grief.
- Being with people who make them laugh.
- Keeping a notebook with jokes, cartoons, pictures, and vignettes of funny events and using this on days when a "laughter-life" is needed.
- Trying to "think funny" by looking at the absurdities in life.
- Being able to laugh at themselves in a nonjudgmental manner.
- "Surprising" a friend or family member once a month.
- Planning an "unusual" fun activity (e.g., sky-diving).

TABLE 11–5. HUMOR IN THE HOSPITAL

The Where-Else-in-Polite-Society-Do-People-Discuss-This? Joke

A patient who is to undergo a colonoscopy needs to have a series of enemas.

Nurse: "I have another 'enemy' for you."

Patient: (sigh) "Enemies, enemies, enemies!"

"Taboo and embarrassing subjects, by necessity, are commonplace in the hospital. In this setting, a patient comes in under great stress and is expected to cooperate with procedures. Very often, joking is the way we get patients to accept what is going on and to trust us. When you laugh together, you've established a bond of friendship."

The Hostile Joke

A patient, alone in an isolation room, puts a sign on her door: "If you're afraid of the bugs, at least knock when you go by!"

"This is one of the most therapeutic uses of humor. The patient can get rid of a lot of his anger and frustration toward things and people by his joking. To express hostility through a joke is acceptable because the target of the hostility can laugh with you, yet he gets the point. It's helpful to the patient, if the nurse can accept that hostile humor, instead of becoming angry.

The Testing-the-Waters Joke

Dying patient to nurse: "I wish we had pop-up thermometers like turkeys, so we'd know when we're done."

"This patient is sending up a trial balloon to the nurse about his feelings. Acknowledge his joke, but then use it as an opportunity to open up a more serious discussion about what's going on."

Gallows Humor

Nurse receiving advice for a dying patient: "Give her a Bible—and tell her to cram."

"The joking among staff can become grim and macabre, the same 'bravado in the face of death' that is seen on the battlefield or in concentration camps. When you're in the midst of a crisis, when stress gets the highest, you find hostile and aggressive kinds of humor increasing among staff. You have to laugh at the horrors because, in a sense, it gives you the objectivity which reduces the overwhelming feeling of having to deal with it day in and day out."

(Reprinted with permission. Interview and jokes from Vera Robinson, as quoted by Lindsay, B. (1988). Bellylaughs—nurses need them as much as patients. *Southern California Nursing News, 1,* (8), 6.)

Nurses can regularly model humor and play in clinical settings. Examples include:

- Providing recreation time for hospitalized clients.
- Maintaining a sense of humor with staff and clients.
- Joking with clients without ridiculing them.
- Collecting things that make others laugh in a book, envelope, or box to share with patients or staff.
- Placing funny cartoons on the unit bulletin board.
- Expressing a balanced perspective about work, showing how it is possible to have fun at work and still take it seriously.
- Encouraging clients to make time for fun and hobbies on a daily basis.
- Using appropriate recreational therapy resources.
- Providing comedy audio/video tapes for all clients.

- Using cartoons in client education materials.
- Using work breaks for fun and rest rather than for paperwork or other clerical tasks.

Nurses who seem spontaneous, joyful, enthusiastic, and creative probably practice play self-care on a regular basis. When clients observe these qualities in nurses, they will begin to value and practice self-care in this area.

CLINICAL APPLICATION

Case Presentation

David is a 40-year-old, married, Jewish upper-middle-class, attorney. Over the last two months, he has visited his internist four times with a chief complaint of "severe neck pain." Medical tests have shown no physical pathology. A variety of treatment approaches, including hot compresses, medication, neck bracing, and massage, have been initiated during this time but have met with little success.

David's life-style during his childhood and adult life has been characterized by traits typical of a type A personality.[7] Both of his parents were physicians, and he grew up with a strong belief that "one plays only after all work is done." All work is never done for David. He is extremely time-pressured, competitive, work-oriented, ambitious, reliable, and restless. He has always been able to get angry at his family and work associates but has difficulty expressing other feelings, such as sadness, joy, or excitement. He is often not aware of these repressed feelings. He does not remember the last time he laughed out loud or had so much fun that he briefly forgot about work.

David's neck pain has been attributed to muscle tension. David has recognized that he allows no fun and playful time for himself. He sees that as a priority self-care problem in view of his extreme tension and states that he would like to explore it in more depth.

Assessment

- self-care demand
- assets
- limitations

David's *developmental level* has a major influence on his present behaviors. At 40, he is approaching the pinnacle of his career and believes that his present actions will either "make or break his future." David's work-oriented and time-pressured behavior is rewarded and reinforced by mainstream society.

David's *family background* and *sociocultural orientation* have reinforced values of achievement and seriousness while discrediting spontaneous and less structured experiences. David also reports that he remembers no playful adult *models* in his childhood and that he has no current peer models for play.

David's *major asset* is his interpersonal relationships. His wife, Yvonne, is interested in helping him work on this self-care area. David's 8-year-old son and 10-year-old daughter provide excellent play models for him.

David completed the play self-assessment tool (see Fig. 11–1). His wife also completed the form. Her responses agreed with David's perceptions of himself. David was encouraged to talk with his nurse about some of his thoughts and feelings about play. His comments included, "Adults look *silly* when they play" and "I have so many more important things to do; I don't know what I'd do for fun. Anyway, my work is fun." David had numerous rigid beliefs that laughter and spontaneous fun should *not* be part of adult life.

David also completed the Time Utilization Worksheet presented in Figure 11–2. He typically spent more than 80 hours per week in work activities. This information had a dramatic impact on him; he began to think about priorities in his life. He agreed that at least some of the work activities that he "perceived" as imperative could be reduced or eliminated.

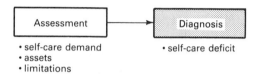

David and the nurse jointly agreed that he had a self-care deficit. In nursing language this was worded as:

Inability to play spontaneously without education and intervention.

His limitations were related to inadequate knowledge, experience, and motivation. His ambivalence and deeply-rooted personality characteristics had a major impact on his difficulty in the area of motivation.

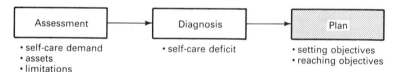

Setting Objectives

Specific methods to help David increase his ability to play were chosen. The nurse and David clarified their roles in this process. David was given reading material about play and was encouraged to use the techniques from Tables 11–2, 11–3, and 11–4.

David decided that this was a good time for him to work on improving this self-care area. He planned to start with "baby steps" and progress after he had a better sense of how this would change his life and his feelings about himself. He completed a self-contract and asked his wife to be his partner (see Fig. 11–3).

PLAY SELF-ASSESSMENT

Complete the following self-assessment to help you look at the role of play in your life. On the scale below circle the numbers which are most true for you and your life during the last year:

	Almost Never	Seldom	Often	Almost Always
1. I have times during the day when I feel free of responsibilities.	①	2	3	4
2. Each week I have time just for me.	①	2	3	4
3. There are times when I find myself playing spontaneously.	①	2	3	4
4. I have fun playing with my family and friends.	1	2	③	4
5. I plan play on a regular basis with friends.	1	②	3	4
6. I play several times each week.	1	②	3	4
7. My family supports my participation in my favorite source of fun.	1	2	3	④
8. I frequently hear myself laughing out loud.	1	②	3	4
9. I play without guilt even when there's more work to be done.	①	2	3	4
10. I am a fun person to be with.	1	2	③	4

Some suggestions for how you might learn from this self-assessment:

1. Connect all the circles down the length of the page. Look at the pattern that your connected line makes. Turn your page sideways to get an even more clear visual picture of the role of play in your life right now. What does it seem to be saying to you?

2. Now add up your total score: _____ 20 _____

   Circle which range it was in:
   10-19   (20-29)   30-40

   If your score was in the 10-19 range you might want to make some changes in how and when you play. Which aspects do you think need the most work? How many "1's" did you mark on this assessment? 4 These might serve as a clue to help you think about making changes in this area of your life.

3. How would you like this self-assessment to look six months from now? Are you interested in working toward those improvements?

4. Remember to congratulate yourself for the ways in which you are playing well. Give yourself a pat on the back, or go out and play as a way to congratulate yourself!

Figure 11–1. Play self-assessment. *(Reprinted with permission from Baldi, S., and others (1980). For your health: A model for self-care. South Laguna, CA: Nurses Model Health, p. 119.)*

Time Utilization Worksheet

Complete this form for how it best represents a *typical weekday* in your life during the *last month*.

Time	What I'm doing	Comments/How I feel about this activity
6:00 a.m.	↓ Sleeping	
7:00 a.m.	Shower/	Wish I had more
8:00 a.m.	Shave/ Breakfast	time
9:00 a.m.	↑	Rushed, anxious
10:00 a.m.	Work meeting	Tense, many
11:00 a.m.	lots of coffee	decisions to make
12:00 noon	Lunch with boss—	
1:00 p.m.	2 martinis	Much pressure
2:00 p.m.	Back at	Inadequate, anxious
3:00 p.m.	work, prepare	Case is difficult;
4:00 p.m.	for trial tomorrow	wish I were more
5:00 p.m.	Pick up car at garage	prepared.
6:00 p.m.	↑ Rotary Club	Asked to be President
7:00 p.m.	dinner	next year
8:00 p.m.	Stop by office to check file for court in AM	Like the power
9:00 p.m.	Read to kids for ½ hr.	Bored, rushed, so much else to do to get ready for Tomorrow
10:00 p.m.	Take out the trash	Angry – wife could have done the trash.
11:00 p.m.	Fix the bathroom toilet. Return call on exchange	Angry
12:00 p.m.	Reading report due tomorrow	
1:00 a.m.	To bed	
2:00 a.m.		
3:00 a.m.		
4:00 a.m.	Sleeping	Restless
5:00 a.m.	↓	

Figure 11–2. Time utilization worksheet *(Reprinted with permission from Baldi, S., and others (1980). For your health: A model for self-care. South Laguna, CA: Nurses Model Health, p. 37.)*

SELF-CONTRACT

MY GOALS:

Short-term — by the end of six weeks I will . . . _Spend 15 minutes 3x/wk doing a play activity that is "just for myself."_

Long-term — by the end of six months I will . . . _Spend 30 minutes 4x/wk at play_

ENVIRONMENTAL PLANNING: (all the steps I will take to reach my goal)

1. Complete a time utilization assessment sheet now and at the end of each week.
2. Make a list of 3 work or work-related activities which I might eliminate.
3. List five activities that will be playful for me.
4. Ask Yvonne and the kids to help me keep a chart of the play I do each week.
5. Spend one minute 4x/wk laughing in the mirror.

THOUGHTS AND ACTIONS

Helpful thoughts:	Helpful actions:
It's good for me to be playful. I felt better when I laughed with the kids last night.	Spend work breaks with Jim — he is a playful person!
Non-helpful thoughts:	**Non-helpful actions:**
This looks ridiculous. I hope no one sees me.	Spend work breaks making additional work-related phone calls.

MY REWARD (if I meet my goal)   Short-term — Dinner with Yvonne at the Chart House   Long-term — Trip to Boston to see college roommate

THE COST: (if I fail to meet my goal) Wash and wax both cars.

REEVALUATION DATE: 7-15 for 6 wk. evaluation. Jan-9 for 6 mo. evaluation

I agree to help with this project:

_____Yvone_____
(Support person)

I agree to strive toward this goal:

_____David_____   _6/1_
(Your signature)   (date)

Figure 11–3. Self-contract. *(Adapted with permission from Baldi, S., and others (1980). For your health: A model for self-care. South Laguna, CA: Nurses Model Health, p. 47.)*

He hoped that eventually he would be able to spend one hour every day in fun activities. He hoped that his ability to be *playful* in his work life as well as his home life would gradually develop.

Reaching Objectives: Nursing and Client Actions.

The specific plans made by David and his nurse are identified in the environmental planning section of his contract and in the nursing care plan (see Table 11–6). David talked by phone with the nurse several times during the first six weeks of his program. His major support person was his wife. The nurse met with David and Yvonne together at least once a week.

David read the material about play that the nurse had given him, but he still found it difficult to translate intellectual understanding into actually changing habits. He would frequently put off his planned time for himself until very late in the evening and then would be too tired for play.

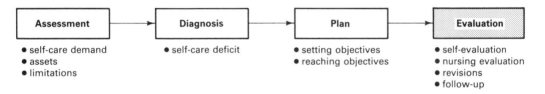

David, his family, and the nurse met formally six weeks after the program began. David's evaluation worksheet (see Fig. 11–4) was used to review his progress. David felt that he had met the goal of his self-contract and was now actually spending 15 minutes three times per week in fun activities.

He reported that his peers at work had been very helpful with his program. Although some friends were somewhat sarcastic and suspicious, most were interested and supportive. Some made suggestions for specific fun activities.

David's family was also supportive of his efforts. One significant family problem, however, had occurred because David was now making more time for personal fun and was at work less often. His wife thought this was wonderful *but* she also believed that it would be better if he spent at least some of that newly found time with the children. She was particularly adamant about this since, as she said: "He was away so much the last few years—they need him."

The nurse was prepared for this complicated issue and helped David and Yvonne to review their life-style. They began to reassess their individual and family priorities. The nurse conveyed a nonjudgmental, open, and hopeful attitude. This tone was adopted by the couple, and they agreed to work on this new issue.

David and Yvonne reported that they were interested in learning more about relaxation and thought that this might be a self-care area they would want to explore in a month or two. The nurse demonstrated some simple relaxation breathing exercises. David began practicing abdominal deep breathing for five

TABLE 11–6. NURSING CARE PLAN

Reason for consultation: "Severe neck pain"   *Client:* David

Assessment	Plan	Evaluation	
		Met	Not met
Self-care demand	*Setting objectives*		
Need for improved play behavior	Six weeks: "Spend 15 minutes three times a week doing an activity that is playful and just for me."	X	
Need for increased joy, spontaneity, and creativity			
Assets	Six months: Spend 30 minutes four times a week at play.	X (not yet time to evaluate	
Intellectual ability to understand the value of play	*Reaching objectives*		
Physical symptoms increase motivation	Client actions		
	Complete a time usage sheet now and at the end of each week.	X	
Financial resources for a wide variety of play activity	Make a list of three work-related activities that could be eliminated.		X (partial list made)
Wife and family are supportive			
Limitations	List five activities that will be playful for me.	X (partial–able to list three activities)	
Chronic history of work-oriented personality	Ask Yvonne and kids to help me play and keep records.		
Lack of playful role models at work	Spend 1 minute three times a week laughing in mirror.		
Developmental crisis at age 40			
Family history of limited value placed on play			

Diagnosis	Nursing actions	
Self-care deficit		
Inability to play spontaneously without education and intervention	Explain and demonstrate record keeping re: time spent in play, daily laughter.	×
	Help client to list five rewards for the self-contract.	× (only listed two)
	Demonstrate laughter exercise.	
	Have client give a return demonstration.	×
	Teach client basic health value associated with laughter, joy, spontaneity.	×
	Ask client's permission to have wife and children at some of the teaching sessions.	×
		Needed revisions
		Major difficulty is in tendency to make play work—to "work at playing"; needs to add techniques to alter this.

Re-evaluation date	Client follow-up
Phone contact during week as needed.	Neck pain has decreased, was able to play 15 minutes three times a week.
Formal meeting on 7/15 for six-week evaluation.	Went to dinner with Yvonne for reward.
Formal meeting on 1/1 for six-month evaluation.	Will contact nurse if needed.

CLIENT EVALUATION WORKSHEET
Reviewed at sixth week follow-up session.

Week No.	Monday	Tuesday	Wednesday	Thursday	Friday	Saturday	Sunday	Thoughts and feelings during this week.
1	Bought my son a balloon. Played 15 min	Practiced laughing		Rode bikes with the kids, laughed some			1 hr. trying to get a kite up in air	Laughing in the mirror is ridiculous
2			Fed birds in park with Jim at noon		Off for 30 min. at noon. Played a record.			
3	In New York on business all week. No time for play — very busy!					Prepared report on trip — due next Monday		I'm exhausted. I just have to get this work done.
4		With Yvonne to amateur comedy night			At work until midnight		Boating with family. Did no work	
5	Practiced laughing		Played cards on plane to Seattle			Movie with Yvonne — Spur of the moment		Yvonne really likes my efforts
6	Practiced laughing			Practiced laughing			Beach alone 1 hr. Took a good book	Guess I am doing better

Figure 11–4. Client evaluation worksheet.

minutes each day and felt this had helped decrease some of the tension he felt at work.

Finally, David stated that the muscle tension in his neck was significantly decreased. It still occurred during particularly stressful times and following long air flights, but he felt that at least 80 percent of the severe pain was gone. He said that it was still hard for him to be "free" and "spontaneous," but when he was he really enjoyed himself. He volunteered that this was the first time he had acknowledged how tense and tight he was. It was hard for him to allow himself the reward, but he did go out to dinner with Yvonne as they had planned in the contract.

David and Yvonne agreed to continue the program for the next month and said that they would then call the nurse and discuss their progress.

SUMMARY

In this chapter, the role of play and laughter in health enhancement and illness prevention has been explored. The history and value of play in human development were presented. Play was differentiated from relaxation and exercise. Utilization of laughter and humor in clinical work was described and techniques to help clients become more playful and spontaneous were provided. The ability of the nurse to *be playful* and to facilitate play in personal and professional interactions was emphasized. The nursing process was then utilized to apply this self-care material to helping clients change behavior. Self-contracting was presented as one mechanism to facilitate change.

STUDY QUESTIONS

Personal Focus

1. Do you play? How often? In what ways? What characteristics does your play most often exhibit?
2. How do you rate yourself as a model of play and playfulness for your family and for your clients?
3. List your most effective models for this area at work, at school, and at home.
4. What helps you to be more playful?
5. Describe how you feel after good play.
6. Demonstrate a deep laughter response.
7. What are your current goals in the self-care area of play? Complete a self-contract in this area.

Client Focus

1. With a group of peers discuss typical client inhibitions in the area of play. Share intervention strategies with each other.
2. Discuss specific educational approaches for teaching about play.
3. Describe how you would differentiate play from relaxation for a client.
4. Practice describing the potential health value of play and laughter to a client. Role-play this with a peer.
5. Describe a play activity appropriate for a hospitalized client.
6. Practice telling a joke to one client.
7. Practice completion of a self-contract for play with one client.

REFERENCES

1. Lehman, C. (1976). *The psychology of play activities*. New York: Arno Press, p. 24.
2. Lieberman, N. (1977). *Playfulness: Its relationship to imagination and creativity*. New York: Academic Press, p. 23.
3. *Webster's new world dictionary of the American language*. (1951). Cleveland, OH: World Publishing Company, p. 708.

4. Harmor, B., & Henderson, V. (1922). *Textbook of the principles and practice of nursing.* New York: Macmillan.

5. Miller, S. (1968). *The psychology of play.* New York: Penguin Books, p. 21.

6. Selye, H. (1976). *The stress of life* (rev. ed.). New York: McGraw-Hill, p. 420.

7. Friedman, M., & Rosenman, R.H. (1974). *Type A behavior and your heart.* New York: Alfred A. Knopf.

8. Murphy, L.B. (1972). Infants' play and cognitive development. In M. Piers (Ed.), *Play and development.* New York: W.W. Norton, p. 120.

9. Judd, H. (1911). *Genetic psychology for teachers.* New York: Appleton, p. 72.

10. Kilpatrick, W.H. (1925). *Source book in the philosophy of education.* New York: Macmillan, p. 5.

11. Hager, P. (1981, June 1). Play becoming a big part of many jobs. *Los Angeles Daily Times,* Sec. IV, p. 3.

12. Krier, B.A. (1982, September 21). The challenge of corporate fitness. *Los Angeles Daily Times,* Sec. V, p. 1.

13. Breuer, J., & Freud, S. (1953). Studies on Hysteria. In *Standard edition of the complete psychological works of Sigmund Freud* (Vol. 2, 1893–1895). London: Hogarth Press.

14. Dewey, J. (1921). *Democracy and education.* New York: Macmillan, p. 241.

15. Harlow, H., & Mears, C. (1979). The power and passion of play. In *The human model: Primate perspectives.* New York: John Wiley & Sons, pp. 141-160.

16. Swinford, P., & Webster, J. (1989). *Promoting wellness: A nurse's handbook.* Rockville, MD: Aspen.

17. Jourard, S.M. (1974). *The healthy personality.* New York: Macmillan.

18. Whitman, R.M. (1969). Psychoanalytic speculation about play: Tennis—the duel. *The Psychoanalytic Review,* 56 (2), 197-214.

19. Curry, N.E. (1971). Consideration of current basic issues on play. In G. Engstrom (Ed.), *Play: The child strives toward self-realization.* Washington, DC: National Association of Child Education, pp. 51-61.

20. Gardner, D.B. (1971). The child as an open system: Conference summary and implications. In G. Engstrom (Ed.), *Play: The child strives toward self-realization.* Washington, DC: National Association of Child Education, pp. 62-68.

21. Lieberman. *Playfulness: Its relationship to imagination.*

22. (1956, July). Experience life *McCall's Magazine,* p. 42.

23. Jourard. *Healthy Personality,* p. 298.

24. Winnicott, D. W. (1971). *Playing and reality.* London: Tavistock.

25. Schwartz, M. (Chair). (1989, February 26). Panel discussion: Winnicott and creativity—Perspective from humanities. Psychotherapy and Creativity Conference, UCLA.

26. Winnicott. *Playing and reality,* p. 54.

27. Cousins, N. (1976). Anatomy of an illness from the point of view of the patient. *New England Journal of Medicine,* 295 (26) 1458-1463.

28. Simonton, C.O., & Matthews-Simonton, S. (1975). Belief systems and management of the emotional aspects of malignancy. *Journal of Transpersonal Psychology,* 7 (29), 29-47.

29. Osterlund, H. (1983). Humor: A serious approach to patient care. *Nursing 83, 13,* 46-47.

30. (1988, November). The healing power of laughter and play—Uses of humor in the healing arts," Conference, Institute for the Advancement of Human Behavior, Long Beach, CA.

31. Elias, M. (1983, December 16). "When we chuckle we show more than our smiles. *USA Today*, 4.0.

32. Robinson, V.M. (1983). Humor and health. In P. McGhee & J.H. Goldstein (Eds.), *Handbook of humor research*. New York: Springer Verlag.

33. Ruston, P. (1988). Humor intervention deserves our attention. *Holistic Nursing Practice*, *2*, 54-62.

34. Blue, B. (1981). "Humorous play in the treatment of grieving patients. Unpublished dissertation. California Graduate Institute, Los Angeles.

35. Leiber, D. B. (1986). Laughter and humor in critical care. *Dimensions of Critical Care Nursing*, *5* (3), 163-170.

36. Kubie, S. (1971). On the destructive potential of humor in psychotherapy. *American Journal of Psychiatry*, *127*, 861-866.

37. Frey, W.F., & Salameh, W. (1987) *Handbook of humor and psychotherapy*. Sarasota, FL: Professional Resources Exchange.

38. Mindess, H. (1971) *Laughter and liberation*. Los Angeles: Nash.

39. Bushnell, D.B., & Scheff, T.J. (1979, August). The effect of laughter on mood, heart rate and skin temperature. Second International Conference on Humor, Los Angeles.

40. Robinson, V. (1977). *Humor and the health professional*. Thorofare, NJ: Charles B. Slack.

41. Swinford & Webster. *Promoting wellness*, p. 202.

PART III: Self-Care Primarily Related to the Body

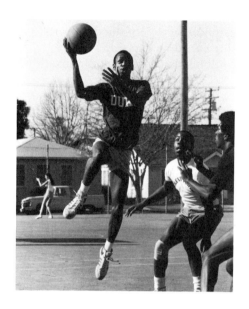

*Every man is a builder of a temple, called his
body . . . we are all sculptors and painters, and
our material is our flesh and blood and bone.*

Thoreau

*Those who think they have not time for bodily
exercise will find sooner or later have to find
time for illness.*

*Edward Stanley,
Earl of Derby, 1893*

12 Movement and Exercise

LEARNING OBJECTIVES

Upon completion of this chapter, readers will be able to:

1. Define movement and exercise.
2. List six benefits of exercise and movement.
3. List and describe the four components of fitness.
4. Differentiate between aerobic and anaerobic exercise.
5. List five major considerations associated with starting an exercise program.
6. Complete a plan for behavior change in exercise or movement.
7. Write an exercise prescription.

DEFINITIONS

Movement   Changes in the spatial configuration of the body and its parts, such as in breathing, eating, speaking, gesturing, and exercising.[1]

Exercise   Active exertion of muscles, involving contraction and relaxation of sets of muscle groups.

Isotonic exercise   Muscle contraction, involving a constant amount of muscle tension, such as in gradually lifting a weight; a term generally used for physical exercise involving body movement.

Isometric exercise   Muscle contraction without major body movement, including tensing and relaxing opposing groups of muscles, or pulling or pushing against stationary objects. Pulling upward on a chair in which one is sitting or pressing one's palms together are examples of isometric exercises.

Aerobic exercise   Sustained muscle activity challenging, but not exceeding, the cardiovascular system's ability to meet the muscles' needs for oxygen.

Anaerobic exercise   Occurs when the body's ability to supply oxygen falls short of the demand from contracting muscles.[2] Usually, this occurs during brief, intense periods of muscle use. If intense muscle action continues beyond a short period of time, the accumulation of unmetabolized lactic acid in the muscles causes pain.

Stretching   Extending body parts to expand the range of motion of muscles and involved joints.

Resting Heart Rate   The rate of the heart when physical activity has been limited to rest. A resting heart rate can be obtained after sleep or an extended rest period.*

Maximal Heart Rate   The rate of the heart at its highest capacity during intense activity. Maximal heart rates are determined during cardiac stress testing. They may also be predicted by the use of standardized maximum heart rate tables.*

Target Heart Rate   A safe range of the pulse or heart rate per minute during exercise. This is a range that will lead, over time, to improved efficiency of the heart, lungs, and muscles.

Fitness   A body state where the heart, lungs, and muscles work together and function optimally, enhancing the physical capacity for play and work. The four components of fitness are:

1. *Cardiovascular conditioning or aerobic conditioning:* Increased efficiency which results from sustained exercise that increases blood flow and decreases heart rate.

   (The American College of Sports Medicine guidelines suggest three to five exercise sessions per week for 15 to 60 minutes at an intensity of 60 to 90 percent of maximum heart rate reserve in order to bring about changes in cardiorespiratory efficiency. Exercising once a week will not improve fitness and may be a greater risk than benefit.[4])

---

*Taking the pulse radially is recommended for client safety.

2. *Endurance:* The capacity to sustain movement or exercise over a period of time.
3. *Flexibility:* The ability to move body parts easily through the full range of motion of the joints.
4. *Strength:* The power of sets of muscles to move, lift, or overcome resistance.[3]

INTRODUCTION

Movement is an integral part of human life and is necessary for survival. Activity and inactivity powerfully influence health. Self-care in this area can make an immediate and easily perceived health improvement.

Most human beings manage quite well to move the necessary muscles to complete daily work tasks such as dressing, eating, and performing routine activities. Many people in contemporary society, however, have relatively sedentary life-styles.

Our ancestors were nomadic hunters and gatherers. They journeyed long distances and frequently used the large muscle groups of their lower limbs for survival.[5] When in danger, they ran or fought. Muscle strength was required to accomplish most tasks. Hunting, agriculture, and other necessary activities depended on vigorous, coordinated upper and lower body movement.

In modern industrialized society the daily activity of most people has been reduced to a minimum. Even though muscles and body structures retain the capacity for strenuous physical activity, low activity levels frequently create imbalances among body systems.

Any frequent muscle movement pattern will cause some temporary or permanent change to occur.[3] Many of these changes are minute and gradual. They may go unnoticed or may not be attributed to the activity that causes them. The same observations may be made with muscle groups that are underused. Nurses recognize atrophy in muscle groups that remain inactive for extended periods of time, such as in clients with neurological deficits.

Conversely, if movement or exercise patterns are maintained over long periods of time, the whole body will reflect these activities. For example, the biceps muscle of the person who does heavy labor will strengthen, enlarge, and have increased endurance. The laborer's total fitness level may be maintained or increased if the exercise has aerobic qualities.[6] Overuse, however, may stress muscle groups, the surrounding tissues, and involved joints. Inflammation and trauma may result and present as "symptoms." *Chronic* changes may also result. These include tissue thickening and hardening and joint degeneration.

Stress can also affect the musculoskeletal system. It triggers muscle tension that accumulates in unique configurations in the body.[7] Stress can be reflected in body posture, muscle tone, gait, flexibility, and so on. Aches and pains in specific body areas are often indicators of stress.

Evidence from the large epidemiological studies, such as the Framingham study, demonstrate a link between biological characteristics and life-style patterns in disease pathogenesis.[8–10] Improper diet and lack of exercise have recently been implicated in the worsening of many degenerative and chronic diseases, such as hypertension, ischemic heart disease, diabetes, and others.[11] There is increasing evidence that appropriate diet and exercise programs can reverse the course of these diseases.[12]

Currently, there are cultural trends toward integrating exercise in daily life. Jogging and swimming have become very popular. Some corporations provide employee fitness centers in the work setting.[13] Communities are building special conditioning courses in parks and often include "mall walks" in the construction of new malls. Senior citizens, as well as children, are finding many opportunities to learn and practice planned movement as a self-care technique.

In summary, the connections among exercise, health, and illness are the subject of continuing exploration and research. While we cannot control risk factors such as sex and heredity, exercise and movement promote health and often provide alternatives and adjuncts to traditional health treatments.[14,15]

TYPES OF EXERCISE AND MOVEMENT

There are many types of exercise or movement that have an impact on health. These include aerobic exercise, anaerobic exercise, stretching activities, strength and endurance exercises, and general movement. Each of these have *specific* health benefits.

Aerobic Exercise

Sustained (often rhythmical) muscle movements that increase blood flow, heart rate, and metabolic demand for oxygen over a period of time are aerobic exercises. Activities that *may* be aerobic are swimming, jogging, cross-country skiing, aerobic dance, bicycling, jumping rope, power walking, and racquetball.

Aerobic activities promote cardiovascular conditioning. Exercise programs which are designed to be aerobic maintain the heart at its target heart rate (or 60 to 90 percent of its maximum rate) for at least 15 minutes, three to five times per week. A formula for calculation of target heart rates is presented in Figure 12–1. Table 12–1 presents data regarding identification of *approximate* target heart rates reflecting 70 percent of maximal heart rates. An individual's *exact* maximal heart rate is determined by a stress test on a treadmill.

Anaerobic Exercise

Anaerobic exercise occurs when the body's ability to supply oxygen falls short of the demand from contracting muscles. Oxygen debt then results, and exercise can occur in short bursts only. Examples of anaerobic activities are sprint-

STEP I
    Take 220 and subtract your age

    220 − _____ = _____
            your age   A

STEP II
    Now subtract your resting pulse rate from the number in A.

    _____ − _____ = _____
            A   your resting pulse   B

STEP III
    Multiply B times 65%

    _____ X 65% = _____
            B   C

ALSO

    Multiply B times 75%

    _____ X 75% = _____
            B   D

STEP IV
    Now add your resting pulse rate to the numbers in C and D, separately

    _____ + _____ = _____
            C   your resting pulse   low target heart rate range

    _____ + _____ = _____
            D   your resting pulse   high target heart range

These two figures are the lower and the upper range of your target heart rate.

Write them in here:
My target heart range while exercising is _____ to _____ beats per minute.

You should aim for this range to get the benefits of aerobic conditioning.

Figure 12–1. Target heart rate calculation. *(Reprinted with permission from Baldi, S., and others (1980).* For your health: A model for self-care. *South Laguna, CA: Nurses Model Health, p. 94.)*

ing and weightlifting. Although these types of exercise may have other self-care benefits, they do not provide the cardiovascular conditioning that comes from regular aerobic exercise.

Stretching Activities
Movements that allow muscles and joints to be stretched gently through their full range of motion increase flexibility. Specific warm-up and cool-down exercises, hatha yoga, t'ai chi, and some forms of dance are examples. Benefits include increased range of joint movement, improved circulation and posture, and relaxation. If breathing patterns are integrated with slow, gentle movement, the relaxation response may occur.

Strength and Endurance Exercises
A variety of muscle-building programs fall into this category. Weight training,

TABLE 12–1 TARGET HEART RATE CHART

Take the necessary safety precautions to check out your own health status before exercising. Since you may have special health conditions this chart cannot be used as a definite target for *your* pulse.

Find your resting pulse rate at the top line, then follow down to your approximate age range and locate the number representing a Target Heart Rate.

Target Heart Rate (70% of estimated maximum rate)

Resting Pulse

Age	50	55	60	65	70	75	80	85	90	95	100
20	155	156	158	159	161	162	164	165	167	168	170
25	151	153	154	156	157	159	160	162	163	165	166
30	148	149	151	152	154	155	157	158	160	161	163
35	144	146	147	149	150	152	153	155	156	158	159
40	141	142	144	145	147	148	150	151	153	154	156
45	137	139	140	142	143	145	146	148	149	151	152
50	134	135	137	138	140	141	143	144	146	147	149
55	130	132	133	135	136	138	139	141	142	144	145
60	127	128	130	131	133	134	136	137	139	140	142
65	123	125	126	128	129	131	132	134	135	137	138
70	120	121	123	124	126	127	129	130	132	133	135
75	116	118	119	121	122	124	126	127	128	130	131
80	113	114	116	117	119	120	122	123	125	126	128

(Reprinted with permission from Baldi, S., and others (1980). *For your health: A model for self-care.* South Laguna, CA: Nurses Model Health, p. 101.)

calisthenics, and specific isometric exercises can build both strength and endurance, increasing the power of the muscular-skeletal system and generally improving the whole body. They may or may not have aerobic benefit.

Movement and Daily Life Activities

General movement as part of a physically active life-style does not fall into one of the specifically defined categories above. Housecleaning, running after playful toddlers, climbing stairs instead of riding elevators, and walking outside during concert intermissions, however, all have an impact on health. Increased fitness does not require a gym.

EFFECTS OF EXERCISE

There are many potential health benefits of exercise and movement. No one type of movement meets all the criteria for conditioning, however, and no one exercise provides all of the potential benefits. The actual benefits of any movement program differ from person to person. Certain types of movement and levels of activity are more likely to produce specific results. The benefits of movement may be transient or long-lasting. It is important to recognize that these benefits cannot be stored; they do not last over long periods of time if regular exercise is not continued. It is not possible to exercise only on a weekend or a two-week vacation period and experience long-term health benefits. Some of the potential benefits of *regular* exercise follow.

Physiological Benefits

Regular exercise can increase:[3,8–10,16–26]

- Peripheral blood flow
- Muscle efficiency and flexibility
- Cardiac efficiency
- Efficiency of nerve impulse transmission
- Efficiency of body temperature regulation
- Circulating fibrinolysin (substance that breaks up small clots)
- Excretion of catecholamines (which facilitate relaxation)
- Metabolic rate
- Endurance

It can also improve:

- Pulmonary functioning
- Coordination
- Lipid, lipoprotein profile
- Insulin-mediated glucose uptake
- Effects and control of diseases such as arthritis, obstructive lung disease, hypertension, cardiovascular disease, osteoporosis, and non-insulin dependent diabetes
- Length and quality of life

Psychological Benefits

Regular exercise can improve:[27–33]

- General sense of well-being
- Self-image
- Appetite control
- Sleep
- Vitality (as fatigue is decreased)
- Depression

INITIATING AND MAINTAINING AN EXERCISE PROGRAM

Initiating and maintaining an exercise program is best done after the client understands the overall value and specific benefits of different types of movement. The client has the responsibility for the initiation and outcome of the program. The nurse's role is that of a resource person who provides guidance and structure. A list of concepts that serve as guidelines in this process follows.

- Choice of activity
- Setting objectives
  Duration and intensity
  Time
  Setting
  Equipment
  Money
- Baseline
- Risk and safety factors, including pre-exercise considerations
- Support systems
- Nutrition
- Negative factors
- Evaluation

Choice of Activity

Activity selection is guided by client motivation, needs, and personal interest. Various exercises develop different aspects of fitness. For example, jogging produces cardiovascular conditioning but does little for increasing flexibility. Hatha yoga enhances flexibility, and in some cases strength and endurance, but does not address cardiovascular conditioning. Depending on the client's health status, personal preferences, and desired result, a combination of movements may be the best choice. Table 12–2 outlines various common movement activities together with some characteristics for each.

Setting Exercise Objectives

Setting a beginning movement or exercise goal will be based largely on the type of activity selected and the client's previous movement level. The nurse may help delineate *one* component of fitness on which to focus the initial plan. A longer-range goal may be gradually to to add combinations of movements that build total fitness.

Exercise or fitness prescriptions are written by nurses and include: activity type, duration, intensity, frequency, and progression of exercise. The prescriptions should be individualized according to client capability, motivation, goals, interests, time, equipment, and facilities.[34,35]

Duration and Intensity. Once an activity has been chosen, the next step is determining the duration of activity and its intensity. Whatever the selected movement, the actual goal needs to describe and limit it. For example, a client might choose one of the following beginning exercise goals:

Walk ½ mile daily in 10 minutes in the first week.
Do stretching exercises for five minutes every other day.
Learn three warm-up exercises within two weeks.
Sign up for a hatha yoga weekend workshop by August 1.

Some people may be able to move to long-term objectives easily and may choose a goal similar to the two listed below:

Bicycle for 10 minutes three times a week, increasing by five minutes each week until reaching 30 minutes.
Swim two laps in the pool four times a week for two weeks, then increase by one more lap each week.

Often clients are too ambitious, starting with much more exercise than they have been used to. The nurse acts as an advocate in these situations by helping to make the goal more realistic and attainable, making sure the target heart rates are maintained. It is much better to have small successes than large failures.

Time. An exercise program takes time. A beginning goal may involve an activity level that requires a brief time. As the client becomes more conditioned and stamina is increased, more time will be devoted to that activity. It is important that the client plan realistically in allowing time for exercise, including warming up and cooling down. Some people may try to squeeze more than is possible into 15 minutes.

Setting. Where the activity takes place is important. Is it close to the client's home or work? Will it involve a trip by car or bus? Are there climate restrictions? If accessibility to the setting is difficult, will the client drop out?

Equipment. What equipment is required? Making sure the client is knowledgeable in this area and has at least the minimal basic, good-quality, safe equipment is essential. For example, a person who plans to walk or jog should wear shoes designed for those activities.[36] Nonbinding clothes and protection from wind and cold (mittens, hats, windbreakers) must also be considered.

Money. Another factor associated with many types of exercise is money. Is there expense involved in getting the necessary equipment? Are there facility expenses that would continue on a regular basis? Is the expense realistic considering the socioeconomic status and priorities of the client? The nurse needs to help the client consider these issues and may also serve as a resource person concerning community facilities, classes, and so on.

Baseline

The current fitness and activity level of the client needs to be considered. If the client has been inactive for a period of time, limited goals and short periods of

TABLE 12–2 EXERCISE ACTIVITIES AT A GLANCE[a]

Exercise	Time Required for Activity[b]	Place	Equipment Needed	Cost	Aerobic Versus Nonaerobic[c]	Advantages	Disadvantages	Precautions and Risks
Walking	Activity range 5–120 minutes	Anywhere; climate may be a factor; can walk through all rooms at home; safety of neighborhood a factor.	Good walking shoes, socks; reflector for shirt if walking at night.	Cost of shoes, wide range: $25–$75.	Nonaerobic as a general rule; some "stress walking" becomes aerobic.	Can be done anywhere and easily integrated into daily life-style. Can do alone or with others.	Generally nonaerobic.	Walking alone in certain areas; dangers at night; need good shoes to prevent strain; walk on smooth surface to prevent injury.
Jogging/ running	Activity range 5–60 minutes	Indoor track; outside—climate and steep hills sometimes a limiting factor.	Good running shoes, socks, shorts, support bra for women, athletic support for men.	None once basic shoes are purchased; wide range for shoes: $25–$75.	Generally aerobic.	Major cardiovascular benefits; excellent for weight control; builds endurance and promotes sleep.	Stretching and flexibility not automatically integrated; limited by area, climate; access to shower. May be lonely for some. Wear and tear on weight-bearing joints.	Build endurance gradually; risks of running alone in certain areas; high risk at night; stress to knees; stay 30–50 feet from edge of road (air pollution); if running on street shoulder, run equal time on opposite sides to ensure balanced stress to joints.
Race-walking	Activity range 5–60 minutes	Can be done anywhere one can jog.	Running shoes, socks.	Only for shoes and socks.	Usually is aerobic.	Less traumatic to lower legs than jogging or running; firms and strengthens buttocks, thighs, upper body.	Need to learn technique. Climate/weather can interfere.	Use warm-up and cool-down stretches to prevent injuries.
Bicycling (including stationary)	Activity range 5–120 minutes	Any outdoor place; climate sometimes a factor; can use stationary bike at home.	Bicycle, shoes, helmet, gloves, toe clips.	Wide range: $75–$500.	Most often not aerobic; must be very rapid and often uphill, to reach aerobic level.	Can be done at home, any hour; excellent for weight control and sleep promotion.	Often is not aerobic; total stretching not incorporated; traffic dangers; air pollution.	Traffic dangers; need helmet, cuff guards, gloves; buy stationary bikes carefully; need at least 40-pound flywheel.
Aerobic dance or Jazzercise	Activity range Records and classes usually require 45–60 minutes two to three times a week	Studio, gym, YMCA, home, health club.	Shoes, socks, shorts, tights, support hose; tights and leotard for Jazzercise	Cost of shoes, class registration ($20–$30 a month); cost of aerobic record/ tape/book if doing at home.	Aerobic component; also includes nonaerobic stretching.	Includes gentle stretching; warm-up and cool-down in the routine; relationships with classmates.	Gets boring for some; may need access to class; may take more time than available; cost.	Need good shoes; learn to avoid falls; build endurance slowly; screen prospective classes to determine safety (i.e., work within target heart rate).

	Activity range	Location	Equipment	Cost	Aerobic	Considerations	Difficulties	Precautions
Rebounding	Activity range 5–30 minutes	Anywhere on flat surface. (If indoors) ceiling must be at least 8 feet.	Mini-trampolines —at least 34 inches diameter.	$50–$200.	May be aerobic if fast pace achieved.	Fun! Can be done indoors or out. Quiet. May be done to music. Some health clubs have equipment. Strengthens leg muscles.	Difficult to achieve target heart rate if in good condition.	May be excessive pronation of ankles; strains, sprains to ankles, knees. Some people have difficulty maintaining balance, can fall off.
Jumping rope	Activity range 5–30 minutes	Indoors or outdoors; requires limited space; can use any room.	Rope, good shoes, socks.	$5–$10 for cost of rope; cost of good shoes.	Generally aerobic.	Can be done anywhere and at any time; can be alone or with others.	Stress to knees; stretching not incorporated; flexibility limited.	Can cause stress to knees, ankles, hips; need good support shoes.
Swimming	Activity range 10–30 minutes	Indoor or outdoor pool, ocean, lake, rivers; climate at times a factor.	Suit, body of water; cap to protect hair.	None if own pool or access to community pool; can be expensive to join club with pool.	Generally not aerobic unless covering long distance in very short period of time.	Excellent for stretching and flexibility; good during pregnancy and for elderly; minimal stress to joints.	Should not be done alone; hair damage; may be limited by climate; access to pool can be expensive.	Dangers of swimming alone; knowledge of CPR; check water sources for safety; free from pollutants.
Tennis	Activity range 60–90 minutes	Indoor or outdoor court; climate at times a factor.	Racquet, balls, clothes, shoes, socks.	Cost to rent court or join club if free resources not available. $5/hour to $200/month for private clubs; cost of shoes, racquet, and balls.	Most often is non-aerobic (unless two excellent players so that running is maintained). Doubles games not aerobic.	Builds relationships. Outdoors for some people; reaching integrates more stretching.	Some find it difficult to find partner; cost; can be limited by weather; often not aerobic.	Strains; falls; need eye protection; warm-up and cool-down; ankle, knee injuries.
Racquetball	Activity range 60–90 minutes	Indoor or outdoor court.	Racquet, balls, eye guards, clothes, shoes, socks.	Same as for tennis.	Most often non-aerobic (unless two excellent players).	Builds relationships; integrates some stretching.	Cost to rent court; need a partner.	Strains; falls; need eye protection; warm-up and cool-down; ankle, knee injuries.

aCriteria for aerobic exercise, pre-exercise considerations, and precautions apply to each exercise.

bFor aerobic benefit: Exercise three to five times a week for 15–60 minutes at an intensity of 60 to 90% of maximum heart rate reserve.

cSee criteria for aerobic exercise

activity will be appropriate. Clients may not feel thay are doing anything *signifi-cant* if they start slowly; the nurse can be helpful in combating this "perfection-ism." Use of diaries and pedometers can help people identify actual levels of current exercise, heart rates, and movement.

Starting up Gradually.   A good exercise program will start with gentleness, using common sense to build up to a higher level of activity based on previous successes, life-style patterns, and health status. Exercise movements should *not* be painful or forced.

Active motion should start and end with warm-up and cool-down move-ments to prepare muscles and joints for the activity to follow. Typically, there should be five to ten minutes of stretching and gentle movement before and after vigorous exercise.

Working within the target heart range is one way to identify a safe pace for the exercise program. Another way that is both simple and quick is the "talk test." If it is possible to *converse normally* during exercise without running out of breath, the pace of the program is probably safe and realistic.[37]

Risk and Safety Factors

Perhaps more than in any other self-care area, safety precautions need to be built into an exercise program. Individual factors such as physical condition, chronic illness, blood pressure, family history, and medications must be taken into account. If *any* risk factors are present, further evaluation by and consulta-tion with a health advisor is warranted.

For those clients with more serious health problems, the American College of Sports Medicine has issued guidelines. The College has listed the following as *absolute contraindications to exercise:* congestive heart failure, acute myo-cardial infarction, active myocarditis, rapidly increasing angina with effort, recent embolism, systemic or pulmonary dissecting aneurysm, acute infections, thrombophlebitis, ventricular tachycardia or other dangerous dysrhythmias, and severe aortic stenosis.[38]

Awareness of possible hazards may prevent injury and physical strain. For example, clients must learn to avoid extreme heat or cold, icy streets, and heavy smog. Good equipment can also prevent injuries. Common sense rules, such as not proceeding with movement when there is pain, must be emphasized. Table 12–3 presents a sample risk assessment tool. Table 12–4 focuses on exercise caution signs and symptoms.

Support Systems

For many people, finding an exercise partner can make a crucial difference to success or failure. Clients without meaningful support systems may need infor-mation and encouragement in attaining this important help. Movement and

TABLE 12-3. RISK FACTOR ASSESSMENT

1. Have you ever had pain or pressure in your chest that occurred with exertion and lasted a few minutes, then subsided with resting?

2. Do you get chest discomfort from climbing stairs, walking against a cold wind, or during any physical (including sexual) or emotional activity?

3. Does your heart ever beat unevenly or irregularly or seem to flutter or skip beats?

4. Do you get sudden bursts of very rapid heart beating or periods of very slow heart action without apparent cause?

5. Do you take any prescription medicine on a regular basis?

6. Has your electrocardiogram at rest or during exercise ever been abnormal?

7. Do you have any respiratory problem, such as emphysema or asthma?

8. Do you have arthritis, rheumatism, gout, or any condition affecting your joints?

9. Do you have any orthopedic problems affecting your feet, ankles, knees, or hips?

10. Do you have a bad back or a sacroiliac or disc problem?

11. Do you smoke?

12. Are you more than 20 pounds overweight?

13. Do you have high blood pressure?

14. Are you over 35 and leading a sedentary life?
(*Note:* Stress testing is mandatory for sedentary people over 35 and for any person with a past or current cardiovascular condition.)

If you have answered "yes" to any of the responses above, it is recommended that you seek consultation from your medical advisor before starting an exercise program. Choose your health consultant or medical advisor wisely. Make wise health choices for yourself.

(Adapted with permission from Zohman, L.R. (1978). *Run for Life.* Pamphlet of Connecticut Mutual Life Insurance Company, p. 8.)

exercise classes provide one way for clients to make new contacts who will support self-care behavior as a long-term life process.

Nutrition

Muscle movement is fueled by food energy, which is measured in calories. The more vigorous and sustained the exercise, the larger the caloric expenditure per hour. When calories burned are greater than calories consumed, weight loss will occur; when more calories are eaten than are used, there will be a weight gain. Exercise and diet can be used efficiently together to reduce body weight. (Approximately 3500 calories equals 1 pound of body fat.[39])

Exercise can leave a person weak and shaky. The quantity, quality, and timing of food intake are important. General principles of nutrition apply to a

TABLE 12–4. EXERCISE CAUTION SIGNS AND SYMPTONS

Stop exercise immediately and consult your health care provider if you have:
- Chest pain or pressure in the center of the chest
- Irregular heart action
- Dizziness, fainting, light-headedness, or blackout

Reduce your program or take more rest periods if you experience:
- Prolonged rapid heart action more than 15 minutes after stopping moderate exercise
- Prolonged breathlessness after moderate exercise
- Nausea or vomiting after exercise
- Insomnia
- Prolonged fatigue

Check your equipment or check with a health advisor if any of these occur:
- Reactivation of old arthritis, knee, or back problems
- Pulled muscles
- Muscle cramps or charley horse
- Shin splints or pain of any type

(Adapted with permission from Zohman, L.R. (1978). *Run for Life*. Pamphlet of Connecticut Mutual Life Insurance Company, p. 18.)

person involved in a movement program. Adequate vitamin intake is essential, as is sufficient protein intake, although there is not an *increased* need for protein during exercise. If stressful, high-pressure circumstances prevail, vitamin intake should be increased.

The body's need for fluids is especially important during exercise. Fluids should be consumed regularly throughout the day (1½ to 2½ quarts per day under ordinary circumstances; more during hot weather or after vigorous exercise). Regular fluid breaks should be scheduled during heavy exercise. Fluids consumed should have less than 2.5 grams of glucose or sucrose per 100 milliliters of water. Plain water is highly preferable to concentrated "sports drinks," which need to be diluted with equal parts of water. Electrolyte-replacement drinks are generally not recommended.[40] Food intake immediately prior to exercising should be limited. (Also see Chapter 14 on nutrition.)

Negative Factors

Many enterprises start grandly, only to fizzle out over time. Exercise and diet programs are notorious for this. Common examples of negative factors that can impair the success of movement programs include:

- Limited rewards or minimal praise from others
- Images of failure from past attempts at "getting in shape "
- Physical discomfort
- Initial overenthusiasm, leading to burnout in type A[41] individuals who compete even in noncompetitive activities
- Negative images based on prejudice or preconception, such as:

I'll sweat too much.
Women don't do that.
There's no shower at work.
It takes too long.
It's too hot or too cold.

The "Four F's" have been suggested as precautionary factors to help clients avoid dropping out of exercise programs:

1. *Flexibility:* Too tight a body leads to injury. Special emphasis on stretching and limbering movements may be necessary.
2. *Feasibility:* The exercise program must not make unrealistic demands.
3. *Faithfulness:* The client must exercise regularly to attain success.
4. *Fun:* Either the activity must be fun or a way must be found to make it so; otherwise, dropping out is likely.[42]

Evaluation

Planned early reevaluation times are part of an effective movement program. Clients can be taught to monitor their own health states at periodic intervals. As clients gain skill in monitoring changes in heart rate, blood pressure, and pulmonary function, they may make needed modifications in their programs independently.

Nutritional patterns should also be reassessed at regular intervals, and the relationship of movement to all health areas should be considered. For example, have smoking or drinking patterns changed? Is the client less depressed?

Recent life changes should be noted and discussed; pregnancy, a death in the family, or increased demands at work could mean that the client would have to alter his or her exercise plan.

EXERCISE IN SPECIAL SITUATIONS: SELF-CARE IMPLICATIONS

Many people have special considerations or needs in regard to exercise. Included here are sections on children, women, women during pregnancy, the elderly, and the physically disabled.

Exercise for Children

Many children perform strenuous exercise naturally—just ask their parents! Many cultures promote physical activity for children. Children sleep better and feel better if they are physically fit. In one study, during a successful fitness program for school-age children, visits to the school nurse declined by 60 percent a year.[43]

Children can easily get out of shape. Parents and caretakers need to be aware both of children's need for exercise and of the limited capacity of young children to regulate their exercise. When structured exercise is involved (e.g., hiking, running, or bicycling with a group), parents need to allow children to rest when they wish, to pay attention to physical complaints, and to provide proper equipment and adequate fluids.

For further asssessment of exercise in the school-age child, *Sports Medicine: Health Care for Young Athletes* and "Counseling and Health Screening for Children Entering Sports and Physical Exercise" are excellent references.[44,45]

Women and Exercise

Women can participate as fully as men in movement, exercise, and sports programs. The following physiological differences between men and women are listed for completeness, but their significance and ultimate limitation on women's physical achievements are unknown. In fact, in many sports, women's world records are approaching those of men.

- *Structural differences:* The ratio of strength to weight is lower in women, owing to a smaller proportion of muscle in relation to adipose tissue.
- *Metabolic differences:* Men have a higher metabolic rate than that of women.
- *Circulation differences:* Men have approximately 15 percent more hemoglobin and 6 percent more red blood cells, providing a higher oxygen-carrying ability in circulating blood.[46–48]

Questions are often asked about women exercising during menstruation. There is no reason why women should not exercise when menstruating. There is evidence that as physical fitness increases, menstrual discomfort lessens in severity. Hatha yoga can be especially helpful in this regard.

Some women who exercise heavily and who have a very low percentage of body fat, sometimes develop amenorrhea. Menstrual cycles return to normal with less vigorous activity and increased body weight. The cause is unclear, but speculations have included physical stress, the pressure of training or competition, and the relationship between body fat and estrogen production.

Some additional self-care factors for women who exercise include screening for iron-deficiency anemia, wearing a good support bra, and remembering ordinary safety precautions such as not running alone at night in unsafe areas.

Exercise during Pregnancy

Pregnancy is an especially important time for good self-care. Unless contraindicated, this will include exercise. "Aerobic exercise appears to have no harmful effects in the majority of pregnant women."[49] Specific contraindications may include preeclampsia and placenta previa. In advanced pregnancy, aerobic exercise may unduly alter heart rate and respiratory exchange requiring a decreased level of activity.[50]

Common sense dictates that physical fitness is a wonderful asset to pregnancy, enhancing an expectant mother's natural glow. Some women continue ongoing exercise programs during pregnancy, and some may choose to start a movement program during this period. There are many activities specifically designed for pregnant women, including classes in swimming and hatha yoga. Stretching and limbering movements may be especially helpful during advanced pregnancy.[51]

Simple guidelines apply in pregnancy:

- Begin by building on the pre-pregnant level of activity.
- Observe and listen to the body's messages. What is fine for one pregnant woman may not be comfortable or wise for another.
- Discuss problem situations with a health advisor familiar with childbearing and women's health.
- Be aware of bodily changes in regard to safety. Balance may be affected, leading to falls. Good shoes are even more important for running.

Exercise and the Elderly

Exercise can benefit the elderly by increasing a sense of independence, permitting greater activity, decreasing fatigue, and combating insomnia.[52] Favorable mood changes associated with exercise have been reported.[53] Movement programs at YMCA's or senior citizens' centers can provide social outlets as well.

The risks associated with exercise in the elderly must be evaluated carefully, especially if a client has been previously inactive. Hypertension, cardiac disease, obesity, osteoporosis, arthritis, degenerative joint disease, and smoking are obvious precautionary factors. Consultation with a health advisor is recommended before the elderly client starts a movement program. It is again worth noting that many chronic diseases affecting the elderly, such as diabetes, hypertension, and anxiety, may be *helped* by various types of exercises.[54,55] Swimming and hatha yoga are especially beneficial for the elderly because at beginning levels there is relatively little physical stress on the body.

Exercise and Physical Disability

Often there is a tendency to limit physical activity during illness (such as by prescribing bed rest), under the misconception that inactivity is harmless. Physical and mental complications of illness and injury can begin in the first few days of inactivity, interfering with the recovery process.[56] The list of acute and chronic problems resulting from immobility is lengthy. Disuse atrophy, osteoporosis, decubitus ulcers, decreased cardiopulmonary capacity, disorientation, and depression are common.

"No matter what limitation there may be, it is possible to enhance the quality of life by tending to the needs of the body, mind and spirit."[57] Movement can be a positive factor for physically disabled people, and ordinarily a variety of types of movement, stretching exercises, aerobics, and so on, are possible. In addition to being joyful in its own right, exercise can raise self-esteem, increase mobility and a sense of independence, and contribute to general health improvement.

There are many ways that exercise can de adapted to meet the needs of physically disabled people; new avenues have been developing rapidly in the past few years. Examples include wheelchair sports such as basketball, races for people in wheelchairs or on crutches, and Special Olympics for the handicapped and developmentally disabled.

By advocating movement programs, nurses can be extremely helpful to those with physical disabilities. To be most effective, however, the nurse must be sensitive to the client's psychological as well as physical difficulties. Shame may be very pronounced; tact, reassurance, and encouragement may be required. The disabled person should also be supported in stopping activity temporarily whenever pain or discomfort occur. There may be special needs for money or equipment (for example, wheelchairs or transportation) as well as simple needs for information concerning programs available in the community. The input of an expert health care advisor regarding contraindications is essential.

NURSES MODEL MOVEMENT AND EXERCISE SELF-CARE

Nurses model attitudes, skills, and approaches to exercise and movement on a daily basis even when they are not directly teaching clients about an exercise plan. Clients cannot help but notice the ways in which nurses:

- Manage their own bodies while moving clients and heavy equipment.
- Use stairs in preference to elevators.
- Use breaks for stretching rather than drinking coffee.
- Seem flexible and fit rather than slow moving and out of breath.
- Attend aerobic dance classes on agency premises before or after work.

Many nurses may be under the impression that they are meeting their movement needs regularly at work. They may be walking, reaching, twisting, and lifting, but it is easy to misjudge the extent to which these motions are sufficient to meet daily movement needs. Nurses need to analyze these daily work activities in relation to the four components of fitness: conditioning, endurance, flexibility, and strength. The routine work of a nurse is usually not varied or extensive enough to maintain or increase cardiovascular conditioning. Simple methods of recording motion, such as the use of a pedometer, can augment other self-assessment tools.

In clinical settings nurses convey that they value movement and exercise in almost all interactions with clients. Examples of this include:

- Positioning intravenous equipment so that clients can continue to move easily.
- Teaching family members to help clients move and exercise even though they may be confined to bed.
- Encouraging usual levels of exercise and movement if possible.
- Using exercise specialists when indicated.
- Helping clients plan for movement self-care upon discharge.

If nurses appear to be fit and flexible and to have good endurance, clients will be more likely to believe that movement and exercise self-care skills have benefits and should be practiced on a regular basis.

CLINICAL APPLICATION

Case Presentation

Jennifer is a 29-year-old unemployed former school teacher. A single parent, she lives with her four-year-old daughter in an urban apartment. She came to the Health Center for a tuberculosis skin test and health clearance as a prerequisite for a new job as a substitute teacher. A brief health history and health risk appraisal indicated that Jennifer's largest health hazards stemmed from being inactive and overweight. The screening physical and lab work all revealed negative findings.

As a child and young adult, Jennifer had been active in women's basketball and bicycling. After her marriage she began her teaching career and became less active. Her free time was devoted to her home and socializing with friends. Daily activity included much "desk sitting," and some walking at home and in the classroom. During that time Jennifer would bicycle or exercise on brief occasions months apart.

Since the birth of her daughter four years ago and the separation from her husband two years ago, Jennifer has become increasingly sedentary. She spends most days at home. Her routine activities provide a busy day but no physical activity that would directly contribute to increasing or maintaining her level of fitness. At the end of most days she is fatigued, with a vague sense of frustration. She reports sleeping poorly most nights and has occasional headaches. During the last three years she has gained 20 pounds; she is increasingly disturbed by her weight and personal appearance.

Assessment

• self-care demand
• assets
• limitations

Jennifer expressed an interest in finding some way to manage her weight and sleep better. She explored her daily patterns and alternatives with the nurse.

In the area of *nutrition*, Jennifer prepares and shares two snacks and three meals a day with her daughter. During her daughter's nap period she treats herself to time alone, snacking while she reads a book or does needlepoint or some other *recreational* or play activity.

To engage in an activity without her daughter, Jennifer would need to establish a support system for child care. It is difficult to arrange this because for the past two years her *social interactions* have been limited. She has few friends from whom she can ask assistance. She also has to be careful about money.

In addition to informal discussion, the nurse and Jennifer used self-assessment tools to review nutrition, sleep, and exercise habits. This helped Jennifer understand the connections among her life-style, limited activity, weight gain, fatigue, and other concerns. Her exercise assessment responses are presented in Figure 12–2. The assessment revealed that Jennifer had few occasions for fitness, stretching, or vigorous exercise.

The self-assessment questions reminded Jennifer that she had often enjoyed exercise in the past. It also reminded her of the barriers that made it difficult to exercise now, including lack of child care, apartment living, limited finances, few friends, and the fear of not being able to compete successfully as she had in the past.

Her *physical screening* had indicated that there were no organic causes for her insomnia, occasional headaches, and weight gain. She had a number of *self-care strengths* in many areas. Jennifer realized that she needed to alter her nutritional and sleep patterns, but her first and primary interest was in pursuing the self-care area of movement and exercise. She though that this would also help resolve her other complaints.

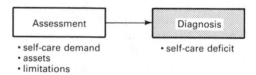

After self-assessment and discussion, Jennifer began to understand that her movement and exercise deficit could be described as:

Inability to engage in movement or exercise on a regular basis without education and intervention

In nursing diagnostic terms, this might be:

Level I activity intolerance related to a sedentary life-style

Her main limitation was knowledge, with lesser limitations in the areas of motivation and skill. Jennifer also had emotional barriers or blocks that were examined as a plan of action was developed.

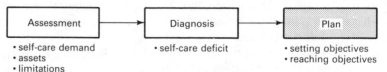

EXERCISE SELF-ASSESSMENT

Complete the following self-assessment to help you look at the role of exercise in your life. On the scale below circle the numbers which are most true for you and your life during the last year:

	Almost Never	Seldom	Often	Almost Always
1. I plan to exercise three times each week.	(1)	2	3	4
2. I end up exercising for at least 20-30 minutes at least three times per week.	(1)	2	3	4
3. I climb stairs rather than ride elevators.	(1)	2	3	4
4. My daily activities include moderate physical activity (rearing young children, working on my feet, etc.).	1	2	(3)	4
5. I know my "target heart rate" range, and I reach it during my exercise periods.	(1)	2	3	4
6. I do some form of stretching–limbering exercise for at least 15 minutes twice a week.	(1)	2	3	4
7. I have the necessary items and facilities to engage in my activity properly.	(1)	2	3	4
8. I look forward to my exercise program.	(1)	2	3	4
9. My family/friends encourage me in my exercise program.	(1)	2	3	4
10. I am willing to make the time to exercise 20-30 minutes a day, 3-5 days per week.	(1)	2	3	4

Some suggestions for how you might learn from this self-assessment:

1. Connect all the circles down the length of the page. Look at the pattern that your connected line makes. Turn your page sideways to get an even more clear visual picture of the role of exercise in your life right now. What does it seem to be saying to you?

2. Now add up your total score: _____ 12 _____

   Circle which range it was in:
   (10-19)   20-29   30-40

   If your score was in the 10-19 range you might want to make some changes in your exercise patterns. Which aspects do you think need the most work? How many "1's" did you mark on this assessment? 9 These might serve as a clue to help you think about making changes in this area of your life.

3. How would you like this self-assessment to look six months from now? Are you interested in working toward those improvements?

4. Remember to congratulate yourself for the ways in which you are providing good exercise patterns in your life. Give yourself a pat on the back; or go out and exercise as a way to congratulate yourself!

Figure 12–2. Exercise self-assessment. *(Adapted with permission from Baldi, S., and others (1980). For your health: A model for self-care. South Laguna, CA: Nurses Model Health, p. 87.)*

Setting Objectives

Jennifer wanted to work on her self-care deficit. The nurse helped her explore the question of whether it was a good time for Jennifer to begin to plan for a change. For a variety of reasons, including her desire to improve her appearance, Jennifer decided that it was time to start.

An agreement was reached about the nurse's role in assisting Jennifer with her plan. They agreed that Jennifer must take responsibility for the actual self-care action and that the nurse would be a resource and support person once the plan was developed.

The nurse introduced Jennifer to the idea of self-contracts. After explaining each section of the contracting tool, the next step was to help her set realistic long-term and short-term goals. Since Jennifer had been inactive for a period of time and was overweight, the nurse helped her understand the importance of beginning with short-term goals. She began by wearing a pedometer to measure how much walking she did during her household and child-rearing routine. She discovered that she was walking 1½ to 2 miles a day and was surprised that she was not walking more.

Jennifer initially selected basketball as her exercise activity because it was familiar from her past. She wanted to practice it for one hour five days a week. Since she had no child care available, the goal of five times a week would lead to failure before she even began the contract. Nor was she able to identify any group with which she could practice. The nurse supported her in exploring other realistic alternatives.

Some of the criteria for establishing a realistic plan included finding movement activities that would:

1. Allow her to participate near home or at home.
2. Be low in cost or expense-free.
3. Fit her home routine with minor alterations.

Jennifer suggested that maybe she should choose a compromise activity instead of fantasizing about playing women's basketball. The nurse reinforced Jennifer's openness, and together they identified three realistic possibilities: jumping rope, brisk walking, and a beginning aerobic dance class.

A dance class at a nearby city recreational center met for two afternoons a week and provided child-care. Jennifer decided to enroll. She also decided that to complete her plan she would take brisk walks on two alternate days. She would ask a neighbor to watch her daughter for those 20-minute periods.

This process allowed Jennifer to plan self-care activities that fit with home constraints. Her program was low in cost and close by. Her short-term goal was:

> By the end of six weeks, I will be walking briskly for 15 minutes two days a week and participating in the aerobic dance class two days a week.

Her complete contract appears in Figure 12–3.

SELF-CONTRACT

MY GOALS:

Short-term — by the end of six weeks I will . . . *Go to aerobics dance 2x per week.*
Walk briskly for 15 minutes 2x a week.
Do aerobic exercise 20 minutes

Long-term — by the end of six months I will . . . *4x per week.*

ENVIRONMENTAL PLANNING: (all the steps I will take to reach my goal)

1. *Neighbor to watch daughter.*
2. *Sign up for aerobics at recreation center.*
3. *Read more about exercise (materials from nurse).*
4. *Keep a calendar of progress beside my bed.*
5. *Buy new shoes.*
6. *Learn to take heart rate radially.*
7. *Calculate target heart rate.*

THOUGHTS AND ACTIONS

Helpful thoughts:	Helpful actions:
I really do sleep better when I exercise like this.	*Set out dance clothes before daughter's nap.*
Non-helpful thoughts:	**Non-helpful actions:**
I have to be with my daughter all the time.	*Eating before exercise.*

MY REWARD (if I meet my goal) *A new tee shirt.*

THE COST: (if I fail to meet my goal) *Wash the garbage can.*

REEVALUATION DATE: *12/10*

I agree to help with this project:

_____Susan_____
(Support person)

I agree to strive toward this goal:

___Jennifer___ ___11/4___
(Your signature)   (date)

Figure 12–3. Self-contract. *(Adapted with permission from Baldi, S., and others (1980). For your health: A model for self-care. South Laguna, CA: Nurses Model Health, p. 47.)*

Reaching Objectives: Nursing and Client Actions

Jennifer made a list of the specific actions she would take to ensure success. These included:

1. Arranging for child care.
2. Signing up for an exercise class.
3. Reading one book on exercise and movement.
4. Learning to take her heart rate radially.
5. Buying proper shoes.
6. Attending reevaluation sessions with the nurse.

Nursing actions relative to the program included:

1. Providing reading resources.
2. Teaching about movement and exercise advantages.
3. Demonstrating stretching motions.
4. Assisting with the detailed assessment process.
5. Providing feedback regarding safety precautions.
6. Teaching about components of fitness.

Jennifer agreed to take primary responsibility for her self-care program. She planned to call the nurse with a report of her progress once a week and more often if necessary.

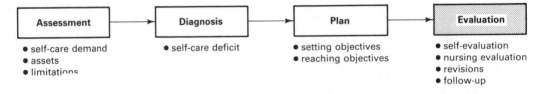

As Jennifer started on her contract some groundwork was necessary. At one point she began to feel guilty for making child-care arrangements with her neighbor. She was afraid that she was putting her own concerns before her daughter's. A brief discussion on the phone with the nurse reminded her that the exercise arrangements would benefit both Jennifer and her daughter.

Jennifer also became skeptical as to whether the exercise would really help her with her self-esteem, sleep, and weight. Again the nurse's role was to help her see its potential value.

Once Jennifer began her movement contract, she met with the nurse several times to reevaluate her overall progress. The instructor in the aerobics class and her neighbor had also become supportive, encouraging her and noting her weekly progress. Jennifer became more interested in the physical and emotional changes she was noticing in herself. She found additional materials on fitness and movement in her nearby library.

At the end of four weeks, there were many "ripple effects." Jennifer's daughter looked forward to the time with the neighbor. In her class Jennifer found two new women friends in similar situations. She began sleeping soundly. Her craving to snack with her daughter subsided. Although her weight did not drop during the first four weeks, she felt more comfortable in clothing that she had not worn in a long time.

After four weeks there was a reevaluation meeting; Jennifer's contract was slightly altered. She opted to include one exercise period of jumping rope and stretching in place of one of the brisk walks.

Jennifer's behavior changes were reviewed at the end of six months. The evaluation worksheets (see Fig. 12–4) revealed both progress and problems. They were used to see what was helpful to her in overcoming barriers. The evaluation process allowed Jennifer to put her progress in perspective. She had forgotten many of her small accomplishments. She had succeeded in building a long-term movement program into her life-style in a realistic manner. She had lost nine pounds. On three occasions she was called on for substitute teaching and had satisfying experiences that boosted her self-confidence. She was proud of her improved appearance. She had bought several new t-shirts and was establishing new rewards on a monthly basis.

				CLIENT EVALUATION WORKSHEET Jennifer				
Week No.	Monday	Tuesday	Wednesday	Thursday	Friday	Saturday	Sunday	Thoughts and feelings during this week.
1		Walked 4 blocks 10 min	First aerobics class 20 min		Aerobic dance 20 min		Walked 4 blocks 20 min	It's fun to be with other people at dance class
2		Rained I walked anyway			Learned warm-up in class 20 min		5 blocks new shoes	I can see some progress
3	Walked 6 blocks with friend		Class cancelled teacher sick	Walked with daughter slowly	Dance 20 min	Brisk walk with neighbors dog 7 blocks		I think I've lost weight. Sleeping much better.
4		Daughter ill	Holiday	Walked 8 blocks in 15 min.	Aerobic class 25 min		Jump rope 2 min	
5	Walked with friend 9 blocks		Dance class Fun! 25 min.	Phone call to nurse	Daughter sick — nothing today	Jump rope and walked		I really can exercise. Basketball might be possible.
6	Friend showed stretching exercise		Dance Class	Walked 10 blocks in 15 min.	Class 25 min		Walked fast 15 min	Re-evaluation with nurse. Glad that I have done this.

Figure 12–4. Client evaluation worksheet.

TABLE 12–5. NURSING CARE PLAN

Reason for consultation: TB skin test, health clearance

Client: Jennifer

Assessment	Plan	Evaluation	
		Met	Not met
Self-care demand	*Setting objectives*		
Need for regular exercise and movement	Six weeks: Will walk briskly for 15 minutes twice a week.	X	
Assets	Go to aerobic dance class twice a week.	X	
Positive past experiences with exercise	Six months: Aerobic exercise 20 minutes four times a week.	(not yet evaluated)	
Community resources available	*Reaching objectives*		
High motivation	Client actions		
Daily moderate activity level	Complete and sign a self-contract.	X	
Treats self to alone time regularly	Have neighbor watch daughter.	X	
Has hobbies and recreation	Join aerobic class at recreation center.	X	
Intelligent, verbal	Read exercise materials from nurse.		
Interested in self-care			
Limitations	Keep a calendar of progress by my bed.	X	
Stress re: single parent and recent divorce	Learn to take heart rate radially.	X	
Economic limitations re: babysitter	Buy new support shoes.	X	
20 pounds overweight	Attend the reevaluation sessions with the nurse.	X	
Employment amount and time not certain	Nursing actions		
Difficulty separating from daughter	Teach physiology of movement and exercise.	X	
Few friends or support systems			
Chronic fatigue			
Fear of success; images of failure			X (partial)

Diagnosis		
Self-care deficit Inability to engage in movement or exercise on a regular basis without education and intervention	Teach emotional and physical benefits of exercise; demonstrate stretching skill.	×
	Initial support person for contract until client makes new friends.	×
	Help client consider risks and precautions of any exercise program.	×
	Facilitate exploration of self-limiting thoughts and actions (help client identify ways in which she might sabotage program).	×
	Model movement self-care.	

Needed revisions
Program is effective.
Continue to revise re: weight loss as needed.

Reevaluation date	Client follow-up
By phone as needed. In four weeks with nurse at clinic. In six months with nurse at clinic.	Goal is to help client build sufficient support system so that program continues without nurse involvement.

At the time of the evaluation she still had dreams of being in a women's basketball league. It was now much closer. She had found that the local community college had a women's basketball class once a week in the evening. Her two new friends traded child care, allowing her additional time away from home. The aerobics instructor introduced her to yoga and other general stretching and movement techniques.

Jennifer agreed that she would benefit from continuing her exercise program. She initiated a new contract on her own, agreeing that she would probably not need nurse support any longer. Jennifer also understood that she could request assistance in the future. Table 12–5 presents a nursing care plan for this clinical situation.

SUMMARY

This chapter has presented the physiological and psychological benefits of movement and exercise. A variety of different movement and exercise activities were explored. Cardiovascular conditioning, endurance, flexibility, and strength were presented as components of fitness.

Considerations in beginning and maintaining an exercise program were outlined. A special emphasis on precautions and risk factors that must be acknowledged in association with any exercise plan was included. Considerations for those with special movement needs were explored. The nurse's role as a health model was emphasized. A clinical presentation underlined the role of both the client and nurse in initiating behavior change in this area.

STUDY QUESTIONS

Personal Focus

1. How do you rate yourself as a model for exercise and movement for your clients? For your family?
2. What are your current goals for personal exercise?
3. List the people at work, at school, and at home who are positive exercise models for you.
4. Describe who or what helps you to be physically active.
5. Describe how you feel after being active or exercising.
6. Write an exercise prescription for yourself.

Client Focus

1. List barriers that would discourage or prevent people from beginning an exercise or movement program.

2. How would you begin to work with a client who was reluctant to exercise?
3. Practice teaching the four components of fitness to a client.
4. How could you assist a client to choose an appropriate beginning exercise level? How would you help clients move safely toward their exercise goals? Describe the screening considerations and precautions for a client beginning a new exercise program.
5. How would you help a client monitor and evaluate progress in a movement or exercise program?

REFERENCES

1. Feldenkrais, M. (1977). *Awareness through movement*. New York: Harper & Row, p. 32.
2. DeVries, H. A. (1974). *Physiology of exercise*. Dubuque, IA: Wm. C. Brown, p. 32.
3. Anderson, G.B., & Johnson, P. (1979). *Physical fitness digest*. Northfield, IL: DBI Books.
4. American College of Sports Medicine. (1986) *Guidelines for graded exercise testing and exercise prescription (3rd ed.)*. Philadelphia: Lea & Febiger.
5. Kostrubala, T. (1976). *The joy of running*. Philadelphia: J.B. Lippincott.
6. Combs, B., Hales, D., & Williams, B. (1980). *An invitation to health: Your personal responsibility*. Menlo Park, CA: Benjamin-Cummings, pp. 305-307.
7. Selye, H. (1975) *Stress without distress*. New York: Signet, p. 14.
8. Patsch, J., & Patsch, W. (1984). Exercise, high-density lipoproteins and fat intolerance. *Comprehensive Therapy, 10*, 19-37.
9. Blackburn, H. (1983). Physical activity and coronary heart disease: A brief update and population view (Part I). *Journal of Cardiac Rehabilitation, 3*, 101-111.
10. Estok, P., & Rudy, E. (1986). Jogging: Cardiovascular benefits and risks. *The Nurse Practitioner, 11*, 21-28.
11. Pritikin, N. (1979). *Pritikin book of diet and exercise*. New York: Grosset & Dunlap.
12. Barnard, R.J., Weber, F., Weingarten, W., Bennett, C., et al. (1981). Effects of an intensive, short-term exercise and nutrition program on patients with coronary heart disease. *Journal of Cardiac Rehabilitation, 1*, (2), 99-104.
13. Celarier, M. (1983, May). Big bucks in the wellness biz. *MS. Magazine*, pp. 127-128.
14. Clark, C., (1981). *Enhancing wellness: A guide for self-care*. New York: Springer, pp. 77-80.
15. Cooper, R.K. (1989). *Health & fitness excellence*. Boston: Houghton Mifflin.
16. Simon, H.B. (1984). Immunology of exercise. *Journal of the American Medical Association, 252*, 19.
17. Kohl, H.W., & Blair, S.N. (1988). Physical activity, physical fitness, and cardiovascular disease mortality in men and women. *American Heart Association Council on Epidemiology Newsletter 43*, 45.
18. Kasch, F.W., & Wallace, J.P. (1976). Physiological variables during ten years of endurance exercise. *Medicine and Science in Sports, 8*, (5), 5-13.

19. Smith, E.L., & Reddan, W. (1976). Physical activity—a modality for bone accretion in the aged. *American Journal of Roentgenology, 126,* 1297.
20. Spirduso, W.W. (1978). Replication of age and physical activity effects on reaction and movement time. *Journal of Gerontology, 33,* (26), 26-30.
21. Carlow, T.J., Appenzeller, O., & Rodriguez, M. (1978). Neurology of endurance training: Visual evoked potentials before and after a run. *Neurology, 28,* 390.
22. Wood, P. (1985). Exercise does promote cardiovascular health. *Contemporary OB/GYN, 125,* 64-70.
23. Fardy, P.S., & Halpenny, C.J. (1982). Normal physiologic responses to exercise. In S.L. Underhill, S. Woods, E. Sivarajan, C. Halpenny. (Eds.), *Cardiac Nursing.* Philadelphia: J.B. Lippincott.
24. Kaplan, N. (1985). Non-drug treatment of hypertension. *Annals of Internal Medicine, 102,* 359-373.
25. Milhorn, H.T. (1984). Prescribing a cardiovascular fitness program. *Comprehensive Therapy, 10,* 46-53.
26. Smith, E. (1985). How exercise helps prevent osteoporosis. *Contemporary OB/GYN, 125,* 105-115.
27. Mirkin, G., & Hoffman, M. (1978). *The sports medicine book.* Boston: Little, Brown.
28. Greist, J., Klien, J., Eischens, R., et al. (1979). Running as a treatment for depression. *Comprehensive Psychiatry, 20,* (1), 41-54.
29. Barnes, L. (1981). Running causes behavior changes in children. *The Physician and Sportsmedicine, 7,* (98), 23.
30. Altshul, V. (1978). The ego integrative (and disintegrative) effects on long distance running. *Current Concepts in Psychiatry.* 6-11.
31. Samuels, M., & Samuels, N. (1988). *The well adult.* New York: Summit Books.
32. Carr, D.B., Buller, B.A., Skrinar, G., Arnold, M., et al. (1981). Physical conditioning facilitates the exercise-induced secretion of beta-endorphin and beta-lipotropin in women. *New England Journal of Medicine, 305,* 560.
33. Monahan, T. (1986). Exercise and depression: Swapping sweat for serenity? *The Physician and Sports Medicine, 14,* 192-197.
34. Gibson, S., et. al. (1983). Writing the exercise prescription: An individual approach. *The Physician and Sportsmedicine, 11,* 87-110.
35. Dunn, M. (1987). Guidelines for an effective personal fitness prescription. *The Nurse Practitioner, 12,* (9), 9-26.
36. Ocker, G., & Rosenbaum, J. (1986). Shape's second annual aerobic-dance shoe survey. *Shape, 6,* 74-79.
37. Friedman, B.J., & Knight, K. (1978). Running for life, health, and pleasure. *American Journal of Nursing, 78,* 602-607.
38. American College of Sports Medicine. (1980). *Guidelines for graded exercise testing and exercise prescription* (3rd ed.). Philadelphia: Lea & Febiger.
39. Blattner, B. (1981). *Holistic nursing.* Englewood Cliffs, NJ: Prentice-Hall, p. 213.
40. Wenck, D.A., Baren, M., & Dewan, S.P. (1980). *Nutrition,* Reston, VA: Reston, pp. 364-365.
41. Freidman, M., & Rosenman, R.H. (1974). *Type A behavior and your heart.* New York: Alfred A. Knopf.
42. Zohman, L. *Run for life.* (1978). Pamphlet of Connecticut Mutual Life Insurance Company (140 Garden Street, Hartford, CT 06105), p. 11.

43. Legwald, G. (1982). Little bodies and healthy hearts: Counseling in the schools. *The Physician and Sportsmedicine, 10*, (5), 128-130.
44. Smith, N.J. (Ed.). (1983). *Sports medicine: Health care for young athletes*. Evanston, IL: American Academy of Pediatrics.
45. Siegel, B. (1985). Counseling and health screening for children entering sports and physical exercise. *The Nurse Practitioner, 10*, 11-21.
46. Haycock, C. (1980). *Sports medicine for the athletic female*. Oradell, NJ: Medical Economics Books.
47. Ullyot, J. (1976). *Women's running*. Mountain View, CA: World Publications. pp. 119-120.
48. Ritz, S. (1981). How to deal with menstrual cramps. *Medical Self-Care, 12*, 19-20.
49. Leaf, D.A. (1981). Exercise and pregnancy compatible. *The Physician and Sportsmedicine, 9*, 22.
50. Hutchinson, P., Cureton, K.J., & Sparling, P.B. (1981). Metabolic and circulatory responses to running during pregnancy. *The Physician and Sportsmedicine, 9*, (8), 55-57.
51. Thompson, J. (1977). *Healthy pregnancy the yoga way*. New York: Doubleday/Dolphin Books, p. 11.
52. Marsiglio, A., & Holm, K. (1988). Physical conditioning in the aging adult. *The Nurse Practitioner, 13*, (9), 33-41.
53. Rechnitzer, P. (1982). Specific benefits of post-coronary exercise programs. *Geriatrics, 37*, (3), 47-49.
54. Barry, H. (1986). Exercise prescriptions for the elderly. *American Family Physician, 34*, 155-162.
55. Gregory S. Thomas, Philip R. Lee, Pat Franks, and Ralph S. Paffenbarger, Jr., (1981). *Exercise and Health* (Cambridge, MA: Oelgeschlager, Gunn & Hain.
56. Talbot, D., Pearson, V., & Loeper, J. (1978). *Disuse syndrome: The preventable disability*. Minneapolis: Sister Kenny Institute, p. 1.
57. Coletti, S. (1982). Exercise and nutritional needs of the physically limited. Unpublished paper. Santa Rosa Community College, Santa Rosa, CA:

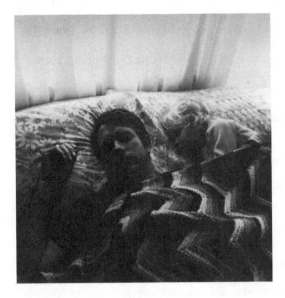

Sleep is the only medicine that gives ease.

Sophocles

13 Sleep and Dreams

LEARNING OBJECTIVES

Upon completion of this chapter, readers will be able to:

1. Define the terms sleep, dreams, and sleep self-care.
2. Identify five stages of sleep.
3. Describe the significance of rapid eye movement (REM) sleep.
4. Differentiate between sleep and relaxation.
5. Describe possible functions of sleep and its relation to health and illness.
6. Describe the function of dreaming and its relation to health.
7. Discuss the influence of sleeping medications and alcohol on sleep.
8. Describe self-care activities that facilitate sleep.
9. Describe changes in sleep that occur throughout the life cycle.
10. Describe the impact of alternating shift work on sleep patterns.

DEFINITIONS

Sleep   A state of repose, characterized by relative unresponsiveness to stimuli; an altered state of consciousness, from which a person nevertheless can be aroused by stimuli of sufficient magnitude. It includes rapid eye movement (REM) and non-rapid eye movement (NREM) stages.

Stages of Sleep

1. *NREM or non-rapid eye movement* [slow-wave sleep (SWS)]: Refers collectively to the first four stages of sleep. Eighty percent of adult sleep is spent in this state. The transition of sleep stages within NREM is gradual, not abrupt.
2. *REM or rapid eye movement* (paradoxical sleep): A fifth stage of sleep (20 percent of adult sleep) during which there is an almost total absence of skeletal muscle tone. EEG waves are fast, desynchronized, and of a low amplitude. Conjugate rapid eye movements occur. Most dreaming occurs during this phase. Activation of sexual organs occurs.[1]

Dreaming   Dreaming is subjectively reported as a memory of a sensory experience during sleep (visual, auditory, and so on). Objectively, it is marked by fast, low-amplitude brain wave activity and rapid eye movements. It occurs during the REM phase. *All* people dream during this stage even if they have no memory of their dreams following sleep.[2]

Circadian Rhythm   Self-sustaining oscillations in body functions (i.e., temperature, pulse, and blood pressure) occurring in predictable, consistent, 24-hour cycles under normal conditions.

Sleep Disturbance   Any discomfort with sleep as defined by the client. Sleep difficulty is often a problem secondary to psychiatric and medical disorders.

Sleep Self-Care   Activities that promote adequate quality and quantity of sleep. These activities include learning to know one's own sleep needs, limiting alcohol and caffeine, exercising regularly, and practicing relaxation. Sleep self-care also involves skills in manipulating one's environment (quiet, dark, minimal interruptions, and so on) to promote sleep.

INTRODUCTION

Most people spend about one-third of their lives in sleep. Although this could amount to as much as 25 years for many people, it is an area of self-care that is often given very little emphasis.

Sleeping and dreaming are among the most powerful organizing factors in life, yet millions of people have trouble doing it properly.[3] Dement has emphasized that sleep requires as much attention as the average American now gives to nutrition and exercise.[4] Sleep self-care is not a new concept, but it has been more strongly encouraged in recent years. Part of this current emphasis results from new findings about the significance of sleeping and dreaming.

Major Characteristics of Sleep

Until recently, scientists dismissed sleep as a time of rest and quiet when absolutely nothing happened. It is now known that the reverse is true—that sleep is a very active state. One stage of sleep, the REM or dreaming stage, is so active that it is considered equivalent to an equal period of jogging.[3] Sleep is more than just the opposite or being awake; it is a period of extensive mental and physical activity.

Sleep periods imply low responsiveness to outside stimuli and little goal-directed activity. Observable behavioral changes during sleep, such as closing one's eyes and breathing deeply, actually reflect important internal bodily alterations. Changes in brain waves are the most dramatic of these.

Stages of Sleep

People undergo different depths or stages of sleep; it is not simply a question of whether a person is "awake" or "asleep." Electroencephalographs, electrooculographs, and electromyographs measure brain activity, eye movement, and muscle movement. Five internationally recognized sleep levels or phases have been discovered. These stages include two major categories: non-REM (or slow-wave sleep), which includes the first four stages, and REM sleep, which is the fifth stage. Transition from one phase of sleep to the next is gradual and not abrupt. Most people cannot subjectively report or measure these transitions for themselves. Table 13–1 presents information regarding each of the five stages of sleep.

Sleep is very different from relaxation. Alpha waves occur during deep relaxation and are also present during the first stage of sleep. Brain waves present during the remaining sleep stages do not occur during relaxation. The relaxation response does not involve the loss of consciousness that is present in sleep.

Sleep and Circadian Rhythms

Sleep is clearly a part of the rhythm of life. There is speculation about the reasons people sleep primarily at night and the types of problems that exist when one's normal sleep time is disrupted.

The term *circadian* refers to the fact that under natural conditions oscillations will occur in predictable, consistent, 24-hour cycles. More than 100 body functions oscillate between maximal and minimal values once a day. Heart rate, body temperature, mood, production of hormones, and intellectual performance, as well as the sleep–wakefulness cycle, are but a few of these functions.[5] Neurotransmitters also show wide circadian variation. The serum level of serotonin, the neurotransmitter most associated with sleep, fluctuates with the sleep–wakefulness cycle.

For most people, these cycles occur during a 24-hour or 25-hour period. Although environmental factors have some influence on these rhythms, the body's basic cycles are self-sustaining and independent. For example, research studies in which people are isolated from clocks and other clues about the time of day have shown that subjects still get sleepy at around the same time that they do in their usual environments.[5] Sleep coincides with low points in one's body rhythm.

"Jet lag" describes the disruptive and unpleasant effects that result from rapid long-distance travel through different time zones. Fatigue and diminished intellectual performance are often associated with this. Nurses who rotate shifts are acutely aware of the disruption that occurs when they are unable to establish consistent sleep periods. Decreased work performance has led many industries to discontinue the practice of shift rotation.

Sleep, perhaps more than any other body process, is disrupted by hospitalization. Sleep interruption because of noise, light, and procedures is most marked in intensive care units. Referral to self-care units and early discharges are now encouraged, in part, to help clients return to their individual rhythms of eating, sleeping, and socializing. This may enhance the healing process.

THE THEORY AND VALUE OF SLEEP

Sleep Theories

Many current theories about the possible functions of sleep are to some degree overlapping and compatible with each other. The two major views that are most different from each other are that sleep occurs as either a recovery or homeostatic process (the need recovery model) or as an instinctive activity (the expressive species activity model) not related to need recovery.

If the specific function of sleep is as yet not clearly determined, there are several important factors about sleep that are agreed upon:

1. The midbrain reticular formation (the waking center) controls wakefulness. Different phases of sleep are connected with different parts of the midbrain reticular formation.[6]
2. The neurotransmitters serotonin and norepinephrine are directly involved in the sleep process.[6]
3. Staying awake indefinitely is impossible even though there is a variation in the amount of sleep that people need to function well.[7]

Value of Sleep

Throughout history sleep has been thought to restore the body in preparation for the next period of activity. In ancient myths and folklore, sleep was a primary treatment for people who were troubled by fits, spirits, or discontent in

TABLE 13–1. THE FIVE STAGES OF SLEEP*

Stages of Sleep	EEG Brainwaves	Time Span	Approximate Percentage of Total Night's Sleep	Affective Aspects	Physiological Alterations
NREM sleep or slow-wave sleep					
Stage 1	Alpha activity	1–2 min	5–10	Fleeting thoughts; may be unaware of being asleep	Light sleep, easily awakened; pulse rate decreased 10–30 beats per min; BMR decreased 10–15%; temperature and respiration decreased; muscle tone minimal; knee jerks abolished; slight decrease in blood pressure
Stage 2	Sleep spindles	5–10 min	50		Transition sleep Easily awakened

Stage	EEG	Time	%		Characteristics
Stage 3	Delta activity appears	10 min	}	10–20	Deep sleep; difficult to awaken; thought to restore, relax, and rest the body
Stage 4	Delta activity predominates	5–15 min			
REM sleep Stage 5	Desynchronized pattern of low-voltage beta activity—similar to waking EEG	10 min, first cycle; 10–12 min, second cycle; 20–30 min as length of total sleep increases	20–25	Dreams believed to occur	Physiologically active; paradoxical muscle movements, rapid eye movements; increase in cerebral blood flow, brain temperature, and body oxygen consumption (most skeletal muscle tone depressed; tendon reflexes depressed)

*The sleeper, on falling asleep, goes through stages 1 through 4, then returns to stage 3, and then to stage 2; followed by a period of REM sleep. This pattern is considered a sleep cycle and usually takes 90 minutes. Further sleep involves stages 2, 3, and sometimes 4, returning to stage 3 and then to stage 2 with another slightly longer REM period.

(Reprinted with permission from Malasanos, L., Barkauskas, V., Moss, M., & Stoltenberg-Allen, K. (1986). Assessment of sleep–wakefulness patterns. In *Health assessment* (3rd ed.). St. Louis: C.V. Mosby, p. 121.)

general.[8] During every age of civilization, parents have probably told their children who were upset that they would "feel better after a good sleep." Athletic coaches continually remind their players to get adequate sleep the night before an important game.

Research has shown that this "common sense" self-care practice is actually based on solid physiological findings. Some of the values of sleep are:

1. Mental efficiency is impaired if sleeping time is drastically reduced. Prolonged sleep deprivation causes irritability and hallucinations.[9]
2. Slow-wave sleep is thought to promote anabolic processes and compensate for catabolic processes. Production of growth hormones increases during sleep.[10]
3. REM sleep may be necessary for brain growth and renewal (for example, premature infants have 50 percent more REM sleep than do normal-gestation infants).[11]
4. Sleep is critical for effective emotional and cognitive functioning. It permits physical and emotional recuperation.[12]
5. Sleep provides people with a subjective sensation of simply "feeling better."

DREAMING AND HEALTH

Dreaming is reported as a memory of a sensory experience during sleep (visual, auditory, and so on). It occurs during the fifth stage of sleep, REM sleep. Infants spend almost 50 percent of sleep in this stage and adults spend approximately 25 percent. *All* people dream during REM sleep every night even though they may not remember their dreams upon awaking.[2]

In ancient civilizations dreams were thought to be visions of future events or links to the supernatural. Examples of the importance and use of dreams are found throughout the Bible. Ancient myths and fairy tales repeatedly use dreams as a mechanism through which oracles receive or deliver messages. More recently, the meaning of dreams has been studied psychologically. Freud considered dreams to be disguised fulfillments of unconscious wishes and "the royal road" to understanding the unconscious mind.[13] Jung emphasized the role of dreams as a path to the unconscious or deeper levels of the personality.[14]

Scientific, musical, poetic, and other artistic endeavors are often dramatically enhanced by dreams. People often fear dreams as statements of what could happen in reality. As Shakespeare reflected,

Merciful powers,
Restrain in me the cursed thoughts that
Nature
Gives way to in repose!

(*Macbeth*, ii, 1, 7)

The Senoi (a Malaysian tribe) use dream material to learn about themselves and the best way to function in daily life.

> Each morning the tribe gathers to share the previous night's dreams. . . . Members reporting dreams of pleasure and happiness are urged to continue having and telling them. Unhappy or incomplete dreams are either interpreted positively or the person is urged to continue the dream the next night so that a resolution can be found. For example, if someone dreams of having an argument with a friend, the dreamer is urged to continue the dream until the disagreement is resolved.[15]

This practice is becoming increasingly popular. In many clinical as well as social settings, people report and interpret their dreams. Friends often form groups to help interpret each others' drawings, notes, and feelings about their dreams. In some families, the Senoi practice is repeated. Children as young as three or four years can be taught to remember and repeat their dreams. They can be encouraged to dream of successful outcomes to their worries and fears. This self-care approach teaches children and adults that positive alternatives exist in the dreaming as well as the waking world. Dreams often play a major role in helping people to understand the spiritual component of life. Difficulties in relationships are also often understood and resolved through dreams.

The ability to remember, understand, and use one's dreams is a cultivated self-care skill. According to LaBerge, "Dream control translates into more self-confidence during the day."[9] Journal keeping is one approach to using one's dreams. Other techniques for developing self-awareness are also helpful in learning about one's dreams (see Chapters 8 and 10).

Recent research has illuminated what LaBerge calls *lucid dreaming*. This is defined as awareness that one is dreaming during a dream. Using this awareness as a starting point, LaBerge has encouraged research subjects to pursue problem solving during dreams.[16,17]

The Function of Dreaming

Many theories attempt to explain the function of dreaming, such as dreaming is necessary for the physiological development of the nervous system,[11] or dreaming is in some way linked to the presence or absence of psychosis.[12] Recent findings about dreams include:

1. Deprivation of REM sleep is manifested by irritability, suspiciousness, apathy, lack of alertness, poor judgment, and increased sensitivity to pain and discomfort. People who are systematically deprived of REM sleep will dream an abnormal amount (up to 60 percent more) to compensate for lost dreams before returning to normal dream phases. This process is known as REM rebound.[7]
2. Dreams are thought to be essential to the process of mental restoration.[18]

3. REM sleep seems to help in the processing and storage of information. According to Cartwright, in animals REM sleep increases after new learning. In human begins REM sleep is highest in infancy—a period when most new learning takes place.[9]

4. Retarded people have shorter-than-normal REM periods. Dreaming is perhaps linked to intelligence (Cartwright).[9]

5. Recovery from emotional trauma, such as an accident or a divorce, seems to be enhanced by dreams (Cartwright).[9]

6. A sharp increase in dreaming usually occurs when people face any difficult situation, such as taking an exam or learning a new skill (Cohen).[9]

7. Dream control may play a major role in physical health. Dreamers may be able to "program" an enhanced physical healing process (LaBerge).[9] (This is similar to the visualization and imagery approaches for healing of cancer used by Simonton and Simonton during waking states.[19])

SLEEP SELF-CARE

Sleep is a self-care activity requiring the same attention as that given to exercise, nutrition, and all other self-care areas. Effective self-care in all areas will inevitably lead to a healthier physical and emotional life; it will also improve sleep. When people sleep well, they have more energy available to devote to self-care. Table 13–2 presents a number of self-care skills that promote sleep.

Sleep Throughout the Life Cycle

The total amount of time people spend sleeping, the distribution of sleep in each 24-hour period, and the length of each phase of sleep, all change throughout normal development.

Many complaints about sleep are secondary to inadequate knowledge or unrealistic expectations. There is a wide variation in what is considered normal.

Nutrition and Sleep

Dietary habits play a significant role in individual sleep patterns. L-Tryptophan is an amino acid thought to aid sleep. Caffeine, on the other hand, impairs sleep for most people.

L-*Tryptophan*

Large doses (up to 4 grams) of the essential amino acid L-Tryptophan have been reported to induce and prolong sleep.[20,21] Since all protein contains tryptophan, it is possible that ordinary diets contain enough L-Tryptophan to enhance sleep. Thus a "warm glass of milk" (which is high in L-Tryptophan) may be scientifically as well as proverbially helpful in inducing sleep.[22] L-Tryptophan is also available in tablet form without a prescription.

TABLE 13–2. TECHNIQUES TO FACILITATE SLEEP SELF-CARE

1. Learn the amount of sleep needed for your optimum functioning. Alter daily routine to allow for this.
2. During illness or other life stress, plan for additional sleep or rest.
3. Reduce caffeine intake slowly. Limit to more than six hours before sleep. Eventually eliminate completely.
4. Exercise strenuously for 20 minutes at least three times per week. Do not exercise right before sleep.
5. Provide for one hour of "quiet time" just before going to bed. Complete a relaxation, yoga, or meditation exercise before sleep.
6. Complete "sleep rituals" as needed (drink glass of warm milk, take hot bath, listen to favorite record, say prayers).
7. Learn which foods seem to promote sleep for you. Include these in your daily diet.
8. Complete a basic relaxation exercise for 10 minutes four times per week.
9. Evaluate all alcohol and medication intake. Reduce and eliminate if possible.
10. Limit frequent shift changes at work; limit travel between time zones.
11. Provide for physical comfort during sleep. Attend to temperature, ventilation, night clothes.
12. Remove telephone from hook if sleeping during unusual times. Leave note asking not to be disturbed.
13. Provide for a nap time if sleep is disrupted by uncontrollable conditions such as sick children.

Caffeine

Caffeine is an effective, long-acting stimulant whose 12-hour to 20-hour duration of action can considerably lighten nighttime sleep, even if taken at lunch.[23] Coffee, tea, chocolate, soft drinks, or any substance that contains caffeine may prevent sleep.[10] The total duration of sleep may not be reduced, but the first three hours of sleep are affected. Slow-wave sleep is reduced by an average of 18 minutes; however, REM sleep is not significantly affected.[24] In addition to caffeinated beverages, many over-the-counter medications contain high levels of caffeine. Table 13–3 presents a list of the caffeine content of certain beverages and over-the-counter drugs. Many people take some of these preparations to aid sleep, when in reality they may have the opposite effect.

TABLE 13–3. COMMON SOURCES OF CAFFEINE

Product	Amount of Product	Amount of Caffeine (mg)
Coffee		
Drip	5 oz	146
Percolated	5 oz	110
Instant, regular	5 oz	53
Decaffeinated	5 oz	2
Tea		
One-minute brew	5 oz	9–33
Three-minute brew	5 oz	20–46
Five-minute brew	5 oz	20–50
Canned ice tea	12 oz	22–36
Cocoa and chocolate		
Cocoa beverage		
(mix with water)	6 oz	10
Milk chocolate	1 oz	6
Baking chocolate	1 oz	35
Nonprescription drugs		
Caffedrine capsules	Standard dose	200
No Doz tablets	Standard dose	200
Vivarin tablets	Standard dose	200
Anacin	Standard dose	64
Excedrin	Standard dose	130
Midol	Standard dose	65
Aqua-Ban	Standard dose	200
Dristan	Standard dose	32
Dexatrim	Standard dose	200
Dietac	Standard dose	200
Prolamine	Standard dose	280
Soft drinks		
Mr. Pibb Diet	12 oz	52
Tab	12 oz	44
Dr. Pepper	12 oz	38
Sunkist Orange	12 oz	42
Pepsi	12 oz	37
RC Cola	12 oz	36
Diet Rite	12 oz	34
Diet Pepsi	12 oz	34
Coca-Cola	12 oz	34
7-Up	12 oz	0
Sprite	12 oz	0
Diet Sunkist	12 oz	0
Fresca	12 oz	0
Hires Root Beer	12 oz	0

(Reprinted with permission from Caffeine: How to Consume Less. (1981, October). *Consumer Reports*, pp. 598-599.)

Medications That Interfere with Sleep

Many prescription and nonprescription drugs alter sleep patterns. The relationship of sleep changes to the initiation of any medication regimen requires careful assessment. This assessment is often difficult because sleep disturbance may be a function of the disorder being treated by the medication or an effect of the medication itself.

Table 13–4 lists a number of medications that interfere with sleep patterns. The first section of the table describes specific drugs that affect REM sleep. The second section lists drugs that affect stage 4 or NREM sleep. Insomnia may result from drug interactions. Medications given specifically for sleep may themselves cause more sleep problems.

Self-care responsibility regarding medications of any type can be taught to

TABLE 13–4. EFFECTS OF PHARMACEUTICAL AGENTS ON THE SLEEP CYCLE

Decrease Time		Increase Time		Allow Normal Time	
Drug	Dosage	Drug	Dosage	Drug	Dosage
REM sleep					
Placidyl	500 mg	Reserpine	1–2 mg	Chloral hydrate	0.5 g
Doriden	500 mg	LSD	30 µg		1.0 g
Seconal	100 mg				1.5 g
Phenobarbital	200 mg				
Nembutal	100 mg			Dalmane	15–30 mg
Quaalude	300 mg			Quaalude	150 mg
Benadryl	50 mg			Librium	50–100 mg
Scopolamine	0.006 mg/kg			Valium	5–10 mg
Morphine					
Heroin					
Alcohol	1 g/kg				
Tofranil	50 mg				
Elavil	50–70 mg				
Miltown	1,200 mg				
Amphetamine	15 mg				
Stage 4 sleep					
Doriden	500 mg	Antidepressants in the presence of depression			
Nembutal	100 mg				
Valium	10 mg				
Librium	50 mg				
Reserpine	0.14 mg/kg				
Chloral hydrate	1.5 g				

(Reprinted with permission from Malasanos, L., Barkauskas, V., Moss, M., & Stoltenberg-Allen, K. (1986). Assessment of sleep–wakefulness patterns. In *Health assessment* (3nd ed.). St. Louis: C.V. Mosby, p. 131.)

clients. Clients can learn to relate changes in sleep patterns to medication and discuss side effects with prescribing health care providers.

Sleeping Medication

Sleep disturbance is a major health problem in this country. Americans spend more than $200 million on a variety of medications to help them sleep.[4,25] Millions of prescriptions for barbiturates and other potent sleeping pills are written every year.

The stress of disturbed sleep seems to make many people rush *first* for medications rather than consider other self-care approaches. The effectiveness and appropriateness of both over-the-counter and prescription medications for sleep are being seriously questioned. Coates and Thoresen strongly state that "almost all drugs now available [for sleeping disorders] actually make sleep *worse* rather than better."[26]

Most sedatives and tranquilizers interfere with REM sleep. The few drugs that do not disturb REM sleep, decrease stage 4 (deep) sleep. No drug has yet been discovered that induces normal sleep.

REM Rebound and Tolerance. A rebound effect occurs when chemical suppression of REM sleep is abruptly stopped. During withdrawal from sleeping medications, people experience excessive REM sleep, in which it is common for dreams to be particularly vivid, frightening, and disruptive. People often wake up in the middle of terrifying nightmares, determine that their sleep is getting worse, and reach for more sleeping pills.

Tolerance to most sleeping medications is another severe problem. As one adjusts to certain drugs, larger and larger quantities are needed to achieve the same effect.

Figure 13–1 depicts the cycle of sleeplessness leading to drug ingestion, followed by dependence, tolerance, more sleeplessness, and increased drug ingestion.

Alcohol and Sleep

Dependence and tolerance also occur with alcohol. Many people drink heavily right before sleep, experience disturbed sleep because of the alcohol, and begin to drink more and more alcohol to help them sleep better. Tolerance develops and even more alcohol is ingested. Alcohol does speed the onset of sleep but interferes with REM sleep and adversely affects many physiological functions.

Client education concerning dependence and tolerance is crucial. Clients need to know why their sleep has become more disturbed during withdrawal from sedatives, tranquilizers, or alcohol. They also need reassurance that normal sleep patterns will eventually be reestablished. This can take weeks or even months.

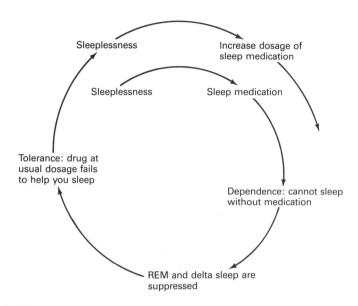

Figure 13–1. Effect of sleeping medications: dependence and tolerance. *Used with permission from Coates, T.J., & Thoreson, E. (1977).* How to sleep better, *Englewood Cliffs, NJ: Prentice-Hall, p. 43.*

SLEEP DISTURBANCE

Most people experience difficulty in sleeping at some point in their lives. Sleep disturbance during periods of emotional stress is particularly common. People trying to make important life decisions, preparing for final examinations, or mourning the loss of someone close frequently report sleep difficulties. Sleep disturbance is also associated with many psychiatric and medical conditions. The most common sleep disorders are insomnia, narcolepsy, and sleep apnea. Common disorders are listed and defined in Table 13–5. This table presents primary sleep disorders (in which disordered sleep is the only problem), secondary sleep disorders (which occur in conjunction with specific clinical disorders), and parasomnias (waking behaviors that appear during sleep).

Sleep disturbance is endemic in hospitals. Clapin-French found that although 71 percent of her sample received sleeping medications, only 54 percent had a sleep history conducted by nursing staff.[27] Many nurses are insecure about this assessment area. The assessment tool provided in Table 13–6 helps nurses to determine the environmental and emotional components surrounding the client's sleep in the hospital. This is an important starting point.

Assessment and Referral

Physiological causes of sleep disorders need to be ruled out *before* behavioral or self-care approaches are initiated. Enuresis, for example, is sometimes the result of delayed nervous system development, allergy, or cogenital abnormalities of the urinary tract. Sleep apnea is sometimes fatal and may require lifesaving measures such as use of an apnea monitor or a tracheotomy. Diagnostic sleep centers are available throughout the country, primarily in large medical centers. Clients may be reluctant to travel long distances at great expense when they think the problem may correct itself spontaneously. The nurse's role in this process is to provide education and encouragement. Self-care approaches are then used concurrently with medical treatment. There is now increasing information on sleep disorders in the nursing literature. Potter and Perry provide an excellent guide to the nursing diagnosis of sleep disturbance in *Fundamentals of Nursing: Concepts, Process and Practice.*[28]

Nursing Diagnosis and Sleep Self-Care

The nursing diagnosis of *Sleep pattern disturbance* is most related to sleep self-care. This diagnosis is defined as a disruption of sleep time that causes client discomfort or interferes with the client's desired life-style. Irritability, disorientation, listlessness, restlessness, and lethargy are some of the objective signs that may point to this nursing diagnosis. *Altered thought processes related to sleep deprivation* and *Potential for injury related to attacks of sleepwalking or*

TABLE 13–5. COMMON SLEEP DISTURBANCES

Primary sleep disturbance	
Insomnia	Inability to fall asleep, frequent or prolonged awakening, or early morning awakening. Most commonly reported sleep disturbance.
Hypersomnia	Tendency to sleep for excessive periods (acute or chronic). Often stress-related.
Narcolepsy	Uncontrolled onset of sleep. Person falls asleep suddenly and immediately enters REM sleep (20-fold higher incidence in family members).
Sleep apnea	Periodic cessation of breathing during sleep; most common in overweight men over age 40.
Sudden infant death syndrome	Sudden crib death of healthy infants. May be related to apnea, immature nervous system, or defect in REM sleep patterns.
Secondary sleep disturbance	
Related to physical disorders: Chronic renal insufficiency Chronic obstructive pulmonary disease	People with these clinical disorders experience alterations in sleep patterns. Non-REM and/or REM sleep may be affected.

TABLE 13–5. (con't)

Pain
Duodenal ulcer
Metabolic disorders
Rheumatoid arthritis
Cardiovascular symptoms
Migraine headaches
Thyroid disorders
Neurological disorders

Related to psychiatric disorders:
Depression
Grief
Schizophrenia
Alcoholism
Mania
Anorexia nervosa
Other:
Pregnancy
Aging

Parasomnias

Somnambulism	Common in children; sleep walking occurs in stages 3 and 4; person has amnesia for the incident; may be dangerous, for example, if person falls.
Sleep talking	Talking generally occurs during non-REM sleep.
Bruxism	Grinding teeth during sleep; in 15% of population; occurs in stage 2 of sleep.
Enuresis	Bed-wetting during sleep; in 5–15% of all preadolescent children.

(Information adapted from Malasanos, L., Barkauskas, V., Moss, M., & Stoltenberg-Allen, K. (1986). Assessment of sleep–wakefulness patterns. In *Health assessment,* (3rd ed.). St. Louis: C.V. Mosby, pp. 124–130).

narcolepsy are other related diagnoses. The sleep self-care skills described in this chapter can be used in the intervention phase of the nursing process.

NURSES MODEL SLEEP SELF-CARE

Many nurses may be accustomed to thinking about sleep only when significant sleep disturbances occur. Self-care regarding sleep and dreams, however, is vital for health even when specific sleeping problems are not present.

Self-assessment helps nurses to acknowledge the value they place on sleep.

TABLE 13-6 SAMPLE SLEEP ASSESSMENT FORM

Aspects of Sleep Pattern	Questions to Elicit Sleep Pattern
Time retired Initial insomnia	"What time do you usually go to bed?" "Do you fall asleep right away?" "How long does it take you to fall asleep?" "How often do you have trouble falling asleep? Does it occur every night? Every other night? Just the weekend? Every Monday?" "How do you feel before you fall asleep?"
Maintenance insomnia	"Do you wake up in the night? How often does this occur?" "What wakes you up once you have fallen asleep? Is there something that helps you get back to sleep?"
Arousal-terminal insomnia	"What time do you wake up? How often do you get up this early? What wakes you up at this early hour?" "What do you do once you wake up?"
Quality of sleep (affective response)	"How do you feel when you get up?" "Do you feel rested after a night's sleep?"
Naps	"Do you nap during the day?"
Dreams, night terrors	"Do you dream at night?" "Are your dreams ever frightening?" "Do your dreams ever wake you?" "How do you feel when you wake up from a bad dream?"
Bruxism	"Has anyone ever told you that you grind your teeth in your sleep?"
Special activities associated with sleep: Bath, massage	"What do you do just before going to bed?"
Food	"Do you eat before you go to bed?" "Do you like to have a snack before bed?"
Drink (warm milk, water)	"Do you like a drink before going to bed?" "What do you prefer as your bedtime beverage?"
Medication	"Do you take any medicine to help you sleep?" "Are you taking any medicine at all?"
Personal beliefs about sleep	"How much sleep do you think you should have to stay healthy?" "What will happen if you don't get enough sleep?"
Impact on others	"How does the way you sleep affect your family?"
Psychiatric disorders (anxiety, depression, schizophrenia)	"How have your spirits been?" "Have you had a lot of worries lately?"
Physical disorders	"Do you have any medical complaints right now?"

Somnambulism	"Has anyone ever told you that you walk in your sleep?"
	"Have you ever awakened in some place different than the one in which you went to sleep?"
	"Have you ever awakened to find furniture or other objects moved around in your home?"
Daytime activity work pattern	"What kind of work do you do?"
Shift change	"What hours do you work?"
Recreation, exercise	"What kind of activity is involved?" "What do you do for fun?" "Do you engage in regular exercise?"
Home responsibilities	"Do you work at home? What kind of work do you do at home?"
Sleep environment:	
Bedding (mattress, pillows, blankets)	"Do you need any special bedding to help you sleep?" "How many pillows do you use?"
Light	"Do you sleep with the lights off?" "Does having a light on at night bother you?"
Noise	"Do you have to have it very quiet to sleep?" "Do noises keep you awake at night? Wake you up?"
Ventilation	"Do you open the window at night?"
Temperature	"Do you need the bedroom to be cold [warm] in order to sleep well?"

(Reprinted with permission from Malasanos, L., Barkauskas, V., Moss, M., & Stoltenberg-Allen, K. (1986). Assessment of sleep–wakefulness patterns. In *Health assessment* (3rd ed.). St. Louis: C. V. Mosby, p. 132.)

Those values are modeled in clinical settings in both covert and in overt ways. The ways in which nurses model sleep self-care in their personal lives include:

- Arranging shift work, days off, and vacation time to provide adequate rest.
- Manipulating their home environments to promote sleep and avoid chronic fatigue.
- Drinking adequate fluids when traveling across times zones; helping children decrease stress of circadian rhythm changes during travel.
- Keeping dream journals.
- Requesting in-service sessions related to sleep self-care.
- Practicing all of the sleep self-care skills presented in Table 13–2.

In clinical settings nurses emphasize the importance of sleep by respecting clients' needs in this area. Nurses promote self-care actions particularly when clients do not seem to respect their own needs for sleep and dreams.

Other ways in which nurses serve as positive models include such actions as:

- Allowing parents to room with hospitalized children.
- Assessing the client's usual bedtime and sleep routines when admitting to hospital.
- Listening carefully when clients report their dreams.
- Providing herb tea or decaffeinated coffee rather than caffeinated beverages with meals.
- Promoting privacy, quiet, and darkness when needed for sleep.
- Limiting amount of contact with hospitalized clients during nighttime hours.
- Planning nursing care around clients' sleep needs.
- Providing for massage, warm milk, hot bath, and other sleep-promoting rituals.
- Teaching and providing self-care alternatives to sleeping medications such as relaxation music tapes.
- Allowing family to be with clients who are trying to fall asleep, promoting touch at these times.

All these nursing actions model sleep self-care in subtle as well as obvious ways. When nurses model the personal benefits gained from sleep self-care, clients are also more likely to value and practice these skills on a regular basis.

CLINICAL APPLICATION

Case Presentation

John is a 70-year-old black male whose wife of 50 years died five months ago. John has three children and eight grandchildren who all live nearby. They visit him once or twice a week. Until five years ago, John worked as a shift supervisor at a local post office. He retired at 65 and since then has supported himself on retirement benefits, social security, and a small savings account.

This is John's first visit to the community free clinic. His initial complaint is that he is having "sleep trouble." He has begun to get more worried about his lack of sleep since he now finds it difficult to nap during the day. His children continue to mention how tired he looks and have encouraged him to come to the clinic to get some "strong sleeping pills." He tells the nurse that this is his expectation also and that he is sure he will be fine after he gets the right medicine. No physical causes for John's sleep disturbance were found when a health history and physical examination were performed.

```
┌─────────────────────┐
│     Assessment      │
└─────────────────────┘
 • self-care demand
 • assets
 • limitations
```

John told the nurse that he had tried a number of self-care approaches to deal with his problem. These included:

- Buying earplugs to decrease outside noise at night.
- Drinking warm milk and eating crackers right before sleep.
- Drinking up to four glasses of sherry right before sleep.
- Buying a sleeping medication at the corner drugstore and trying one pill.

None of his efforts were successful in improving his sleep.

Using material from Table 13–6 as a guideline, the nurse helped John to assess his current sleep difficulty. Together they determined that John had no physiological reason for his sleep disturbance. He was in good health; in fact, he had had only two brief contacts with a health care provider when he was a young man and had had pneumonia.

John had a long history of practicing *self-care*. He had *strengths* in the areas of exercise, nutrition, and spirituality. His routine practices in these areas, however, had decreased in the last two months. Since his wife's death, John had not been taking his daily walks or eating quite as well. He had stopped going to church because that activity reminded him so much of his wife. He had also neglected his woodworking hobby.

John's self-care *limitations* were in the area of relaxation. He did not know what it was or how to do it. He did, however, consider himself a "relaxed" person and said that most of his life had been "easy" and "smooth."

There were several important events associated with John's sleep complaints, including:

- The recent death of his wife.
- His concerns about retirement and aging.

- Changes in his relationships with his children, grandchildren, and peers. ("Everyone seems so busy now—no one has time for me.")
- Predictable sleep changes associated with normal aging.

In exploring his *specific sleep patterns*, John and his nurse learned that for the last two months John has had trouble falling asleep, woke up frequently, and often was unable to get back to sleep. He had no family history of sleep disturbance. All of his family members had been quite healthy. He did remember that once in a while his father would take a drink if he had trouble sleeping. John completed the self-assessment tool presented in Figure 13–2.

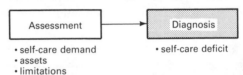

John agreed that he had a self-care deficit in the area of sleep. He had an:

Inability to obtain adequate sleep without education and intervention

His current limitation was primarily related to a lack of knowledge about the way in which the recent events of his life had probably influenced his sleep.

A more traditional medical diagnosis would identify John's problem as *insomnia*. His present difficulty was partially linked to unresolved grief following his wife's death. John was himself at high risk of sudden death in connection with his wife's death.[29]

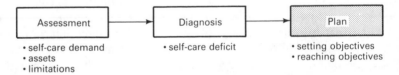

Setting Objectives.

John was reluctant to work on self-care methods to improve his sleep that did not involve medications. He was worried that he would become ill if he did not get some sleep, and he felt desperate to have a "quick cure."

John did agree, however, to try a self-care approach first. His self-contract is presented in Figure 13–3. He thought that he could evaluate his success by whether or not he began to feel more rested when he got up each day. John set the following goals for himself:

Short-term: Keep a sleep diary four out of seven nights.
             Talk about my wife for 10 minutes each time the children come over.
Long-term: Fall asleep within 10 minutes and sleep soundly for five hours at least five times a week.

SLEEP AND DREAMS SELF-ASSESSMENT

Complete the following self-assessment to help you look at the role of sleep and dreams in your life. On the scale below circle the numbers which are most true for you and your life during the last year:

	Almost Never	Seldom	Often	Almost Always
1. I plan regular sleep periods for myself.	1	2	3	(4)
2. I enjoy my sleep periods.	(1)	2	3	4
3. I fall asleep easily without using drugs or alcohol.	1	(2)	3	4
4. I fall asleep within 10-15 minutes of when I lay down for sleep.	(1)	2	3	4
5. I remember my dreams without fear (and learn from them).	1	(2)	3	4
6. I feel that I get adequate sleep.	(1)	2	3	4
7. I am able to go back to sleep quickly when my sleep has been disturbed.	1	(2)	3	4
8. I am able to sleep well even if my environment or schedule changes.	1	(2)	3	4
9. I find it easy to start my day when I wake up.	(1)	2	3	4
10. My family and friends support my need for sleep.	1	2	3	(4)

Some suggestions for how you might learn from this self-assessment:

1. Connect all the circles down the length of the page. Look at the pattern that your connected line makes. Turn your page sideways to get an even more clear visual picture of sleep in your life right now. What does it seem to be saying to you?

2. Now add up your total score: _____ 20

   Circle which range it was in:
   10-19   (20-29)   30-40

   If your score was in the 10-19 range you might want to make some changes in your sleep life. Which aspects do you think need the most work? How many "1's" did you mark on this assessment? 4 These might serve as a clue to help you think about making changes in this area of your life.

3. How would you like this self-assessment to look six months from now? Are you interested in working toward those improvements?

4. Remember to congratulate yourself for the ways that you are providing sleep for yourself. Give yourself a pat on the back.

Figure 13–2. Sleep and dreams self-assessment. *(Adapted with permission from Baldi, S., and others. (1980).* For your health: A model for self-care. *South Laguna, CA: Nurses Model Health.)*

SELF-CONTRACT

MY GOALS:

① Keep a sleep diary 4 out of 7 nights.
② Talk about my wife for 10 minutes

Short-term — by the end of six weeks I will . . . each time the children come over.

Fall asleep within 10 minutes

Long-term— by the end of six months I will . . . and sleep soundly for 5 hrs.
5x/week

ENVIRONMENTAL PLANNING: (all the steps I will take to reach my goal)

1. Read all of the materials about sleep that the nurse gave me.
2. Show my sleep diary to my grandson every afternoon.
3. Complete a "new thought worksheet" and talk about it with my grandson.
4. Do a 10 minute "relaxation exercise" every evening.
5. Plan one pleasant activity to look forward to each day.

THOUGHTS AND ACTIONS

Helpful thoughts:	Helpful actions:
I am really able to learn how to sleep better.	Hot bath, warm milk, soft music.
Non-helpful thoughts:	**Non-helpful actions:**
I'm so old — maybe I should just accept that I'll never sleep well.	① Watch a mystery T.V. program. ② Stay in bed and toss and turn for hours when I wake up.

MY REWARD   (if I meet my goal)   Short term: Dinner with Arnie at Bob's each Saturday
Long term: Trip to Las Vegas with Arnie.

THE COST: (if I fail to meet my goal)   Wash Arnie's car for him.

REEVALUATION DATE: July 1

I agree to help with this project: I agree to strive toward this goal:

Arnie (grandson)   John   May 16
(Support person)   (Your signature)   (date)

Figure 13–3. Self-contract. *(Adapted with permission from Baldi, S., and others. (1980). For your health: A model for self-care. South Laguna, CA: Nurses Model Health, p. 47.)*

Reaching Objectives: Nursing and Client Actions.

John's specific actions to reach his goal are identified in his self-contract. His self-care efforts were completed in three phases. In the *education phase*, he:

- Completed his self-assessment tools.
- Bought and learned to use a sleep diary (Fig. 13–4).
- Learned about normal sleep patterns involved with the aging process.
- Learned about the normal grieving process; recognized that he did not need to be stoic about his wife's death.
- Enlisted the help of his 21-year-old grandson, Arnie, as a support person.

Figure 13–4. Sample client sleep diary. *Form used with permission from Coates, T.J., & Thoreson, C.E. (1977).* How to sleep better. *Englewood Cliffs, NJ: Prentice-Hall, p. 62.*

In the second phase of *cognitive restructuring*, John:

- Learned that many of his thoughts when he was unable to sleep were about his wife and his loneliness.
- Identified his cyclical ways of talking to himself—by telling himself that he could *never* get back to sleep at night, he increased his anxiety and created a "self-fulfilling prophecy."
- Learned new ways of talking to himself during his night waking periods— telling himself that he *would* be able to get back to sleep and that if he did not sleep for one night he would still be able to manage his life.
- Learned that positive changes in behavior often follow positive thoughts; learned that he could relabel and restructure his thoughts.

John began to understand that many psychosocial factors could be influencing his sleep. In the third phase of *long-term planning*, he agreed that he needed to complete a number of specific self-care actions that would promote sleep. These included:

- Getting up and working on a wood project when unable to fall asleep within 20 minutes.
- Having a glass of milk, reading one page of a book, or listening to a record when up during the night.

Enhancing his general self-care activities was also central to his plan. He agreed to:

- Learn a relaxation exercise and practice it with his grandson for 10 minutes each evening.
- Begin to walk one mile with his grandson's dog each evening.
- Plan for one pleasant activity for each week so that he would have something to look forward to.
- Go to the Senior Citizen center once a week to develop new relationships.
- Go to church at least once a month.

During all of these self-care phases, the nurse provided education, consultation, and support. By modeling self-care the nurse helped John to regain his past skills in taking care of himself. Specific nursing actions are outlined in Table 13–7.

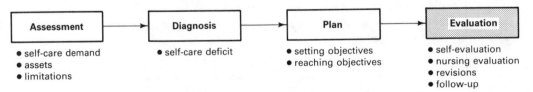

John continued to keep sleep diaries and go over them with his grandson and the nurse each week. During the six-week follow-up session, he reported that he was able to fall asleep quickly (within 15 minutes) four out of seven nights but rarely got five hours of uninterrupted sleep. He said that he did wake up during the night but was able to fall back asleep quickly. He was still troubled by waking up early (5:30 to 6:00 A.M.) but was pleased that he had been successful in setting up a ritual in which he did his deep breathing, got up and did some gentle stretching exercises, and then started on his current project—rather than trying to force himself to go back to sleep. In this way he was less upset about waking up and was able to nap in the afternoon if he was still tired.

An important part of the evaluation process was that during each session he talked about his wife a little more. He had renewed a friendship with one person who had been a mutual friend of theirs; this friend had agreed to go to Las Vegas with John and his grandson to fulfill the contract reward. John said that he would call again if he needed to, but he did not think it would be necessary.

SUMMARY

This chapter presented theories of the function and value of sleep and dreams in promoting health throughout life. A brief discussion of sleep disturbance was provided and specific factors that interfere with sleep were explored. Self-care actions that promote sleep were presented.

The role of the nurse as a model of sleep self-care was described. Ways in which nurses can promote sleep self-care in hospital settings were also explored. A clinical presentation demonstrated integration of these concepts within the nursing process. Self-contracting provided the mechanism to facilitate sleep self-care behavior change.

STUDY QUESTIONS

Personal Focus

1. How do you rate yourself as a model for the practice of sleep self-care?
2. Write down one of your recent dreams. Discuss it with a friend. What can you learn from that dream about enhancing your health?
3. Complete a self-care plan to facilitate your own sleep needs. Evaluate your plan with a friend. What activities can your practice on a regular basis to ensure adequate sleep for yourself?
4. Review your family history regarding sleep and dreams. Were these self-care activities emphasized? Ignored? How can you change current family patterns regarding sleep?

TABLE 13–7. NURSING CARE PLAN

Reason for consultation: Sleep trouble for the last two months

Client: John

Assessment	Plan	Evaluation	
		Met	*Not met*
Self-care demand	*Setting objectives*		
Need for improved sleep	Six weeks:		
Assets	Keep a sleep diary four out of seven nights.	X	
Support of family	Talk about wife for 10 minutes when the kids come over.	X	
Positive history of self-care in other areas	Six months:		
Highly motivated	Fall asleep in 10 minutes and sleep soundly for 5 hours at least five times a week.	(not yet evaluated) but has already reported success.	
Good physical health	*Reaching objectives*		
Life hobbies	Client actions		
Past history of friends and support systems	Short-term:		
Limitations	Buy the diary, talk with the nurse about how to keep it.	X	
Current use of alcohol for stress	Talk to Arnie about being my partner.	X	
Life stress re: recent death of wife	Return to see the nurse in five days.	X	
Developmental changes in sleep patterns secondary to the aging process	Read all the materials about sleep.	X	
Expectation for a "quick cure" through medication	Show the diary to Arnie in the afternoon.		X (only part done)
Recent loss of church as support system			
Recent decrease in exercise patterns			

Diagnosis		
Self-care deficit Inability to obtain adequate sleep without education and intervention	**Long-term:** Complete a "new thought" worksheet and talk to Arnie about it.	x (once)
	Do a 10-minute "relaxation exercise" in afternoon.	x (do know deep-breathing)
	Plan a "pleasant activity" for every day.	x (did four days)
	Nursing actions	
	Explain and demonstrate record-keeping methods.	x
	Teach normal sleep patterns for age.	x
	Teach substitute activities for night waking periods.	x
	Work with grandson as needed.	x
	Model own values regarding sleep.	x
	Rule out physical causes for sleep troubles.	x
	When appropriate help client to continue grieving process.	x
		Needed revisions Subjective report that sleep is better; needs to continue with same process.
	Reevaluation date Formal meeting with nurse for ½ hour each week for six weeks.	**Client follow-up** Plans to use family and friends for additional support.

Client Focus

1. Evaluate your current clinical placement regarding the ways in which the environment either facilitates or limits sleep for clients. Look at sound, light, disturbances, privacy, use of sleeping medications, and so on. Keep a list of your assessment of these issues. Discusss it with your peers.
2. Role-play and practice describing the process of REM rebound to a client.
3. Complete a role-play activity with another student in which you teach a client about the health value of both sleep and dreams.
4. List nursing activities that can facilitate sleep in hospital settings. Discuss them with your peers. Which ones could you implement immediately?
5. Practice teaching a client how to relax before sleep. Consider the use of calming music tapes (see Chapter 9).
6. Complete a self-care/nursing process worksheet with a client. Utilize a self-contract to facilitate sleep self-care behavior change. Discuss your project with your instructors and peers.

REFERENCES

1. Malasanos, L., Barkauskas, V., Moss, M., & Stoltenberg-Allen, K. (1982). Assessment of sleep–wakefulness patterns. In *Health assessment* (2nd ed.). St. Louis, C.V. Mosby, p. 115.
2. Dement, W.C. (1974). *Some must watch while some must sleep*. San Francisco: W. H. Freeman, pp. 35-53.
3. Swerdolff, A. (1981, July). The body's busy night shift. *Science Digest*, p. 68.
4. The Mystery of Sleep. (1981, July 13). *Newsweek*, p. 54.
5. Dement. *Some must watch*, p. 18.
6. Schneider, A.M., & Tarshis, B. (1980). *An introduction to physiological psychology* (2nd ed.). New York: Random House, pp. 316-331.
7. Dement. *Some must watch*. p. 55.
8. Mora, G. (1975). Historical and theoretical trends in psychiatry. In Freedman, A.M., Kaplan, H.I., & Sadock, B.J. (Eds.), *Comprehensive textbook of psychiatry* (Vol. 1). (2nd ed.). Baltimore: Williams & Wilkins, pp. 1-75.
9. Glassman, C. (1981, July). Sleep on it: Using dreams. *Science Digest*, pp. 64-65.
10. Adam, K. (1980, March 6). A time for rest and a time for play. *Nursing Mirror*, p. 18.
11. Roffwarg, H.P., Muzio, J.N., & Dement, W.C. (1966). Ontogenetic development of the human sleep–dream cycle. *Science, 152*, 599-609.
12. Schneider & Tarshis. *Introduction to physiological psychology*, p. 324.
13. Freud, S. (1958). The interpretation of dreams. In J. Strachey (Ed.), *Standard edition of the complete psychological works of Sigmund Freud* (Vols. 4 & 5). London: Hogarth Press.
14. Jung, C.G. (1961). *Memories, dreams, reflections*. New York: Vintage.

15. Coates, T.J., & Thoresen, C.E. (1977). *How to sleep better—A drug-free program for overcoming insomnia.* Englewood Cliffs, NJ: Prentice-Hall, p. 18.
16. LaBerge, S. (1985). *Lucid dreaming.* Los Angeles: J.P. Tarcher.
17. LaBerge, S. (1987, April). Power trips: Controlling your dreams. *OMNI,* p. 1.
18. Hayter, J. (1980). The rhythm of sleep. *American Journal of Nursing,* 457-458.
19. Simonton, C.O., & Simonton, S. (1975). Belief systems and management of the emotional aspects of malignancy. *Journal of Transpersonal Psychology, 7,* 29.
20. Hartmann, E. (1977). L-Tryptophan: A rational hypnotic with clinical potential. *American Journal of Psychiatry, 134,* 366-370.
21. Weilburg, J.B., & Donaldson, S.R. (1988). L-Tryptophan for sleep. *Massachusetts General Hospital Newsletter Biological Therapies in Psychiatry, 11* (4), 13-16.
22. Sleep disorders: Help for the patient who can't sleep. (1976). *Patient Care, 10,* 98-133.
23. Egestein, Q.R., & Barbiasz, J. (1980). Sleep disorders: Recognizing them in patients. *The Journal of Practical Nursing,* 22.
24. How diet affects sleep. (1978, November 16). *Nursing Mirror,* p. 32.
25. Coates & Thoresen. *How to sleep better,* p. 41.
26. Coates & Thoresen. *How to sleep better,* p. 42.
27. Clapin-French, E. (1986). Sleep patterns of aged persons in long-term care facilities. *Journal of Advanced Nursing, 11* (57).
28. Potter, P.A., & Perry, A.G. (1989). *Fundamentals of nursing: Concepts, process and practice* (2nd ed.). St. Louis: C.V. Mosby.
29. Lynch, J. (1977). *The broken heart: The medical consequences of loneliness.* New York: Basic.

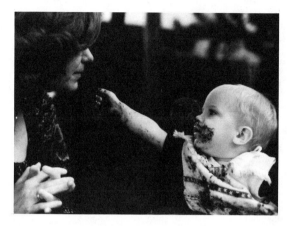

Feed me! I'm yours.

Vicki Lansky, Feed Me! I'm Yours *(New York: Bantam Books, 1974)*

14 Nutrition

LEARNING OBJECTIVES

Upon completion of this chapter, readers will be able to:

1. Define the following terms: food, diet, food habits, nutritional self-care.
2. Describe two self-care activities relative to nutrition at each developmental stage of the life cycle.
3. List the Surgeon General's guidelines for promoting health through nutrition.
4. Identify how the "meaning of food" can affect nutritional behavior.
5. Discuss three nutritional self-care skills.
6. Complete a plan for nutritional self-care behavior change.

DEFINITIONS

Food   Any substance that is eaten. Food is usually for nourishment but may have little or no nutritive value.

Diet   A particular pattern or grouping of foods that are eaten regularly; food considered in terms of its effect on health.

Food Habits   The way in which an individual eats that becomes a typical pattern.

Nutritional Self-Care   Encompasses all of the ways in which people nurture their bodies with food. Nutritional self-care includes *positive* uses of foods to promote health throughout the life span.

Recommended Dietary Allowances (RDAs)   "Levels of intake of essential nutrients which, based on current knowledge, are considered to be adequate to meet the nutritional needs of most healthy persons in the United States."[1]

INTRODUCTION

Americans are bombarded with many specific diet plans that supposedly promote health. Examples of these include the Pritikin, Atkins, Weight Watchers, Nutri-Systems, Cambridge, and Beverly Hills diet. Each has its followers who believe that their particular diet plan is *the* answer to all of their nutritional (and often emotional) needs. Some of these programs include exercise. Some advocate "quick weight loss" but offer no direction for long-term behavior change. Others advocate life-long weight management. All need to be scrutinized closely for nutritional soundness before being adopted.

Nutritional self-care encompasses all of the ways in which people nurture their bodies with food. Self-care implies *positive* uses of food to promote health throughout the life span. Examples include the use of nutrition to promote:

- Growth.
- Parenting, love, and concern.
- Relationships.
- Healing.
- Positive self-images.

Self-care also implies an awareness of how and what one eats and why. This often includes the meaning that food has for each person.

In every society, food and eating behavior is accompanied by many rituals, customs, and beliefs. These are passed on through generations. Children generally model their eating habits after those of their parents. These patterns, once established, frequently persist throughout life. For example, "dinner must include meat and potatoes."

Many mental health specialists believe that a central part of the infant's personality is formed through intimate mother–child interactions that take place around food. The way in which the mother interacts with her child during feeding times communicates to the infant that he or she is special and valued, contributing to the infant's self-esteem and self-concept.

Food is often used in idiosyncratic ways in individual families; for example, as a symbol of love, approval, punishment, or status. An example of its use as a reward is a banana split for good grades; as a punishment, going to bed without supper. Because food can be such a powerful symbol of love and nurturing, many strong feelings and prejudices occur in this area.

Jelliffe developed a classification of foods based on observation of food behavior. It includes:

1. *Cultural superfoods:* Foods that are dominant staples. Their importance is usually reflected in the religion and history of a people. Wheat and corn might be considered cultural superfoods in the United States.
2. *Prestige foods:* Foods that are expensive, difficult to obtain, and generally reserved for special occasions. Lobster tails are an example of a prestige food.
3. *Body-image foods:* Foods identified with the workings of the body to provide optimal health. The "Basic 4" are body-image foods.
4. *Sympathetic magic foods:* Foods that have perceived magical properties. An example is a belief that eating raw meat will make the person's blood stronger.
5. *Physiological group foods:* Foods designated for a particular age, sex, or condition within the society. Many people feel that milk is only for children.[2]

NUTRITION AND HEALTH

Nutritional requirements have been formally defined by the Committee on Dietary Allowances of the Food and Nutrition Board of the National Research Council. They are organized by age groups and are referred to as Recommended Dietary Allowances (RDAs) for a particular age group.[1]

The RDA tables are long and too complex for the average person to use on a daily basis. Nutrition educators have suggested a variety of systems to organize food groups to facilitate self-care education. During World War I, the "Basic 5" were introduced. During World War II, a "Basic 7" became popular. The system in use today, the "Basic 4," evolved as a simplified method to assist people in planning a balanced diet by dividing foods into four groups (Table 14–1; children's portions are listed in Table 14–2).

Criticisms of the Basic 4 include: There is no provision for sufficient caloric intake; nutrients can be missed if only a single food from a group is selected; and some vitamins and minerals are not taken into consideration with this system. These deficiencies can be met by:

TABLE 14–1. THE FOUR FOOD GROUPS

Food Group	Nutrients	
	Good Source of:	Poor Source of:
I. Milk group: milk, cheese, yogurt, cottage cheese, ice cream	Calcium, vitamins A and D, riboflavin, protein	Iron, vitamin C
Servings: Adults: 2 each day, 8 oz or equivalent Teenagers: 4 each day Children: 2–3 each day Pregnancy and lactation: 4–5 each day		
II. Meat group All meats, fish, poultry, eggs Dry beans and dry peas (legumes), nuts, peanut butter	Protein, B vitamins, iron, fats	Vitamins A, C, and D
Servings: 2 each day, 2–3 oz servings		
III. Vegetable–fruit group All vegetables *Deep yellow:* carrots, squash *Dark green:* green peppers, broccoli, spinach, kale, endive, asparagus *Other:* tomato, lettuce, peas, onion, corn, lima beans, beets, potato, cabbage, cauliflower, celery Fruit *Citrus:* orange, grapefruit *Other:* apple, banana, peach, pear, plum, apricot, grapes, berries, prunes	Vitamins A and C, carbohydrate and fiber, iron	Fat
Servings: 4 each day, ½ cup serving		
IV. Bread–cereal group (These should be whole grain or enriched) Bread Cereal (ready to eat) Cereal (cooked) Noodles Macaroni Spaghetti Rice Grits Crackers	Carbohydrate (starch, fiber), B vitamins, iron	Vitamin C
Servings: 4 each day, 1 slice or 1 oz		

(Reprinted with permission from Wenck, D.A. et al. (1980). *Nutrition.* Reston, VA: Reston, p. 10.)

TABLE 14–2 CHILD-SIZE SERVINGS

Daily Need	Serving Sizes for Children	
	2–3 Years Old	3–6 Years Old
3 servings milk	4–6 oz	6 oz
2 servings		
Eggs	½ medium	1 medium
Meat, poultry, fish	1–2 oz	2 oz
3 servings		
Cereal	2 T cooked	¼ cup cooked
	⅓ cup ready to eat	½ cup ready to eat
Bread	¼–½ slice	½ to 1 slice
3 servings		
Vegetables	1–2 T	2–4 T
Fruit	¼–½ of whole fruit	½ of whole fruit
Juice	3–4 oz (⅓–½ cup)	4 oz (½ cup)

(Reprinted with permission from Wenck, D.A. et al. (1980). *Nutrition*. Reston, VA: Reston, p. 332.)

1. Selecting a wide variety of foods within each food group.
2. Using primarily unprocessed foods, such as whole grains rather than enriched white flour products.
3. Selecting dark green leafy vegetables for their high nutritive value.
4. Increasing serving sizes to meet caloric requirements.
5. Using vegetable oil as a fat source to supply vitamin E.[3]

In addition to the Basic 4, the American Dietetic Association and the American Diabetes Association developed another system of food exchanges. These six food exchange lists have become quite popular even among nondiabetics for their simple, easy-to-use format. This new system differs from the Basic 4 in that:

1. It has a separate category for fats.
2. The vegetable–fruit group is two groups: one for vegetables and another for fruits.
3. The vegetable list does not include starchy vegetables such as potatoes and corn. These are included in the bread list.
4. Meats are divided into three groups: lean, medium-fat, and high-fat.

Because of the more specific divisions, many of the criticisms of the Basic 4 are eliminated. Specific information regarding these exchange lists may be found at local offices of the American Diabetes Association.

The benefits to health from good nutrition are becoming better known. These include reduced risk of death and disability from specific diseases. The Surgeon General has documented that 75 percent of all deaths in the United

States are related to degenerative diseases such as heart disease, stroke, and cancer—diseases whose incidences have been linked to dietary factors. This report states that Americans would probably be healthier if they consumed:

- Only calories sufficient to meet body needs and maintain desirable weight (fewer calories if overweight).
- Less saturated fat and cholesterol.
- Less salt.
- Less sugar.
- Relatively more complex carbohydrates, such as whole grains, cereals, fruits, and vegetables.
- Relatively more fish, poultry, legumes, and less red meat.[4]

These guidelines are very general and do not point to a specific diet or program. Instead, they address areas in the "average American diet" that can be changed to promote optimum health and to reduce the risk of degenerative disease.

Using the Surgeon General's guidelines as a base, this chapter identifies nutritional components for self-care as:

- Carbohydrates and fiber
- Fats and cholesterol
- Sugar
- Salt
- Water
- Vitamins and minerals
- Additives and caffeine
- Alcohol

For each area, the following information is included: sources, positive and problematic effects, recommendations, assessment questions, and self-care activities. These tables have been created to provide *beginning* points for the development of nutritional self-care programs. *They are not intended to be comprehensive but only to provide beginning information.*

These topics are reviewed in Tables 14–3 through 14–10.

NUTRITION ACROSS THE LIFE SPAN

There are a variety of factors that influence nutritional requirements at different points throughout life. Age, sex, genetic makeup, activity level, and specific states such as pregnancy, lactation, and illness all play a role in establishing nutritional needs. In addition, there are self-care activities that promote wellness at each developmental point. A brief overview of these self-care activities is found in Table 14.11 (pp. 314–317).

TABLE 14–3 COMPLEX CARBOHYDRATES AND FIBER

Sources	Self-care activities
Whole-grain flours, breads, crackers, cereals, brown rice, fresh fruits, fresh vegetables, legumes, nuts.	Eat whole-grain products: cereals, breads, brown rice.
Positive effects	Read labels to determine if *whole* wheat, *whole* grain.
Mechanically smooths function of large bowel; absorbs water; decreases transit time.	Grow some vegetables—eat from the garden.
May improve irritable bowel syndrome.	Encourage children to participate in seed selection, planting, tending, harvesting, preparation of home-grown foods.
Slow, even energy source; high source of vitamins, minerals, fibers.	Purchase foods as close to "natural" as possible (e.g., fresh squash is preferable to canned or frozen).
Decrease incidence of elevated serum cholesterol; colon, rectal, and breast cancer.	Use an "air popper" to pop corn for an easy snack; do not add butter or salt.
Problematic effects	Use whole-grain flours to make pancakes, waffles, cookies.
Excessive calories if guidelines are exceeded.	Add high-fiber items like wheat germ, bran, oatmeal to "hold together" foods such as burgers, meat loaf, meatballs.
Some conditions (e.g., diverticulitis) might be aggravated by high-fiber diets.	Use special techniques to increase appeal of whole foods to family (e.g., smell of bread baking before dinner, fresh-sliced strawberries on oatmeal).
Recommendations	Provide appetizers with "whole" foods in mind: fresh fruits, raw vegetables, whole-grain crackers.
Four servings whole-grain products per day.	
45–55% of calorie intake from complex CHO.	
Vegetables as desired; three servings fresh fruits.	

The following references were used in the compilation of Tables 14–3 through 14–10:

AHA Committee. (1982). Rationale of the diet–heart statement of the American Heart Association. *Nutrition Today, 17* (5), 17.

Council on Dental Therapeutics. (1979). Prescribing fluoride supplements. In Dosage recommendations for dietary fluoride supplements. *American Journal of Diseases of Children, 133,* 683-684.

Food and Nutrition Board, National Research Council. *Recommended dietary allowances* (9th ed.). Washington, DC: National Academy of Sciences.

Meneely, G.R., & Battarbee, H.D. (1976). Sodium and potassium. In *Nutrition reviews, Present Knowledge in Nutrition* (4th ed.). New York: The Nutrition Foundation, pp. 270-273.

National Advisory Committee of Hyperkinesis and Food Additives. (1977). *Statement summarizing research findings on the issue and relationship between food additive-free diets and hyperkinesis in children.* New York: The Nutrition Foundation.

National Research Council. (1982). Executive summary: Diet, nutrition, and cancer. *Nutrition Today, 17,* (4), 22-23.

U.S. Department of Health, Education and Welfare. (1979). *Healthy people: The surgeon general's report on health promotion and disease prevention.* Washington, DC: U.S. Government Printing Office.

Wenck, D., Baren, M., & Dewan, S.P. (1980). *Nutrition.* Reston, VA: Reston. High blood pressure: Newer treatments. (1989). *Harvard Medical School Health Letter, 14,* (3).

Gleser, R. (1988). *The healthmark program for life.* New York: McGraw-Hill.

Lang, S., (1987, August). Beyond bran. *American Health,* 110-112.

Phillipson, B., Rothrock, D., Connor, W., Harris, W., et al. (1985). Reduction of plasma lipids, lipoproteins, and apoproteins by dietary fish oils in patients with hypertriglyceridemia. *New England Journal of Medicine, 312,* 1210-1216.

Kromhout, D., Bosschieter, E., & deLezenie Coulander, C. (1985). The inverse relationship between fish consumption and 20-year mortality from coronary heart disease. *New England Journal of Medicine, 312,* 1205-1209.

Schommer, N. Nutrition news: Fake fats are on the way. *Longevity, 1,* 8.

TABLE 14–4. FATS AND CHOLESTEROL

Sources

Oils, fats used in cooking, red meats, nuts, organ meats, eggs, shellfish, salad dressings, cheeses, whole dairy products, processed foods, fat substitutes.

Positive effects

Necessary for fatty acid supply; high-density lipoprotein protective of heart, blood vessels.

Problematic effects

Decrease oxygen supply to tissues.

Disturbance in CHO metabolism; low-density lipoprotein atherogenic in increased amounts; effect on very low density lipoprotein unknown.

Recommendations

Decrease overall fat intake; increase of unsaturated over saturated; limit to less than 20% overall calorie intake (5% saturated, 15% unsaturated).

Self-care activities

Use no oil and nonstick skillets for pan frying. If desired, use pump sprayer with commercial nonstick preparation.

Watch content of new fat substitutes.

Use chicken broth to "stir-fry" vegetables, meats.

Use ground turkey instead of ground beef.

Limit intake of red, cured, canned, and processed meats.

Try more alternate protein sources, such as tofu or beans.

"Brown" ground meat in a colander in microwave to allow fat to drain.

Read labels on "basted with butter" poultry for added fat and chemicals.

Eat foods that contain lecithin.

Skin poultry before cooking.

Use polyunsaturated oils, margarine instead of lard, bacon grease, butter.

Limit egg consumption to two per week or cholesterol intake to 300 mg/day.

Use two egg whites instead of one whole egg.

Consume fish high in Omega-3 fatty acids (i.e., salmon, albacore tuna).

Use tuna canned in water (low or no salt) instead of oil pack.

Use nonfat dairy products: milk, hoop cheese, sapsago cheese, yogurt.

Use low-fat, low-carlorie mayonnaise.

Replace use of sour cream with low-fat or nonfat yogurt.

Know serum cholesterol level and all lipoprotein levels.

Maintain your cholesterol–HDL ratio below 3.5 (total cholesterol divided by HDL).

Maintain total cholesterol below 200 mg/dl.

Maintain HDL levels;
  Men $>$ 45 mg/dl
  Women $>$ 55 mg/dL.

Maintain LDL $<$ 130 mg/dL.

Maintain VLDL $<$ 150 mg/dl.

Maintain triglycerides $<$ 150 mg/dl.

(Sources: See Table 14–3.)

TABLE 14–5. SUGAR

Sources	Self-care activities
Sources Added sugars, some baked goods, processed foods, salad dressings, condiments, soft drinks, cereals, canned fruits, canned vegetables, honey, fresh fruit. **Positive effects** Energy source. **Problematic effects** Lack of vitamins, minerals, fiber in "empty calories." Contributes to cardiovascular disease, diabetes mellitus, obesity, dental caries. Increases serum triglycerides. Associated with hyperactivity in children and depression in adults. **Recommendations** Decrease overall intake.	Sweeten baked goods with unsweetened apple juice concentrate or dried fruits. Read labels for hidden sugars: sucrose, lactose, glucose, maltose, corn syrup, turbinado, molasses, honey. Sweeten cereals with fresh fruit or chopped dried fruit; add small amount of apple juice concentrate to milk. Limit intake of simple refined sugars found in baked goods, candies, soft drinks, and so on. Use fresh fruits instead of those canned in syrup; many fruits are available packed in fruit juice with no added sugars. Use unsweetened applesauce on pancakes or waffles instead of butter or syrup; "syrups" made from cooked dried fruits such as apricots, apple juice concentrate, almond extract, and cardamom are good alternatives. Use fresh or dried fruits for snacks. Substitute diluted, unsweetened fruit juice for soft drinks; *initially* mix with carbonated water to provide fizzy effect, then delete carbonated water.

(Sources: See Table 14.3)

VARIATIONS IN NUTRITIONAL PRACTICES

There are a variety of nutritional practices that differ from "common" food habits. These practices need to be considered when helping clients learn sound nutritional self-care.

- *Vegetarianism:* There are two types: pure or true vegetarians, who consume no animal products, and lacto-ovo vegetarians, who may consume milk, milk products, and eggs. True vegetarians must be skilled at combining vegetable products to ensure consumption of complete proteins.[5]
- *Fasting:* A variety of liquids may be consumed during a fast according to specific guidelines. The period of fasting may vary widely. Adequate nutritional intake may be very difficult to maintain over time, even if periods of fasting are very limited. Medically supervised fasts are also becoming commonplace. Fasting may be related either to health or religious practices.

TABLE 14–6. SALT

Sources	Self-care activites
Added salt, processed foods, canned foods, cured meats, frozen foods, some seasonings. Naturally found in most foods in safe amounts.	Use spices, vinegars, lemon, lime to provide taste instead of salt.
Positive effects	Read labels for hidden salt, sodium content; most canned, processed, cured meats, and frozen foods contain high amounts.
Needed for fluid and electrolyte balance.	Buy canned items with no salt or low salt.
Problematic effects	Avoid spices such as "lemon pepper" or "seasoned pepper" with *salt* listed as their primary ingredient.
May exacerbate hypertension or precipitate edema.	Remove salt-shaker from the table and cooking area.
Recommendations	Put shakers of spices or dried chili peppers on the table.
Limit intake to 2–3 grams a day unless specific sodium restriction is given; adequate sodium contained naturally in foods.	Start an herb garden; encourage children to participate in tending and then using fresh herbs to season foods.
	Use low-sodium baking powder or yeast as leavening agent; yeast contains many B vitamins.
	Read drug labels; many over-the-counter drugs, particularly antacids, have high sodium content.

(Sources: See Table 14.3.)

Special diets are also used to treat various illnesses and chronic diseases. Examples of these conditions include: diabetes mellitus, colitis, hypertension, cholecystitis, renal disease, allergies, and hypoglycemia. Specific information regarding nutritional requirements for these conditions may be found in therapeutic nutrition or nursing texts. The primary role of the nurse in working with clients who have special dietary needs is to assist them in practicing nutritional self-care within the constraints of their condition or illness.

NUTRITIONAL DISORDERS

Although the focus of this text is on health promotion, there are several nutritional disorders that deserve mention. Nurses often recognize these problems when working with supposedly well clients. Additional information about these disorders can be obtained from nursing and therapeutic nutrition texts.

- *Anorexia nervosa:* A preoccupation with "thinness" occurs, resulting in a lack of food intake. Fluid and electrolyte and cardiac disorders are

TABLE 14–7. WATER

Sources	Self-care activities
Drinking water, coffee, soda, tea, milk, fruits, vegetables.	Drink 6-8 glasses of water per day. Flavor with lemon, lime, or herb tea to vary taste and increase appeal.
Positive effects	
Required for all chemical reactions in body that convert food to energy and body tissue.	Make self-contract to drink 8 ounces every two hours for first week when changing this behavior.
Cells bathed in solutions containing vital nutrients and oxygen.	Find *content* of water supply from water company; be aware of pollutants such as lead, asbestos, mercury and additives such as fluoride. Inform pediatrician of levels.
Primary component of blood.	
Aid to temperature regulation of body.	
Problematic effects	Have emergency supply of water stored for drinking.
Toxic reactions to contaminated water.	Eat fresh fruits and vegetables that have high water content.
Persons with certain disease processes can become over-hydrated.	Provide children with adequate water; pay particular attention to this with increased exercise, illness (fever and diarrhea), in summertime, and in hot weather.
Water intoxication from drinking massive amounts (exceeding the kidneys' filtration ability).	Increase water consumption with vigorous exercise, warm weather, fever, or diarrhea.
Recommendations	
Drink from healthy water supply.	
One glass of fluid with meals, at least one in between each meal; 6-8 glasses daily; pregnant, lactating women may require 8 or more glasses daily.	

(Sources: See Table 14.3.)

common with this condition. Starvation is possible. It occurs most commonly in adolescent women.[6]

- *Bulimia:* Food habits involve "gorging" or "binging," then inducing emesis to prevent weight gain. This also occurs most often in adolescent and young adult women.[6]
- *Pica:* Involves the persistent eating of nonnutritive substances, such as paint, plaster, string, sand, cigarette butts, leaves, or rocks. For pregnant women, the most common substance is constarch. This occurs primarily in infants and children, although it may occur in pregnant women.[6]

TABLE 14–8. VITAMINS AND MINERALS

Sources 　Most foods, supplements. **Positive effects** 　Strengthening of bones; forma- 　tion of blood, oxygenation; aids 　metabolism, vision, integrity of 　epithelial tissue; minerals part of 　intracellular enzymes. **Problematic effects** 　Toxic in excessive doses. **Recommendations** 　Refer to Recommended Dietary 　　Allowances (RDA)*. 　Fluoride supplement in children. 　Iron supplement for women in 　　childbearing years.	**Self-care activities** 　Eat balanced diet of fresh, unprocessed 　　foods. 　Steam or stir-fry vegetables to prevent 　　vitamin loss. 　Eat vegetables and fruits raw. 　Select supplements carefully; use guidance 　　of health care professional skilled in this 　　area. 　Select whole-grain foods. 　Make a game out of developing vitamin in- 　　take assessment with family. 　Make children aware of vitamin/mineral 　　function through pictures—feature a dif- 　　ferent food with its good ingredients each 　　week on refrigerator door. 　Have home reference with specific develop- 　　mental needs (e.g., pregnancy, adolescence, 　　menopause, etc.). 　Ask health care provider about supplements 　　needed to counteract effects of certain 　　medications, such as birth control pills, 　　diuretics, etc. 　Take additional vitamin C when ill.

(Sources: See Table 14.3.)
*Food and Nutrition Board, National Research Council. (1980). *Recommended dietary allowance* (9th ed.).
Washington, DC: National Academy of Sciences.

Medical interventions are usually required for these disorders. Self-care approaches can then be encouraged in conjunction with medical treatment.

NUTRITIONAL SELF-CARE SKILLS

There are a number of general self-care skills that apply to all aspects of healthy nutrition. Learning and practicing these skills is a life-long process.

1. Reading labels
   - Ingredients are listed in order of the amount contained in the prod-uct, with the largest amount listed first.
   - Contact manufacturer regarding products with unlisted ingredients.
   - Standardized products are not required to list ingredients (for exam-ple, ice cream).
2. Making meal times pleasant

TABLE 14–9. ADDITIVES AND CAFFEINE[a]

Additives	Self-care activities: Additives
Sources Processed, packaged foods, vitamins and minerals, over-the-counter drugs. **Positive effects** Provide color, make foods and drugs resistant to spoilage, enhance flavor, provide consistency. **Problematic effects** Associated with impaired learning performance in children. May provoke disturbed behavior in children. May be carcinogenic. **Recommendation** Consume as little as possible.	Read labels to determine types of additives used; know which are safest (i.e., beta carotene is a natural colorant). Consume *fresh* vegetables, fruits, meats. Avoid excessive quantities of any single processed food. Become knowledgeable about different types of additives and their effects. Teach children to be label readers and aware of additives, risks, functions. Write manufacturers of unlabeled products to determine additives used. Reduce animal fat intake (pesticides accumulate here). Refrigerate fresh foods immediately after purchase. Grow own fruits and vegetables when possible.

Caffeine	Self-care activities: Caffeine
Sources Coffee, tea, cola drinks, some non-cola soft drinks, over-the-counter drugs. **Positive effects** Used clinically as a stimulant. **Problematic effects** Stimulant; insomnia; elevation of blood pressure; implicated in birth defects, fibrocystic breast disease (although this is controversial), PMS. **Recommendation** Consume as little as possible.	Withdraw from caffeine slowly; decrease 1 cup per day per week until consumption at desired level (rapid withdrawal is associated with severe headache). Have noncaffeinated beverages available: herb teas, decaffeinated coffees, juices, mineral waters. Limit caffeine intake 3–4 hours before sleep. Read labels for hidden caffeine consumption.

[a]Additional information on caffeine is contained in Chapter 13.
(Sources: See Table 14.3.)

- Promote a calm, pleasant atmosphere (for example, use quiet music, conversation, candles, flowers).
- Recognize each individual present in a positive way.
- Turn TV set off to promote conversation.

3. Shopping
   - Prepare menus for the coming week.
     Saves money.
     Allows for thoughtful nutritional planning.

TABLE 14–10. ALCOHOL (ETOH)

Sources	Self-care activities
Liquor, wine, beer, medications.	Celebrate with sparkling fruit juices; they are festive for children also.
Positive effects	Drink dry white wine, mineral water, or exotic fruit drinks without alcohol.
Relaxation, vasodilation.	Be aware of effect of ETOH on your body; validate with spouse, friends.
Problematic effects	Know alcohol content of beverages.
Danger of addiction; damage to liver, nervous system; congenital birth defects; precipitates hypertension in some people; continued overindulgence can destroy relationships, physical health.	Keep an ETOH diary for six months to determine drinking patterns.
	Use a "stop drinking program" if needed.
	Do not drink and drive.
Recommendations	Do not mix medications with alcohol.
Do not use alcohol for insomnia or pain control.	Role model responsible behavior with ETOH to children; show them it is easy to have fun socially without drinking.
Limit to two servings/week.	Learn and teach concepts of tolerance, dependence, intoxication.
Measure intake by the ounce— not by glass.	Learn withdrawal symptoms, potential dangers.
	Take turns being the driver for the evening when drinking with friends.

(Sources: See Table 14.3.)

> Involves entire family in a unified approach to the nutritional self-care process.
- Eat before going shopping to prevent impulse purchasing.

4. Eating out
   - Read menus carefully.
   - Ask waiter about ingredients.
   - Order meat broiled instead of fried or sauteed.
   - Ask for salad dressing on the side.
   - Order baked potato "dry" (without butter or sour cream).
   - Top salads and potatoes with other condiments: vinegar, salsa, lemon, chives.
   - Eat out at restaurants that serve foods known to be prepared with low fat, low sodium guidelines (Pritikin, Health Mark, etc.).
   - Order decaffeinated coffee or herb tea.
   - Order fresh fruit for dessert.

5. Snacking
   - Prepare "old standards."
     Pre-cut fresh vegetables and leave in refrigerator.
     Dip vegetables in salsa or dip made with hoop cheese instead of sour cream.

TABLE 14–11. NUTRITIONAL SELF-CARE ACTIVITIES THROUGHOUT THE LIFE SPAN

Developmental Stage	Nutritional Considerations	Self-Care Activities
Infancy	Feeding experiences promote bonding with significant others.	Hold baby close during feeding. Feed promptly when hunger noticed.
	Iron stores are depleted by 4–5 months.	Add iron supplement 4–5 months.
	Primary teeth begin erupting at about 6 months.	Introduce solid foods 4–6 months. Begin with strained, mushy foods. Progress to bite-size by 10–12 months.
		Introduce new foods one at a time at weekly intervals to screen for allergy.
		Offer foods from six exchanges by end of first year.
	Overweight infants have increased incidence of lower respiratory infection and an increased number of fat cells.	Allow child to determine quantity of foods. Allow, encourage child to self-feed when able.
	Underweight infants have: slow bone growth, delayed calcification, slow fat deposition, retarded growth of lean body mass, smaller reserve, and higher susceptibility to illness.	Encourage physical activity.
	Infants who drink cows' milk are subject to dehydration during hot weather, or during illness with vomiting, fever or diarrhea.	Give fluid supplements: water and/or electrolyte solution.
	Skim milk lacks calories, linoleic acid, and results in an increased renal solute load for infants.	Limit use of skim milk before 1 year of age.
Toddler	Toddlers eat less than infants because of change in rate of growth.	Use "serving size rule:" one teaspoon or bite of each food for each year of age.
	Coordination can be poor and eating messy.	Offer finger foods.
		Offer praise for self-feeding.
	Molars may not have erupted.	Avoid inappropriate foods: tough, stringy foods, nuts, popcorn, peanut butter, raw carrots, hot dogs.
	Iron is often deficient in diet.	Offer iron supplements, foods high in iron.
	Toddler begins to identify and model food habits.	Provide good modeling of nutritional self-care.

314

Stage	Characteristics	Interventions
Preschool	Activity level strongly influences amount of foods consumed. May "play too hard to eat." Likes to make choices and help prepare foods. Suspicious of new foods. May dislike "strong-tasting" foods.	Make nutritious snacks. Offer foods cut in finger-sized pieces. Have child help prepare meal, set table. Begin nutrition education. Arouse interest in foods. Talk about it when buying, storing, preparing. Model good nutritional self-care. Introduce small amounts of spicy foods, broccoli, cabbage, and so forth.
School-age	Appetite may be low or fluctuate. Sedentary children become overweight. Beginning to eat away from nuclear family. Stable mealtimes may be difficult to maintain as activities increase. Nutrition may affect school performance. Some nutritious snacks such as peanut butter or dried fruit may also promote tooth decay.	*Child:* Gain new skills in balancing own energy input and output. Learn to avoid foods with caffeine and stimulants. Choose healthy snacks. *Parent:* Provide for dental self-care. Provide nutritious snacks. Model nutrition self-care. Praise wise choices. Encourage physical activity.
Adolescence	Most common nutritional problems are tooth decay, anemia, and obesity. Key period in acquiring adult habits. American obsession with thinness may precipitate fad diets, bulimia, or anorexia nervosa. Strenuous physical activity requires additional calories, fluids. Growth spurts and periods of heavy appetite vary widely. Many adolescents have sound nutritional knowledge.	*Adolescent:* Provide for own iron intake. Balance own energy input/output. Model nutrition self-care for peers/family. Provide for adequate fluid/caloric intake. *Parent:* Provide for dental self-care. Support self-care activities. Continue nutrition education. Praise wise choices. Allow to budget, plan, shop, and prepare family foods.

Table 14–11 cont.

Young adulthood	Leaving home for college, job, marriage. New responsibility for budgeting, planning, preparing foods. Metabolic rate leveling off. Caloric intake tied to activity level.	Model nutrition self-care for peers/family. Plan eating out carefully. Increase skills in budgeting and shopping. Alter intake in response to changes in exercise and stress levels.
Pregnancy/ lactation	Mother's nutritional status affects the health of fetus, infant. Adequate calories, fluid, nutrient intake to meet demands of developing fetus and nursing infant.	Increase water intake to 6–8 glasses per day, more in hot weather. Eat regularly 5–6 times per day to develop regular supply of nutrients, fluids, calories. Balance energy input and output. Avoid alcohol, caffeine, over-the-counter drugs. Use LaLeche League for additional information, support.
Middle age	Nutrition-related conditions may surface during this time: cardiovascular disease, diabetes mellitus, gallbladder disease, liver disease. Changing life-style: decreased child-care responsibilities, career involvement, slower physical pace. Metabolic rate decreasing. Body image changing.	Maintain exercise program to offset decreasing metabolic rate. Keep alcohol, caffeine intake at a minimum. Provide for regular mealtimes and break times. Balance energy input and output. Maintain calcium intake to prevent osteoporosis.

Later adulthood	Aging process affects nutritional planning: decrease in taste sensitivity, decrease in gastric secretion, decrease in metabolic rate, declining body mass.	Balance energy input and output. Limit fatty, spicy foods as needed. Limit sugar intake. Eat small, more frequent meals.
	Food selection may be attached to memories: e.g., may like dill pickles because of the memory of growing and canning cucumbers.	
	Food purchases are influenced by: changing financial status, ability to get to and from marketplace, physical stamina to prepare foods, interest in food preparation (particularly if living alone), ability to chew and digest foods, and beliefs of nutritional models.	Use available services such as: meals-on-wheels, senior centers, food stamp programs to provide supplementary assistance.
		Consider strengths and limitations when planning diet.
	Aging adults generally need: more protein, iron, calcium, vitamins A and C, folic acid, and fiber. They usually need less fat, sugar, sodium, and fewer calories.	Use selected convenience foods when necessary. Encourage eating with another, sharing of food preparation.

(Sources: Jelliffe, D.B. (1977). Protein in cow's milk. *Nutrition and the M.D., 3* (4), 2; Kandzari, J., & Howard, J. (1981). *The well family: A developmental approach to assessment.* Boston: Little, Brown, pp. 167-222; Knittle, J.L. (1972) Obesity in childhood: A problem in adipose tissue cellular development. *Journal of Pediatrics, 81,* 1048; Neumann, C.G. (1975). Obesity in infancy—prevention and management. *Nutrition and the M.D., 1* (9), 1; Wenck, D.A., Baren, M.., & Dewan, S.P. (1980). *Nutrition.* Reston, VA: Reston; Winick, M. (1977). Nutrition and aging. *Contemporary Nutrition, 2* (6).)

Leave basket of fresh fruit on counter.

Use air-popped popcorn as a TV snack (no butter or salt); season with paprika, ground garlic, or parmesan cheese.

Make pots of herb teas, herb sun teas, and pitchers of fruit juices.

- Encourage children and their friends to help prepare snacks.
- Make cookies with whole-grain flours, grains, nuts, dried fruits, and sweeten with unsweetened apple juice concentrate.

6. Cocktail hour
   - Order dry white wine if drinking at all.
   - Order exotic fruit drinks without alcohol.
   - Order mineral water with a twist of lime.
   - Serve unsalted nuts, vegetables, air-popped popcorn.
   - Keep sauces separate for those who like ungarnished foods.
   - Offer alternatives to liquor: mineral water, fruit juice, sugar-free soda.

7. Support systems
   - Group together with family and friends to exchange recipes.
   - Use food clubs to order bulk goods.
   - Purchase unprocessed foods.

8. Family projects
   - Teach children about food selection and preparation.
   - Make a family project to take turns selecting and cooking foods.
   - Have children make their own sandwiches, cut up fruit salads, assist in tending the family garden.

9. Food diaries
   - Keep a food diary (food habits and patterns are easier to see when written down).
   - Learn to pay attention to how your body works and reacts to foods. (For example, notice if you feel sluggish after eating certain foods. Are you more active? Unable to sleep? Do you get headaches?)

10. Exercise
    - Regulate food intake with activity level.
    - Learn about fluid supplements during periods of strenuous exercise (see Chapter 12).
    - Exercise strenuously 20 to 30 minutes three to five times per week.
    - Use stairs rather than elevators.
    - Walk instead of driving whenever possible.
    - Develop indoor exercises for inclement weather.
    - Teach children the value of exercise and its relationship to food intake.

11. Relaxation
    - Substitute relaxation techniques for an emotional urge to eat or avoid eating.
    - Practice relaxation 15 minutes every day.

12. Knowledge of food needs
    - Become knowledgeable about food needs, amounts, and quality.
    - Update this knowledge regularly.
    - Develop knowledge base for special nutritional needs during illness, stress and specific developmental periods.
13. Self-awareness
    - Learn to know when you are full, hungry, or in need of additional fluids.
    - Learn the ways in which anger, joy, tension, and depression influence your nutritional habits.
    - Use a food journal and self-contracting to build and maintain self-awareness.

NURSES MODEL NUTRITIONAL SELF-CARE

Nurses have an important role as models of nutritional self-care. Traditionally, they have been involved with ordering diets and bringing trays to the bedside. Do clients perceive that this is what the nurse believes is best for them in the way of foods? Are snacks of Jello, sugared custard, whole milk, and sugared soft drinks nutritionally sound?

Ambulatory clients, families, and peers frequently have the opportunity to observe firsthand the nurse's nutritional habits. Coffee breaks and meals are frequently taken in the cafeteria. Some hospitals now have fast-food restaurants such as McDonalds.[7] Do drinking coffee, smoking cigarettes, and eating sweet rolls model good nutritional self-care? It is often thought that having a cup of coffee will provide a "minute to relax" and will reduce the stress of work. In fact, the caffeine produces the same physiological response as work stress.

In their personal and professional lives, nurses act as role models for families and friends. Figure 14–1 presents a nutritional self-assessment tool that nurses can use in assessing personal self-care skills in this area. In their personal lives, modeling of nutritional self-care may include:

- Avoiding the purchase of potato chips and sodas "for the kids."
- Eating fresh fruits and vegetables rather than "empty calorie" snack foods.
- Purchasing only healthful foods.
- Planning for personal nutritional behavior change.
- Supporting family and friends involved in food behavior change.
- Limiting intake of caffeine and alcohol.
- Teaching children about reading labels and other nutritional self-care skills.
- Avoiding dangerous fad diets.

This modeling also occurs in nurses' professional lives. This can be facilitated by:

- Offering healthful bedtime snacks instead of Jello or sugar-laden custard.
- Providing caffeine-free and sugar-free beverages.
- Asking families to bring healthful snacks from home for clients.
- Making wise choices in the cafeteria.
- Providing herb teas and fruit for meetings or classes instead of coffee and doughnuts.
- Making mealtimes pleasant for clients.
- Taking nutritious food to potluck suppers.
- Advocating for low-fat, low-sodium, high fiber foods in the cafeteria and served to clients.

CLINICAL APPLICATION

Case Presentation

John is a 35-year-old who holds a middle-management position in a large business concern. He is a typical type A personality. After experiencing a great deal of stress over a pending promotion, he felt the need to have his annual physical examination two months early. He is married and has no children, although his wife, Laura, is currently six months pregnant. He works 60 hours per week and has to squeeze playtime and rest around his work schedule. Their family is upper-middle-class and live in a surburban area.

During the appointment with his health care professional, John was identified as being a diet-controlled, adult-onset diabetic and as having mild hypertension. It was suggested that he lose 10 to 15 pounds. In a collaborative role, John's physician referred him to both a registered dietician and a nurse for work in these self-care areas. The *dietician* worked specifically with John on his *diabetic diet* and communicated frequently with the nurse.

The *nurse* practitioner decided to develop a *self-care program* with John. Particular attention was to be given to self-care activities that would influence his mild hypertension.

Assessment

- self-care demand
- assets
- limitations

The nutrition self-assessment in Figure 14–1 was used as a starting point with John. His particular areas of difficulty were label reading, eating at fast-food restaurants, salting his food, using whole dairy products, consuming up to 10 cups of coffee daily, and eating a lot of meat; he infrequently ate fresh fruits and vegetables.

NUTRITION SELF-ASSESSMENT

Complete the following self-assessment to help you look at the role of nutrition in your life. On the scale below circle the numbers which are most true for you and your life during the last year:

	Almost Never	Seldom	Often	Almost Always
1. I read the labels for ingredients of food I consume.	1	②	3	4
2. I have two meatless days a week.	①	2	3	4
3. I eat food without salting it.	①	2	3	4
4. My meals include nonfat or lowfat milk and dairy products.	①	2	3	4
5. I limit my meals at fast food restaurants to twice a week.	1	②	3	4
6. I limit myself to three alcoholic drinks per week (including wine or beer).	1	2	3	④
7. I limit my caffeine use to three times per week (coffee, tea, cola drinks, etc.).	①	2	3	4
8. I limit sweet desserts to three times per week.	1	2	3	④
9. My typical meals include fresh fruits and raw vegetables.	1	②	3	4
10. Meal times are pleasant to me.	1	2	3	④

Some suggestions for how you might learn from this self-assessment:

1. Connect all the circles down the length of the page. Look at the pattern that your connected line makes. Turn your page sideways to get an even more clear visual picture of your nutritional habits. What does it seem to be saying to you?

2. Now add up your total score: _____ *22*

   Circle which range it was in:
      10-19   (20-29)   30-40

   If your score was in the 10-19 range you might want to make some changes in which you play. Which aspects do you think need the most work? How many "1's" did you mark on this assessment? *4* These might serve as a clue to help you think about making changes in this area of your life.

3. How would you like this self-assessment to look six months from now? Are you interested in working toward those improvements?

4. Remember to congratulate yourself for the ways in which you are providing good nutrition for yourself. Give yourself a pat on the back; go out and eat something "good" as a way to congratulate yourself!

Figure 14–1. Nutrition self-assessment. *(Adapted with permission from Baldi, S., and others. (1980). For your health: A model for self-care. South Laguna, CA: Nurses Model Health, p. 54.)*

John was unaware that these nutritional habits could be contributing to his disease processs; his nurse felt that it was essential that he understand the relationship between these practices and his physical condition.

John also identified his strengths. They included limiting intake of alcohol and sweets and finding mealtimes pleasant. His other self-care activities included playing racquetball once a week and an occasional game of golf on weekends. He had two new sources of motivation: his newly diagnosed diabetes and a new baby on the way. Laura was willing and eager to help in any way possible.

It was also necessary that John look at his food habits in the context of his past social, cultural, and economic life. John revealed that his parents had been very poor during his childhood and that food had played an important role in his life. As a consequence, he enjoyed doing business while eating at gourmet restaurants. He did this at least four times a week. It was on these occasions that he consumed five to six cups of coffee at a single dinner meeting. John wanted to address the problem of his caffeine intake before working on the other acknowledged self-care deficits.

Further assessment of John's caffeine consumption revealed that he had been drinking 8 to 10 cups of coffee per day for the last two years. He also:

- Had had some caffeine intake since age 14.
- Valued coffee as part of all social settings.
- Only drank other types of caffeinated beverages once per week.
- Liked fresh-ground, drip-brewed coffee.
- Did not add sugar or cream.
- Had a coffee maker on his desk at work.
- Had tried to stop four times in the last year. His stopping was abrupt; he got terrible headaches and drank coffee to relieve them.

The nurse talked with John and Laura to facilitate self-exploration, determine the significance of his coffee intake and identify associated problems. At the completion of the interview, John took the Nutrition Diary (Fig. 14–2) home with him to record additional dietary information to be utilized in later sessions.

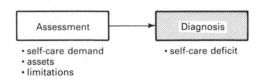

In a collaborative decision, John and the nurse agreed that he had a self-care deficit:

Inability to limit caffeine intake due to inadequate education and motivation

Meal	Monday		Tuesday		Wednesday		Thursday		Friday		Saturday		Sunday	
Breakfast	Eggs 2 Toast O.g. Coffee x2	1 5 5	none		none		Coffee x 3	5	Cereal Coffee	5	Waffles Eggs 2 Coffee	1 5	Coffee Rolls Juice	5 3
Lunch	Steak sandwich Coffee x2	1 2 5	Salad Coffee	5	none		Burrito Chips Coffee x2	1 2 5	Fried chicken Salad Coffee	1	none		none	
Dinner	none		Baked Chicken Broccoli with butter milk	1 1	Prime Rib Baked pot w/sour cream Salad w/oleo Pie, Wine Coffee x 3	1 2 5 1 3	Spaghetti Salad Garlic bread Coffee x1	1 2 5 5	none		Bar-b-qued steak Salad Beer	2 1	Ham and Cheese Sand. Coffee	4 1 5
Snacks what eaten:	Coffee x 5	5	Coffee apple	5	Coffee x 5	5	Coffee Roll x 6	5 3	Coffee Roll x 5	5 3	Coffee x 4	5	Beer	2
Other self-care activities (e.g. relaxation, exercise, etc.)					Racquet-ball x 1 hr.				Read book on relaxation skills for 30 min.				Golf 18 holes	
What were you doing or feeling?	Worked late				Planning big dinner meeting		Kids on my nerves today		Fell asleep after work				Anxious. Boss is demanding	

IDENTIFY FOODS: 1. High fat or cholesterol 2. High salt 3. High sugar 4. Highly processed 5. Caffeinated beverage

Figure 14–2. Nutrition diary. *(Adapted with permission from Baldi, S., and others. (1980). For your health: A model for self-care. South Laguna, CA: Nurses Model Health, p. 71.)*

A nursing diagnosis might read:

Alteration in nutrition related to excess caffeine intake

The deficit was related to his past social, cultural, and economic experiences.

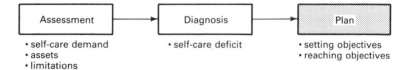

Assessment	Diagnosis	Plan
• self-care demand • assets • limitations	• self-care deficit	• setting objectives • reaching objectives

Setting Objectives

John's initial response had been to tackle the problem and stop using all caffeine immediately. He felt that the 8 to 10 cups of coffee daily were affecting his life in many ways. He was aware that his physician felt that excess caffeine might be contributing to his mild hypertension.

Some of the considerations in setting objectives for caffeine reduction were:

- Gradual reduction of caffeine intake to prevent withdrawal symptoms.
- Assessment of other stimulants consumed.
- Plans for substitution in situations where coffee was previously consumed.
- Identification of physical and emotional benefits of a lowered caffeine intake.
- Provision of a resource person for problems and questions.

John and the nurse agreed on a short-term goal:

To limit coffee to two cups per day by the end of six weeks

To accomplish this, John was to eliminate one cup of coffee per day each week (see Fig. 14–3), thus making the withdrawal gradual and more comfortable.

John was not willing to eliminate coffee totally from his life. There were business and social functions when drinking coffee was too important to him. His long-term goal of:

Eliminating coffee five days a week (allowing one cup two days a week)

was flexible enough to avoid predetermined failure.

Reaching Objectives: Nursing and Client Actions

Laura served as John's support person. A conference call with the nurse once a week for the first three weeks to discuss feelings and problems surrounding these issues was planned.

John's environmental planning included:

- Having herb teas and caffeine-free sodas to drink at work and at home.
- Brewing caffeine-free coffee and tea in his coffee maker at work.
- Arranging in advance to have brewed decaffeinated coffee at his favorite restaurant.
- Attending university extension classes regarding nutritional self-care.
- Marking on his calendar when he drank coffee, how much, and in what situation.
- Recording on a calendar his physical and emotional symptoms when he had caffeine.

The nurse's support of John included:

- Providing information about courses available through university extension.
- Being available for conference calls.

SELF-CONTRACT

MY GOALS:

Short-term— by the end of six weeks I will . . . *Limit coffee to 2 cups every day.*

Long-term— by the end of six months I will . . . *Eliminate coffee 5 days a week, (Allow 1 cup 2 days / week).*

ENVIRONMENTAL PLANNING: (all the steps I will take to reach my goal)

1. Have herb tea and caffeine-free sodas to drink at work and home.
2. Complete diary.
3. Arrange to have brewed decaffeinated coffee at my favorite restaurant.
4. Weekly conference call.
5. Talk to Laura about above.

THOUGHTS AND ACTIONS

Helpful thoughts:	Helpful actions:
I sleep better without so much coffee.	Buy teapot for the office.
Non-helpful thoughts:	**Non-helpful actions:**
My grandfather always drinks 6 cups and he's 86!	Going to business meetings unprepared without anything to drink.

MY REWARD (if I meet my goal) Short-term – A play in town, 6/16 Long-term – Weekend in mountains, 10/28

THE COST: (if I fail to meet my goal) Do all of the grocery shopping for three weeks.

REEVALUATION DATE: 6/15

I agree to help with this project: *Laura* (Support person)

I agree to strive toward this goal: *John* (Your signature)   4/28 (date)

Figure 14–3. Self-contract. *(Adapted with permission from Baldi, S., and others. (1980). For your health: A model for self-care. South Laguna, CA: Nurses Model Health, p. 47.)*

- Educating John and Laura regarding:
  Signs and symptoms of caffeine withdrawal.
  Safety measures.
  Times to call the nurse.
  Relaxation techniques to use in lieu of caffeine intake.
- Providing blood pressure baselines to evaluate the effect of caffeine reduction.

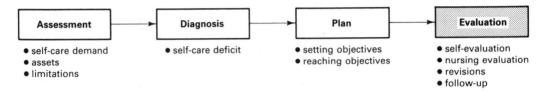

In each weekly conference call, the progress of the plan was reviewed. John had headaches the first couple of days and was tempted to take an over-the-counter analgesic for it together with an extra cup of coffee. He remembered the questions on his assessment tool about label reading and discovered that there was caffeine in his favorite analgesic. Frustrated, he left the office, took a long walk, and stopped in the park to practice his deep-breathing exercises. After about 15 minutes, his headache was nearly gone, and he was able to return to work.

His nurse pointed out that he needed to feel free to call whenever he reached one of these points of frustration and not wait until the next weekly call. John experienced the most difficulty when taking business associates to his favorite restaurants for long luncheons. Drinking many cups of coffee during discussions had become a habit for him, and he needed to find out *before* scheduling a lunch whether or not decaffeinated coffee was available. He also experimented with fruit juice spritzers and mineral water with a twist of lime for those long discussions.

The formal six-week evaluation appointment provided a structured mechanism for evaluating John's progress. John was pleased that he had met his goal. The nurse also confirmed that both his systolic and diastolic blood pressure had dropped 10 points. This time also allowed for discussion of other self-care areas, particularly exercise and relaxation. John had read about the relevance of these areas to his health care and felt that they were important in relation to his hypertension.

The evaluation also identified important issues between John and Laura. Because of his heavy work schedule, she was skeptical of the amount of time he had to devote to his health. After much discussion, it was felt that a joint exercise program would provide them with the exercise they needed and also give them time together.

Finally, John stated that he was actually feeling better physically as a result of the caffeine reduction. He felt that this change contributed to attaining a

TABLE 14–12. NURSING CARE PLAN

Reason for consultation: Diabetes, hypertension, need for self-care program   *Client:* John

Assessment	Plan	Evaluation	
Self-care demand	*Setting objectives*	*Met*	*Not met*
Need for decreased caffeine intake	Six weeks: Limit caffeine intake to 2 cups of coffee every day.	X	
Assets	*Reaching objectives*		
Intellectual ability to understand benefits of decreased intake.	Client actions		
Label reading skills.	Complete diary.	X	
Supportive wife.	Have noncaffeinated drinks available at work.	X	
High-level motivation.	Purchase decaffeinated coffee at restaurant.		X
Limitations	Have weekly conference calls.	X	
Type A personality.	Nursing actions		
Lack of knowledge re: effects of caffeine.	Be available for conference calls.	X	
Lack of physical symptoms, except stress, diabetes, hypertension.	Provide written materials, provide safety/withdrawal information.	X	
Continued exposure to coffee at business meetings, long history of 8–10 cups daily.	Give information on university relaxation extension courses.	X	
	Provide blood pressure baselines.	X	
Diagnosis		*Needed revision*	
		None	
Self-care deficit			
Inability to limit caffeine intake without education and behavioral intervention	Reevaluation date	Client follow-up	
	6/15, six weeks	Concurrent medical follow-up. Weekly conference call. Other self-care skills that would influence blood pressure (i.e., relaxation, exercise).	

more positive outlook and sleeping better. Laura bought tickets and took John to a play in town as his six-week reward.

Both John and Laura agreed to work on the new goal together and continue the weekly conference calls with the nurse. Laura made an appointment with her health care professional in order to start her own self-care program. John continued his follow-up appointments with his physician and effectively used his self-care program together with medical care. Table 14–12 presents a nursing care plan for this clinical situation.

SUMMARY

Nutrition has been identified as an important area of self-care both in terms of creating a sense of well-being and in illness prevention. The most common deficits in this area are knowledge and motivation.

The meaning of food for the individual was discussed. In addition, assessment areas and self-care activities for the following nutritional topics were presented: carbohydrates and fiber, fats and cholesterol, sugar, salt, water, vitamins and minerals, additives, caffeine, and alcohol.

Nutritional guidelines for various developmental periods throughout the life span were presented. Nutritional variations and disorders were also discussed. The role of the nurse as a model of nutritional self-care was explored.

In a clinical case presentation, an illustration of self-contracting as a means of facilitating behavior change was given. The case also emphasized the use of self-care practices in conjunction with medical care.

STUDY QUESTIONS

Personal Focus

1. Rate yourself as a model of nutritional self-care.
2. Look in your kitchen cupboard or on a supermarket shelf at three packaged foods you normally eat. Is sugar listed as an ingredient? Is it listed first, second, or third? Is there more than one type of sugar listed?
3. What types of flours are used in the breads and bakery products you buy? Look at three labels and list the flours.
4. What percentage of your diet is fat? Carbohydrates? Protein?
5. What is your serum cholesterol level? Triglycerides? High-density lipoprotein? Low-density lipoprotein?
6. Complete a self-contract for behavior change involving nutrition.

Client Focus

1. Ask one client to complete a nutritional diary for a period of one week. What self-care deficits can you identify?

2. With your peers, discuss typical client nutritional problems in your clinical setting.
3. Practice teaching one client self-care actions to manage one of the following nutritional components: carbohydrates, fats, salt, sugar (or any of the components presented in Tables 14–3—14–10).
4. Interview one client regarding the emotional significance of food in his or her life.
5. Practice teaching a client at least four general nutritional self-care skills.
6. Complete a self-contract with one client to change one nutritional self-care behavior.

REFERENCES

1. Food and Nutrition Board, National Research Council. (1980). *Recommended dietary allowances* (9th ed.). Washington, DC: National Academy of Sciences.
2. Jelliffe, D. (1967). Parallel food classifications in developing and industrialized countries. *American Journal of Clinical Nutrition, 20,* 279.
3. Cooper, L. (1989). *The health & fitness cookbook.* Bernidji, MN: Advanced Excellence Systems.
4. U.S. Department of Health, Education and Welfare. (1979). *Healthy people: The surgeon general's report on health promotion and disease prevention.* Washington, DC: U.S. Government Printing Office.
5. Wenck et al. *Nutrition,* pp. 199-208.
6. American Psychiatric Association. (1987). *Diagnostic and statistical manual of mental disorders* (3rd ed.). Washington, DC: American Psychiatric Press, pp. 67-72.
7. George, M. (1988, June 30). McWhat! Burgers 'n' fries served up at DGH outlet. *Denver Post,* pp. A1, A10.

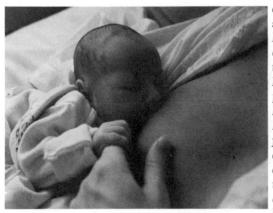

*A cantaloupe sky signals the nearness of dawn
as the two bare bodies again stretch upon the
satin comforter. He nuzzles her skin, breathes
her racy scent, and quickly rouses. He inhales
deeply, presses urgently against her, and unwit-
tingly pinches her nipple in the process.
Flinching slightly, she rubs his nose and whis-
pers softly. He fixes his eyes on her, and
kneads one delectable tidbit with his fingers as
he relishes the other with his lips. She pushes
firmly on his nates as he forces his hips
against hers. An ancient rhythm oscillates and
ebbs. Gradually his grip relaxes and he drifts
toward a deep, refreshing slumber. She ten-
derly disentangles her hair from beneath his
body. Then she covers him with the comforter,
and carries him to his crib.*

Alayne Yates, Sex without Shame (New York:
William Morrow, 1978), p. 11

15 Sexuality

LEARNING OBJECTIVES

Upon completion of this chapter, readers will be able to:

1. Define sexuality.
2. Describe the components of sexual health.
3. Describe the significance of sexuality in promoting health and general well-being.
4. Assess one's own comfort with sexuality.
5. List at least five ways to nurture sexuality.
6. Describe the role of the nurse in facilitating sexual self-care.
7. Develop a nursing care plan in the area of sexual self-care.

DEFINITIONS

Sexuality   A normal human process that provides for reproduction, pleasure, play, relaxation, and tension reduction. Narrowly defined, sexuality refers to the attitudes and behaviors directly associated with sexual and reproductive activity. A broader definition includes attitudes and behaviors associated with bodily sensuality. It is involved in all human relationships and includes all aspects of interaction and communication.

Sexual Health   "The integration of somatic, emotional, intellectual, and social aspects of sexual being in ways that are enriching and that enhance personality, communication and love."[1]

Sexual Disturbance   Discomfort with sexuality as defined by the client.

Sensual   Describes appetites and pleasures connected with gratification of the senses (touch, sight, smell, hearing, and taste).

Erotic   Describes thoughts and behaviors that initiate and maintain sexual arousal.

Sexual Self-Care   All of the activities engaged in to promote sexual health. These include attention to self-concept, body image, relationships, and specific nurturing of one's sexual self.

INTRODUCTION

Sexuality in the United States has the unique distinction of being both blatantly public and intensely private. Although it appears as a public preoccupation on billboards, television, and in magazines, for many individuals sex remains a very private matter, not easily discussed at social gatherings. Shame is often felt by clients who seek health care services for symptoms of a sexually transmitted disease, and clients who undergo infertility screening often are in the midst of a midlife crisis.

Health care professionals have often felt uncomfortable "probing" into their clients' sexual lives. Most nurses are familiar with the discomfort that can be experienced by both nurse and client when sexual questions are asked.

Over the last 20 years, there has been an increasing openness about sexual matters. More and more individuals have begun to discuss their sexual concerns with professionals. Despite this, health care providers need to be more responsive to their clients' sexual needs. Health care professionals can be effective only when they are comfortable with their own sexuality and its integration into their lives.

Defining Sexuality

Johnson and Klein, in their work with cancer patients, bring a new perspective to the definition of sexuality.

> Sexuality refers to all the feelings we have about ourselves as sexual beings and the ways we express those feelings to others. Sexuality and intimate rela-

tionships transcend pure physical sex. And the intimacy that people experience as sexual beings can mean the physical bond that exists between lovers as well as the closeness of family and friends. A definition can be divided into three parts.

Love of Self. You have to love yourself first. If you don't like who you are, it is hard to move outside yourself and like somebody else or appreciate the fact that the other person likes you. Very often, when people go through a major life change, they are unsure of how much they like themselves. When someone says, "I like the way you look," but you have just gained an extra ten pounds and are feeling fat, it is hard to accept the compliment as truthful.

Love of self is not difficult for children. Due to immaturity, they indulge in their own pleasures and consume the love you offer, but are quite restrictive about giving love back. When parents go away, children ask, "But who will take care of me?" instead of saying, "I will miss you." Once people are secure enough to like themselves, it is possible to move outward and consider the second part of sexuality.

Love of Others. People who are secure and comfortable with themselves are then capable of reaching out to care for others. They learn the satisfaction that comes from giving love to other people. Selfish desires for personal happiness are tempered by a desire to also want others to be happy. Now, when a loved one leaves for a few days, the individual can honestly say, "I will miss you," rather than "What about me?" When a person is sick, however, it is easy to regress and once again become consumed with self. Reaching out and caring for other people's wants and needs is difficult when you are preoccupied with your own health.

Loving Together. This third dimension of sexuality, mutual love, is usually the most rewarding for mature adults. Sexual intercourse is, of course, an important part of loving together. But loving together means much more than intercourse. It encompasses all of the social interaction that goes on in an intimate relationship—touching, holding, hugging, sharing intimacies, and accepting all of the loved one's weaknesses as well as strengths. Loving together means both a giving and receiving of love and is a vital part of every person's life.[2]

The Concept of Sexual Health

The World Health Organization considers sexual health to include three basic components. The *first* is the capacity to enjoy and control sexual and reproductive behavior in accordance with social and personal ethics. The *second* is freedom from fear, shame, guilt, misconceptions, and other psychological factors that inhibit sexual response and impair sexual relationships. The *third* is freedom from organic problems that can interfere with sexual or reproductive functioning.[3]

Lion lists the following characteristics of a sexually health person:

1. A positive body image (not necessarily a beautiful or whole body, but one that works); acceptance of sexual and body functions as normal and natural.
2. Reasonably clear knowledge about human sexuality and sexual functioning.

3. Good feelings about psychosocial identity: actions are consistent with own self-concept.
4. Awareness and appreciation of own sexual feelings.
5. Reasonably effective interpersonal relationships.
6. A usable value system that is still developing and allows for acceptance of mistakes without assigning blame or making excuses.[4]

With this same focus, Jourard has identified a number of factors that "foster a *health-engendering* sex life," including:

1. Sensible sexual instruction.
2. Early nontraumatic sexual experiences.
3. A generally satisfying life.
4. The ability to establish healthy relationships.[5]

A sexually healthy person feels comfortable in the expression of his or her sexual drive and accepts that drive as a natural expression of human need. A sexually health person is neither preoccupied with nor denies this need but incorporates it as an aspect of his or her total being. Sexual health involves a balance between seeking immediate gratification and delaying gratification when appropriate, between giving and receiving pleasure. It also involves experiencing the body and its sensations positively.

Sexual satisfaction is frequently, but not necessarily, associated with orgasm, and undue focus on orgasm can lead to performance anxiety.[6] Sexual satisfaction can perhaps best be obtained through an openness to experiencing the values of the moment, whether they be pleasure, tension reduction, expressions of love, connectedness, sharing, or intimacy. It is important to avoid stereotypes and to realize that sexuality can be enjoyed alone or shared.

Benefits of Healthy Sexuality

"Adequate sexual relationships promote a person's ability to function satisfactorily in his work, his leisure, and all of his non-sexual relationships with people."[7] A healthy person is able to reconcile sexual needs with other values, leading to a sense of self-esteem.[8] Sexuality can provide intense pleasure, as well as reduction of tension.

Another important benefit of sexuality is that its expression can be a form of play. It shares with play the characteristics of humor, spontaneous laughter, and freedom of choice, and it is noncumulative (it cannot be "saved up").

Sexuality may also provide benefits associated with spirituality. A special sense of sharing and connecting with another person is often present. Awareness of a force greater than the self may also accompany sexual interactions.

SEXUALITY: A DEVELOPMENTAL PROCESS

Sexuality is a life-long process. In each of its developmental stages, organismic, interpersonal, and psychic components influence and interact with each other in a circular fashion. Certain psychosexual tasks are prerequisites to healthy adult sexual functioning. They include the needs to:

1. Develop trust.
2. Develop positive feelings for bodily contact.
3. Understand that one has a right to one's body and to genital feelings.
4. Value one's body and lose the fear that it is or could be sexually damaged.
5. Find that each sex (male, female) is of equal value.
6. Cope with the biological surge of puberty.
7. Solidify one's sexual identity by becoming confident that one is acceptable to the opposite sex.*[9]

A certain degree of success in the completion of psychosexual tasks is central to healthy adult functioning. Few individuals actually experience a smooth transition from one stage to the next, however, and most individuals grow to adulthood with many tasks never completely resolved.

Sarrel and Sarrel describe the developmental process in adulthood as one that has a very direct relationship to life events. They identify seven stages of adult sexuality as "sexual turning points."

1. Sexual unfolding—taking the first steps toward adult sexuality
2. Making (or breaking) commitments
3. Marriage—for better or worse (in bed)
4. Making babies, making love
5. Parenting—new roles, new challenges
6. Making love the second time around
7. Keeping sex alive (and lively)[10]

Butler and Lewis, in *Love and Sex after 40*, focus on issues for people in their mid and later years.[11] Many people struggle with sexual issues throughout life, a phenomenon that may be more prevalent in complex and multidimensional societies like our own. Table 15–1 presents information regarding the sociological, psychological, and physical components of sexual development.

Sexuality and Learning

Human sexual desire is innate, but sexual behavior is strongly influenced by *learning*. This is apparent from the striking diversity of sensual and sexual behavior within U.S. society and in cultures around the world. What has been learned can presumably be unlearned and modified; thus sexual attitudes and behavior can be changed.

Tiny infants are exquisite creatures of sexual expression. Male infants respond to stimulation of the penis with erections, and infant girls can be ob-

---

*The authors would add, or acceptable to one's choice of sexual partner, not necessarily of the opposite sex.

TABLE 15–1. PSYCHOSEXUAL DEVELOPMENT

Stage	Tasks Common to Both Sexes
Infancy (0–18 mo)	Critical period for body acceptance Close physical contact establishes attitudes (pleasant or unpleasant) toward body Touching vital for survival Expresses all needs with mouth Tendency for infants to stimulate themselves genitally
Toddler (18 mo–3 yr)	Critical period for mastery of body functions and solid-core gender identity Differentiates between sexual and excretory organs Sphincter control—symbolizes autonomy and body control Strives for release of tension through genital manipulation Warm relationship with both parents increases acceptance of own sexuality Spontaneous internal and external genital sensations as a result of completion of myelinization of nerves
Preschool (3–6 yr)	Critical period for identification with same sex and resolution of oedipal issues Genital sensations, fantasies, drives for gratification reach a level of preoccupation Increased intensity of genital sensations become focused on parents Sex role identification with same sex
Early school years (6–9 yr)	Critical period for role identification Preoccupation with social interactions and fascination with world gives *impression* of diminished sexuality Seeks to explore and acquire increasing anatomical knowledge Major sexual activity still remains solitary masturbation
Middle childhood (9–12 yr)	Critical period for beginning acceptance of changes occurring in body at puberty Body begins to prepare itself for sexual maturity Solitary masturbation still the predominant mode of sexual release Sexual experimentation is usually homoerotic Begins separation from emotional ties with parents
Early adolescence (12–15 yr)	Critical period for shift of sexual feelings from parents to peers Beginning to move emotionally away from family of origin

TABLE 15-1. (con't).

	Ability to work and to love develops Preoccupation with body: concerns, delights, disappointments Sexuality has adult procreative potential Major sexual outlet is masturbation, which serves to gain mastery and knowledge of body Learns to identify with one's parents as sexually functioning people
Late adolescence (16-20 yr)	Critical period for identity consolidation Capacity for intimacy develops hand in hand with adult sexual identity Parents are major role models for future capacity to experience intimacy Petting and intercourse common Masturbation and all heterosexual activity increases
Adulthood (21-40 yr)	Critical period for interdependence and the capacity to invest both sexual and tender feelings in the same person Familiarity with own body and varieties of responses and emotions of sexual partner Love—confluence of innate drives and unfinished business of earlier psychosexual development
Middle and later years (40+ yr)	Critical period for expanded sexual freedom and function Peak years of productive and creative endeavors Previous sexual experiences allow for realistic approach to sexuality Faces possibility of chronic illness Fear of losing one's sexual attractiveness and capacity

(Adapted from Gadpaille, W. (1975). In L. Freeman (Ed.), *Cycles of Sex.* New York: Charles Scribner's Sons. © 1975 by Charles Scribner's Sons, adapted with permission.)

served inserting their fingers into their vaginas. Touching and exploring one's body as well as having it touched is comforting and soothing. In some cultures genital manipulation is an accepted method for calming irritable infants.[12] In U.S. culture exploration and touching is often encouraged, but an exception is made for the genitals. Parents often play a game of "naming" with their infants: "Where are your toes?" or "Show me your ears." Generally, however, parents do not say: "Where is your penis?" or "Where is your vagina?"

Sexual exploration of one's body is natural. If unmodified by learning it would be prominent throughout childhood and probably throughout life. It is also natural for children to be curious about other people's bodies and all aspects of sexual and reproductive functioning.

Parents and family members play a major role in the development of individual sexuality. If children are criticized for exploratory sexual behavior or made to feel ashamed or guilty for having sexual curiosity, sexual inhibitions may result that can persist throughout their lives. Furthermore, those repressive attitudes toward sex will be passed on to the next generation. If children have positive experiences exploring their own bodies, experience pleasure in bodily contact with parents, and see examples of comfortable bodily contact, they will have a much better chance of developing a healthy, joyful attitude toward their own sexuality.

Social and cultural *values* also contribute to individual sexual development. These values are communicated in many overt and covert ways: through peers, media, authorities, leaders, laws, religion, and so on. Some cultures are much more publicly tolerant and supportive of sexuality than is contemporary U.S. society. For example, in this country menarche is considered a private matter. It is dealt with by the individual and, sometimes, her family. In some societies, the onset of a young woman's menses is a rite of passage celebrated by a community gathering.[13]

Similarly, sexual intercourse between adults in the United States is rarely witnessed by children and considered to cause problems of anxiety and guilt for children who do witness it. On Mangara, a South Pacific island, children routinely witness nudity and parental intercourse, reportedly without the development of guilt or anxiety.[14]

With increasing numbers of people carrying HIV, in U.S. society there has recently been a more conservative trend toward sexuality. Formal sex education has increased at all levels of schooling. There has also been greater family acceptance of the need to educate children. "Good touching" and "bad touching" are discussed as early as kindergarten. Birth control is readily obtainable by sexually active adolescents. Some college campuses have installed vending machines for condoms. In spite of this trend, many people carry lifelong burdens of sexual inhibition. A current resurgence of fundamentalist religious groups in the United States may enhance sexual guilt and anxiety. It is important for the nurse to explore each client's attitudes about sexuality with an open mind.

The sense of touch plays a valuable role in early sensual and sexual development. For the infant, touching is crucial for survival. Without sufficient touching, babies who are otherwise well cared for fail to thrive and eventually die.[15] Positive experiences with touching and being touched provide the infant with a sense of security, warmth, and connectedness. For adults, touching can be sensual or erotic. Sensual touching provides pleasure but is not arousing in the manner of erotic touching. Both are self-care activities designed to enhance sexuality.

Body image is another example of the effect of learning on sexuality. A person's body image, the "mind's-eye view" of his or her body, is learned and is an important determinant of healthy sexuality. "One of the more pervasive obstacles to achieving a relaxed and conducive posture in sexual relationships is physical self-depreciation or negative body image."[16]

In the United States, an increasingly high value is placed on a rather narrow definition of physical attractiveness. This results in extreme pressure to conform to certain rigid standards. As a result, many individuals find themselves outside the boundaries, feeling depreciated and devalued. Since men are generally considered to be attracted first and foremost by "good looks,"[17] women are extremely vulnerable in this regard.

Body image changes markedly with age. For most people, perceptions of what is sexually attractive change over time. An individual's view of what is sexually attractive at age 16 will probably be quite different when that person is 50 years old. Cultural groups and subgroups also have different perceptions of body image and sexual attractiveness.

PHYSIOLOGICAL ASPECTS OF SEXUAL FUNCTIONING

In 1966, Masters and Johnson published *Human Sexual Response*, a monumental contribution to the understanding of human sexual physiology.[18] With sophisticated measures of physiological changes during sexual arousal, they were able to divide the continuum of sexual response into four phases: excitement, plateau, orgasm, and resolution. These phases primarily relate to the organismic level of sexuality described earlier. More recently, an additional phase has been identified, the transition phase. This phase is characterized by the time it takes to move from a state of nonarousal to arousal; this fluctuates for each individual. Many activities that can facilitate the transition period are discussed in a later section on nurturing sexuality.

Current understanding of the complex brain processes controlling the human sexual response is limited. There is a hierarchical nature to the neurophysiological aspects of sexuality. The limbic cortex and midbrain are thought to influence sexual desire and response. The lower centers of the spinal cord and brain stem are responsible for the reflex responses of erection, lubrication, ejaculation, and orgasm.[19]

Learned experiences, memories, thoughts, and emotional states (which originate in the higher centers) thus become powerful determinants of sexuality. As a result of this hierarchical effect, one can enhance sexual experience by fantasy. Thoughts (attitudes, beliefs, values, and information) are crucial to successful sexual functioning. Sexual functioning can be blocked by negative or nonerotic thoughts, such as worries about work or home. Negative labeling of personal attractiveness ("I'm not a very sexual person" or "I'm not attractive to others") will lead individuals to act in nonsexual, unattractive ways. Changing negative labels is an important aspect of sexual self-care and all self-care areas.

SEXUAL DIFFICULTIES

Nurses must be able to differentiate between healthy sexual functioning and sexual difficulty, making referrals when necessary. Since so much of sexuality is subjective, it is hard to say with any degree of certainty what constitutes sexual difficulty or inadequacy. If a man desires and enjoys sexual intercourse once a month, is he considered sexually inadequate? What criteria would one use to make this judgment? In the final consideration, what may be adequate for

TABLE 15–2. TRADITIONAL CLASSIFICATION OF SEXUAL DIFFICULTIES

Male Difficulties

Premature ejaculation: (1) ejaculation during a process of foreplay understood by both partners to be leading to intercourse; (2) ejaculation just before or during the act of penetration; or (3) ejaculation any time during the first 15 penile thrusts after intromission.

Impotence: inability to achieve or maintain an erection–prior to ejaculation–sufficient for penetration and completion of the sexual act. This definition includes loss of erection during coitus, but prior to ejaculation.

Retarded ejaculation: very slow ejaculation or virtual inability to ejaculate. This condition is usually limited to an essential inability to ejaculate intravaginally, with ejaculation by masturbation not being problematic.

Female Difficulties

Dyspareunia: vaginal or pelvic pain associated with penetration and coitus, very often leading to termination of the sexual encounter.

Anorgasmia: episodic or relatively continuous inability to reach orgasm in situations judged to be appropriately stimulating. There may be anorgasmia with both coitus and masturbation or just with coitus.

Vaginismus: spasm of the perivaginal musculature rendering penetration difficult or virtually impossible to accomplish.

Male and Female Difficulties

Nonspecific sexual withdrawal: withdrawal from sexual activities or decrease in sexual frequency by either or both partners without evidence of one of the specific disorders listed above. It is nonspecific in that sense only; psychologically, the causes of withdrawal may be quite specific.

(Meyer, J.K. (1976). Special problems in office practice: Guidelines for identification and management. In J.K. Meyer (Ed.) *Clinical management of sexual disorders.* Baltimore: Williams & Wilkins, p. 10. Reprinted with permission of Jon K. Meyer, MD, Director, Sexual Behavior Consultant Unit, Halsted 500, The Johns Hopkins Hospital, Baltimore, MD 21205.)

one individual may constitute a difficulty for another. Ultimately only the client can determine when a sexual difficulty exists.

The basic tool for identifying sexual problems is the assessment process. If the client is involved in sex with a partner, it is usually best if the partner is included in the assessment process. A one-sided presentation rarely allows for an accurate assessment.

Sexual difficulties are usually labeled in two different ways. Table 15–2 presents the most common male and female sexual difficulties according to medical teminology. Table 15–3 presents a different classification system that considers both physiological and psychological aspects of sexuality. This system provides for a subjective expression of sexual difficulties.

Treatment and Referral

Clients are increasingly seeking sexual counseling. Nurses need to be able to provide basic sex education. Part of this educative focus is to provide information regarding normal sexuality. A second focus is to teach clients how to be aware of themselves and communicate their needs to partners.

When lack of information or misinformation is causing a problem, the nurse may be effective in a brief educational discussion with a client. It is not unusual, for example, for a woman to think that the removal of her uterus will cause her to quit lubricating during sexual arousal. As a result she may avoid

---

TABLE 15–3 CLASSIFICATION OF SEXUAL PROBLEMS*

1. *Interest (desire):* refers to problem with how often the person wants to have sex. This category generally refers to a persistent and pervasive inhibition of sexual desire when organic causes are not present.
2. *Arousal:* denotes how excited or "turned on" one gets *during* sex.
3. *Physiological readiness*
   a. *Vaginal lubrication:* refers to physical state of vaginal secretions that occur during excitement phase of sexual response cycle.
   b. *Erection:* refers to physical state of penile tumesence that occurs during excitement phase of sexual response cycle.
4. *Orgasm:* refers to physical state of genital muscular contractions that occur during the orgasmic phase of the sexual response cycle.
5. *Satisfaction:* refers to subjective state of feeling either satiated or content or both. Satisfaction is self-reported and therefore has variable criteria.

*This classification implies that no organic cause is present in each problem identified.
(Adapted with permission from Zilbergeld, B., & Ellison, C.R. (1980). Desire discrepancies and arousal problems in sex Therapy. In S. Leiblum and L. Pervin (Eds.), *Principles and Practice of Sex Therapy.* New York: Guilford Press, pp. 70–71.)

sexual situations. Correcting this misinformation may be all that is necessary to resolve the problem.

Brief counseling usually involves several sessions in which sexual concerns can be verbally explored in private. It is designed to help the individual or couple enhance awareness of sexual needs and ability to communicate those needs. In these sessions the nurse must be able to provide the necessary time to explore the problem. If circumstances or environment prevent this, the nurse should make a referral to a specialist.

The national organization that certifies competency and training in the area of sex education is the American Association of Sex Educators, Counselors, and Therapists (AASECT).* AASECT publishes a directory of therapists and educators certified by their organization (an excellent resource for referral purposes).

LIFE-STYLE ASSESSMENT: AREAS INFLUENCING SEXUAL HEALTH

There are numerous areas that are important in helping clients and nurses assess sexual self-care strengths and deficits. If people are chronically fatigued, in pain, working too much, playing too little, have poor body images or have self-care deficits in any area, their sexual health may be influenced.

Examples of important assessment areas include the client's:

- Knowledge of and self-care actions regarding birth control.
- Knowledge of the dangers of sexually transmitted disease and willingness to take self-care measures for prevention.
- Current use of medications or substances that influence sexual functioning.
- Recent or past traumatic experiences with sexuality.

Birth Control
Until the last two decades there were no reliable, easy methods of birth control. Although there are drawbacks to any method of contraception, the ability to prevent unwanted pregnancy is a factor that has greatly influenced sexual behavior in our culture.[20]

Table 15–4 describes common birth control methods and how each affects sexual relations. The nurse should be familiar with various methods and their influence on sexuality. Many people feel stigma when purchasing or asking questions about birth control devices. The self-care implications of each option should be discussed with clients.

Diaphragms need to be changed, cleaned regularly, and periodically checked for size. Clients need to know the potential side effects of birth control pills or use of an intrauterine device. Teaching clients how to recognize and

---

*AASECT, 2000 N. Street, N.W., Washington, D.C. 20036.

TABLE 15–4. BIRTH CONTROL METHODS AND THEIR EFFECTS ON SEXUALITY

Method	Description	Sexual Effects
Rhythm	Abstinence from coitus during fertile period (pre- and post-ovulation), usually 8–12 days.	Hampers spontaneity. Limits sexuality to specific time periods. Lack of reliability causes anxiety and may interfere with sexual desire.
Billings method or cervical mucous method	Recognition of changes in cervical mucous that occur during the menstrual cycle. Abstinence from coitus during fertile period (8–12 days).	Limits sexuality to specific time periods. Lack of reliability may cause anxiety. May need to practice with method for several months before relying on it.
Condom	Thin disposable sheath worn over the penis during coitus.	Requires planning in order to have available. Some men complain about discomfort and decreased sensitivity. Can be used as a part of lovemaking and act as an erotic activity.
Contraceptive foam, jellies, vaginal suppositories	Chemical in aerosol, jelly, or solid form which is inserted inside vagina to act as a spermicide.	Requires planning in order to have available. May hamper spontaneity since must be used prior to each coitus. Some complaints of messiness may inhibit desire. May also irritate sensitive tissues. If used as part of lovemaking may serve as erotic activity.
Diaphragm	Saucer-shaped device made of rubber stretched over a flexible ring. Inserted in the vagina and fitted over the cervix, blocking the entrance to the uterus. Used in conjunction with a spermicide.	Properly fitted, it is not felt by either the male or female. Must be inserted prior to intercourse and may inhibit spontaneity. Some women dislike messiness. Requires planning to have available. If used as part of the sex act, may serve as erotic activity.

Vaginal sponge	Polyurethane sponge saturated with a spermicide that is activated when moistened with water. Inserted to rest in front of the cervix.
	Effective for up to 24 hours, so increases spontaneity. Easier to insert than the diaphragm.
IUD	Intrauterine device. Small plastic or metal device placed inside the uterus by a health care professional. Replaced periodically.
	Not felt by either partner. Does not require preplanning and may relieve anxiety and increase sexual desire.
The pill	Combination of synthetic hormones taken orally to prevent ovulation.
	Requires taking pills cyclically. May relieve anxiety and thus increase sexual desire. Allows for spontaneity. May decrease sexual response secondary to somatic side effects.
Sterilization	Female technique is tubal ligation. It is an operative procedure which cuts or ties the fallopian tubes to prevent ova from entering the tubes and uterus. Male sterilization involves an operative procedure which cuts the vas deferens and prevents sperm from leaving the male reproductive tract.
	Is permanent and therefore relieves anxiety, does not require preplanning, and allows for spontaneity. May increase sexual desire. May be perceived as a threat to sexual identity resulting in impotence and frigidity.
Orgasmic, non-coital sex	Physical stimulation to orgasm by means other than coitus.
	Society's view that penetration is the only mature, moral, and natural way to experience sex often eliminates this method as an option for couples.

monitor symptoms related to birth control methods is an important nursing role. Although none of the methods directly influence sexual satisfaction, each method may indirectly affect one's feelings.

Termination of pregnancy (abortion) is increasingly being used by some as an alternative to preventive birth control. Since it is not a method that involves preventing conception, it is not included in Table 15–4.

Sexually Transmitted Disease

Sexually transmitted diseases (STDs) are caused by organisms that live in warm, moist areas of the body (genitalia, rectum, mouth, or eyes) and are passed from one person to another through direct contact. Some of the STDs are merely nuisances and some have serious consequences. Nurses must be aware of the diseases, their signs and symptoms, and the various ways in which the risks of contracting them can be reduced. Table 15–5 describes self-care practices that help to protect against sexually transmitted disease. Table 15–6 lists the most common STDs and typical treatment approaches.

The industrialized world had grown quite comfortable in the belief that communicable diseases had been conquered, and, therefore, probably no other recent development has had as great an impact on sexual practices than the onset of AIDS. Caused by the human immunodeficiency virus (HIV), the first case of AIDS was diagnosed in 1981.[21] It is the current belief that 1.5 million people in the United States are infected with HIV, and by 1992 there will probably be 365,000 cases of AIDS in the United States.[22] It is also apparent that AIDS has become a threat to global health with over 250,000 cases reported and between five and ten million people infected with HIV worldwide.[23] Transmitted through a variety of mechanisms, that include direct contact, intravenous drug use, blood and blood products, and childbirth, this disease has produced more educational efforts at prevention than any in recent memory. The U.S. Surgeon General completed a mass mailing to every postal address in the country in 1988 with a booklet entitled, "Acquired Immune Deficiency Syndrome." This mailing contained not only basic information about HIV, ARC (Aids-Related Complex), and AIDS, but also educational material about prevention and safe-sex practices.[24]

Substance Use and Sex

For centuries there has been a never-ending search for an aphrodisiac, a drug that would enhance sexual desire. Today, many people take recreational, illicit, or therapeutic drugs on a regular basis. To determine the exact ways in which drugs affect sexual function and performance requires further research. With the knowledge available today it is clear that most drugs, including alcohol and nicotine, adversely affect sexual behavior. Only a few drugs seem to exert a positive effect on sexuality—generally through the indirect methods of tension reduction and release of inhibitions.[25]

TABLE 15–5 REDUCING RISKS OF GETTING SEXUALLY TRANSMITTED DISEASES

Prevention of sexually transmitted diseases is one goal of sexual self-care. There are many self-care practices which can *help* to prevent contraction of these diseases.

1. Practice self-care in all areas (nutrition, exercise, relaxation, etc.) to promote general wellness and increase immune response.
2. Limit number of sexual partners.
3. Decline contact with person who has sexually transmitted disease or symptoms of a sexually transmitted disease.
4. Have an HIV test if you have engaged in risky behavior. Also have new partners tested.
5. Always use condoms.
6. If you or your partner are at high risk, avoid oral sex.
7. Avoid all sexual activity that could cause cuts or tears in the linings of rectum, vagina, or penis.
8. Avoid sex with prostitutes or intravenous drug users.
9. Reduce intake of sugars and refined carbohydrates.
10. If diabetic, maintain control.
11. Practice good hygiene: wash perianal area daily with soap and water, do not use hygiene sprays or deodorant tampons or pads.
12. Wear cotton underwear. Avoid tight-fitting pants, pantyhose.
13. Make sure that sexual parnters are clean. Shower, bathe before sex. Condoms can provide additional protection.
14. Use water-soluble jellies for lubrication. Contraceptive jellies, foams, creams *may* assist in the prevention of infection.
15. Douching after intercourse and at the end of menses (2 T vinegar in 1 qt. warm water) may prevent infection.
16. Some women use plain yogurt with active culture vaginally to maintain normal flora.
17. Void before and immediately after intercourse.
18. For women, after voiding and defecation, cleanse from front to back.
19. If in doubt about exposure to a sexually transmitted disease, go to a health care provider and obtain diagnostic test. (Oral lesions may be transmitted to the genitalia, and vice versa. They may also be transmitted to other parts of the body. Lesions from sexually transmitted diseases are not limited to the genitalia.)
20. If taking antibiotics or steroids, use preventive measures carefully to maintain best possible pH.
21. Some STDs may be transmitted through direct contact with contaminated objects. Hygiene precautions are thus indicated.
22. Notify your partner(s) if you do get an STD. Otherwise, you may become reinfected, and others may as well.
23. Use imagery techniques to prevent STDs.

Sources: See Table 15–6

Table 15–7 illustrates drugs known to have an effect on sexual behavior. If a client is on drugs of any type, self-care teaching must be included in ongoing nursing care. When therapeutic medications are prescribed, clients need to be informed of their influence on sexuality as well as all other side effects. Learning to recognize and monitor these side effects is a basic sexual self-care activity.

Referral to a physician may be indicated when clients wish to change medications because of difficulties with sexual functioning. Information in this

TABLE 15–6 SEXUALLY TRANSMITTED DISEASES

Type	Symptoms	Treatment
Candida albicans (Monilia)	Itching, burning, redness, swelling. Vaginal discharge: milky, creamy, cheesy. Male lesions in groin, scrotal area. Red, itchy, weepy.	Treat both partners. Nystatin or Monistat cream or suppositories. Gyne Lotrimin. Acidic douche (2 T vinegar/ 1 qt. warm water). Decrease sugar, refined CHO intake. Insert yogurt intravaginally.
Trichomonas	Malodorous. Itching, burning, redness, swelling, superpubic tenderness. Thin, foamy, yellow-gray-green vaginal discharge.	Treat both partners. Flagyl orally (do *not* consume alcohol while taking Flagyl). Trichofuron suppositories. Acidic douche (2 T vinegar/ 1 qt. warm water).
Herpesvirus types I, II	Lesions may be anywhere on body. Primarily oral or genital. Painful, thin-walled vesicle followed by ulcer. May be inside vagina, external genitalia, thighs, anus, under foreskin, or on shaft of penis.	Symptomatic treatment: topical anesthetics, sitz baths, analgesics. Increase all self-care skills (sleep, nutrition, exercise, etc.) to reduce chance of recurrence. May be linked to increased incidence of cervical carcinoma. Herpes type II vaccine now in developmental phase.
Gonorrhea	Itching, burning, redness, swelling, dysuria, anal irritation, painful defecation, pelvic inflammatory disease, fever, malaise, nausea, pharyngitis, swollen neck glands. Women often asymptomatic. Men often have thick, milky urethral discharge, pain, dysuria. Infection may be pharyngeal if oral sex.	Treatment of both partners. Probenicid 1 gram p.o., aqueous procaine penicillin I.M., oral ampicillin or tetracycline. Two negative cultures 1–2 weeks apart, including rectal culture before considered cured.
Hemophilus	Malodorous, creamy, white, grayish discharge. May be tender nonindurated ulcer with gray/yellow exudate. Women may be asymptomatic.	Treat both partners. AVC, Sultrin cream, or Furacin cream/suppositories for women. Tetracycline or ampicillin for men.
Condyloma acuminatum	Pale, irregular clusters of raised fleshy lesions. May be on labia, perineum, anus, penis, or scrotum. May also be	Partner should be treated simultaneously if he or she has condylomata. Podophylline 20–25% in tincture of ben-

(continued)

TABLE 15–6 (con't)

	internal: cervix, walls of vagina. May be asymptomatic.	zoin applied to lesions. Must be washed off 3–6 hours after application. Cryotherapy and surgical excision are alternative treatments.
Syphilis	Primary: chancre at site of infection; oral, genital, or other site. Secondary: diffuse rash on palms, soles; fever; alopecia; mucous patches on mouth and throat; papular lesions on vagina/cervix. Tertiary: Any organ of the body may be affected. May be asymptomatic.	Probenicid 1 gram p.o. followed by long-acting penicillil I.M. 30 minutes later. Two follow-up serologies. If treated for gonorrhea, four serologies 1 month apart to allow for 90-day incubation. Transmitted by physical contact—not necessarily sexual.
Pediculosis pubis	Intense genital itching. May also be in chest hair, axillae, eyelashes, eyebrows.	Kwell 1% over body. Dry cleaning/boiling clothing, bed linen. Organism will die within 24 hours after separation from human body. Eggs will live for six days. Treat all family members.
Hepatitis type B	Onset insidious. Vague abdominal discomfort, nausea, arthralgia, anorexia. Fever may or may not be present. Anicteric hepatitis may occur.	Symptomatic only. Individuals may become carriers.
Chlamydia	Primary lesion on genitalia. Painless vesicle or nonindurated ulcer. Painful lymphadenopathy of regional nodes 1–4 weeks after lesion. Purulent proctitis may indicate rectal involvement. Dysuria may be present. May be asymptomatic in women.	Tetracycline 500 mg orally q.i.d. for 2-3 weeks. Sulfasoxazole may also be used. Glandular masses may require aspiration.
Scabies	Linear burrows 1–10 mm. May be red papules. Intense itching, prominent at night. Finger webs, wrists, elbows, ankles, penis common sites.	Kwell 1% lotion/shampoo. Treat family, sexual partners. Dry clean/boil clothing, bed linen.
Nongonococcal urethritis (NSU)	Urethral discharge varies from profusely purulent to small amounts of mucous. Dysuria may or may not be present.	Tetracycline 500 mg q.i.d. for 7 days or Erythromycin 500 mg q.i.d. for 7 days.

TABLE 15–6 (con't)

	NSU is a colloquial term for symptoms caused by a variety of organisms, including *Chlamydia, Ureaplasma Urealyticum, Trichomonas, Candida,* and Coliform bacteria.	
Acquired immune deficiency syndrome (AIDS)	Swollen glands, fever, night sweats, weight loss, diarrhea, fatigue, loss of appetite. Initially mimics flue symptoms, but complaints persists for several weeks. Loss of immunity results. May be due to virus. Occurs most often in homosexual and bisexual men, Haitians, hemophiliacs, and in drug addicts who use needles.	No treatment now available.[a] Symptomatic treatment of infections. Self-care actions include: Limit sexual contact to one partner. Ask partner to limit other sexual contacts; report any AIDS symptoms. Avoid exchange of body fluids/blood. Avoid anal intercourse. Use condoms. Avoid cross-use of needles for drug injection.

[a]AIDS Hotline: 800-342-AIDS (USPHS). NATIONAL GAY TASK FORCE: (800) 221-7044. National Sexually Transmitted Disease Hotline (American Social Health Association): (800) 227-8922.
SOURCES: Women's Health Care Nurse Practitioner Program, Harbor-UCLA Medical Center, Torrance, CA; Boston Women's Health Book Collective. (1979) *Our bodies, ourselves.* New York: Simon and Schuster; Martin, L.L. (1978). *Health care of women.* Philadelphia: J.B. Lippincott; Campbell, C.E. & Herten, R.J. (1981). VD to STD: Redefining veneral disease. *American Journal of Nursing, 81* (9), 1629–1635; Surgeon General's report on acquired immune deficiency syndrome. (1988). Washington, DC: U.S. Government Printing Office.

area is regularly updated, and nurses continually need to review current data about physiological influences of drugs.

Trauma Related to Sexuality

Trauma related to sexuality may occur in both subtle and overt ways. Most people are aware of the overt sexual traumas experienced by men and women. Child abuse, incest, and rape are the most common tragic examples of assaults on a person's sexual self. The effects of these experiences can be long-term and damaging to anyone's sexual and emotional health.

More subtle trauma can also influence sexual health. Although many women report no long-term psychological sequelae of abortion, others report that feelings of guilt interfere with ongoing sexual relationships. Religious and political controversy about this issue exacerbates the situation.[25]

Subtle sexual trauma (or often not so subtle) occurs in cases of sexual harassment. This can include demands that an employee "sleep with the boss," a student "sleep with the teacher," or social group pressures for a person to be or not be homosexual, heterosexual, bisexual, and so on. Although some individuals and social systems are slowly becoming more tolerant, the trauma to sexual health that occurs through harassment must be continually recognized.

In many communities, self-care support groups deal with these issues, Although sex education, preventive measures, and individual counseling are all important, peer-group support is often the most powerful element in alleviating guilt, depression, and withdrawal following sexual trauma.

NURTURING SEXUALITY

There are many self-care activities that promote and nurture sexual health. Skills that nurture sexuality can be conceptualized in a variety of ways. The activities presented below have to do with sensual and erotic skills (which relate to the organismic component of sexuality) and communications skills (which relate to the interpersonal and psychic levels). Sample activities associated with each of these areas include:

Sensual Activities	**Erotic Activities**	**Communication Activities**
Identifying sensual situations	Sexual Fantasy	Values clarification
Grooming	Masturbation	Communication with partner or partners
Relaxation	Erotic touch	
Getting to know your anatomy	Sensate Focus III	
Partner Sensate Focus exercises		
Sensate Focus I		
Sensate Focus II		

As essential criterion to all these activities is *time*. They must be completed in nonhurried, relaxed, private settings. Pushing oneself to do these activities as if they were "work" is self-defeating. Many clients have found that using imagery to picture success improves outcome.

Sensual Activities

Identifying Sensual Situations and Settings
For one week keep track of the times and places you feel most sensual. Identify the cues that seem consistently to trigger *your* sensuality (for example, after a hot bath, walking on the beach, while dancing, in the early mornings). Cues that

TABLE 15-7 DRUGS THAT AFFECT HUMAN SEXUAL BEHAVIOR[a,b]

	Drugs that Enhance Libido and Sexual Functioning	Transient Effect or Questionable Effect	Drugs that May Decrease Libido and/or Sexual Functioning
Recreational drugs			
Legal and socially approved	Caffeine (small amount)	Caffeine may initially overcome fatigue	Caffeine
	Alcohol (small amount)	Alcohol initially lowers anxiety	Alcohol
			Nicotine
Illicit	Amyl nitrate	Marijuana and hallucinogens alter perception but do not actually alter the sexual response; enhance sensation	
	Marijuana		
	Hallucinogens		
	Lysergic acid diethylamide (LSD)		
			Opiates (codeine, opium, etc.)
			Amphetamines (moderate to chronic use)

| Therapeutic drugs | Oral contraceptives
Hormones (androgens,
progesterone, estrogen)
Levo-Dopa | Depression may be a
side effect of some
contraceptives and
may lead to de-
creased sexual
functioning. | Antabuse
Antidepressants
Antihypertensives
Antiadrenergic drugs
Antihistimines
Antispasmodics
Anticholinergic drugs
Antipsychotics
Sedatives
Hypnotics
Narcotics
Corticosteroids
Diuretics
Cytotoxic drugs |

[a]Any drug could influence sexual functioning. This list is not considered inclusive.
[b]For further information on the mechanism of action of each of these drugs, see Woods, N.F. (1979). *Human sexuality in health and illness* (2nd ed.). St. Louis: C.V. Mosby, pp. 378–379; and Lion, E.M. (1982). *Human sexuality in nursing process.* New York: John Wiley & Sons. pp. 331–339.

enhance sensuality might include candlelight dinners, fresh flowers, certain perfumes, music, or specific clothing. Learn to acknowledge and value cues and settings that intensify your sensuality. Nurture your sexuality by promoting these experiences.

Grooming

It is helpful to experience body sensations that accompany normal grooming activities. Take your time bathing, washing and combing your hair, putting on body lotions, choosing clothing, and so on. Experience the pleasure and sensations involved in these "required" activities rather than hurrying through them as if they were work.

Relaxation and Imagery

Learn to relax and communicate with your body. Assume a comfortable position on a bed or chair. Use music or relaxation tapes if you choose. Take 10 to 15 deep breaths and notice your breathing. Close your eyes and focus on a particular body part. Notice if it is tense or relaxed. Focus on relaxing the muscle until it feels limp. Go on to different muscle groups until your entire body is relaxed. Learn to relax your entire body (see Chapter 9).

Getting to Know Your Anatomy

Become familiar with your body and its sensations. Learn how it responds to touch. Get undressed completely; you may want to take a shower or bath and do some relaxation exercises first. Study your body in the mirror from all angles (without being critical). Notice the contours, shapes, details of your skin and coloring, your particular hair distribution patterns, and so on. Identify the parts of your body that you find most sensual. Mark those parts on a full body drawing of yourself.

   Look closely at your genitals. (Women will need to place a small mirror between their legs and spread their labia majora.) Get to know the particular qualities, marks, moles, and hair patterns of your genitals. Exercise your levator ani and coccygei muscles (pelvic muscles). Strengthening these muscles can increase sexual responsiveness. For details on how to locate and exercise these muscles, refer to the book *Super Marital Sex: Loving for Life*[26] or *How to Make Love All the Time*.[27]

Partner Sensate Focus Exercises [28]

Sensate Focus I. These exercises are done with a partner—each person is nude. Learn to experience and focus on the sensation of touch. Each partner takes a turn being both the giver and the receiver—each turn lasts 20 minutes. The giver is to touch the receiver on all parts of the body except the genitals and breasts, experimenting with different strokes, pressures, and so on. The receiver's job is just to relax and enjoy the feeling of being touched in different ways and on different parts of the body. No particular feeling is expected; the receiver just concentrates on feelings.

Sensate Focus II. This activity repeats Sensate Focus I, but this time the receiver guides the giver's hand to demonstrate what kinds of touch feel best. For further information about sensate focus exercises, refer to the book *Human Sexual Inadequacy*.[28]

Erotic Activities

Sexual Fantasy

Facilitate your ability to use fantasy to increase erotic feeling. Take 15 minutes three times a week to concentrate on sexual fantasy. A good time may be after you have relaxed or groomed. In a relaxed, unhurried setting, spend time either writing or mentally developing sexual scenes that are erotic. Get to know what "turns you on."

Reading sexual fantasies in books or magazines may help develop your imagination. Watching movies or plays that you find erotic may also enhance fantasy. Readings might include a favorite magazine (such as *Playgirl* or *Playboy*) or book (such as *My Secret Garden*,[29] *Men in Love*,[30] or *Shared Intimacies*).[31]

Experiment with different approaches. Acknowledge and value your unique ways to nurture sexuality through fantasy. There is no need to enjoy methods used by other people.

Masturbation

Get to know your genital response to erotic touch and increase your comfort with your own sexuality. Advantages of this activity are that you do not need a partner and can choose your own time. Focus entirely on pleasing yourself. Relaxed, nonpressured time is essential. Often it can follow grooming, relaxation, or fantasy experiences. If desired, use a lotion or cream (water soluble). Pay attention to self-care needs related to the choice of creams, including possible allergies, urethritis, and vaginitis. Wash hands well before initiating this activity.

Using your hands, stimulate your genitals with different touches and strokes. Find out what areas are most sensitive and what feels best. Enjoy the feelings. If desired, continue the momentum and intensity until an orgasm occurs. For further details on masturbation, refer to the books *Male Sexuality*[26] or *For Yourself*.[32]

Erotic Touch

Excluding your genitals, identify parts of your body that respond most erotically. Take your time. Note the sensation in each part of your body. Identify the parts of your body that consistently seem to respond erotically (e.g., feet, ears, neck).

Sensate Focus III

This is a continuation of Sensate Focus I and II described under sensual activities. In this activity genital stimulation is included. The purpose is now to focus on the feeling of your body, including genital sensations. Since the focus is on sensation, orgasm is prohibited. Guided touching is used to advise the giver exactly how and where the receiver likes to be touched. Identify the parts of your genitals that feel most erotic under different circumstances.

Communication Activities

Values Clarification

Learn to increase your ability to talk with *yourself* about your sexual values. Make a list of the values of sexuality from *your* perspective. Clarify the priority on sexual health in your life. Think about the value you place on body image, physical attractiveness, seductiveness, touch, specific language, and so on.

Journal keeping and dream analysis can be utilized to keep track of and learn about how your values may shift over time. Sexual problems are frequently symptoms of other conflicts. Figure 15–1 provides one tool for values clarification. Decide if you want to talk about any of these values with friends or a sexual partner.

Communicating with Partner or Partners

Table 15–8 presents a partner questionnaire that can be used to discuss issues of sexuality that are usually not talked about openly between partners. The questionnaire should be completed by one partner, then the other, then followed with a discussion of how each person felt about answering the questions. Partners need to pick a time and place (not during sexual experience) that will allow for adequate expression of feelings and concerns.

NURSES MODEL SEXUAL SELF-CARE

The nurse is often seen as a person who has medical information, a caring attitude, and more time than a physician to listen to personal concerns about sexuality. Clients, however, will not feel free to talk about sexuality unless there is a secure feeling that the nurse is comfortable with the topic, will take the concern seriously, will not make judgments, and will not give glib advice. That secure feeling comes primarily from subtle client observations of the nurse's comfort with his or her own sexuality. Figure 15–2 provides one assessment tool that can help nurses explore their values, feelings, and levels of sexual comfort (see also Figure 15–1 and Table 15–8).

SEXUAL SELF-ASSESSMENT
Values Clarification

Answering the following questions will help clarify your beliefs and attitudes toward sexuality:

1. My definition of sexuality is:

2. The purpose of sex in my life is:

3. I received my information about sex from:

4. I found my first sexual experience to be:

5. I feel sexual when:

6. The messages I got from my parents about sex were:

7. My first experiences with dating were:

8. Asking for what I want in sex is:

9. I remember my experiences with puberty to be:

10. Initiating sexual relationships is:

11. When I have concerns about sex I talk to:

12. I think nudity is:

13. What I like best about my sexuality is:

14. Sexual expression should be limited to relationships which:

15. Sexual satisfaction means to me:

16. Different standards of sexual behavior for men and women are:

17. Virginity before marriage is:

18. Promiscuity is:

19. Erotic material (magazines and movies) is:

20. Sex is best when:

Figure 15–1. Sexual self-assessment—values clarification. *Adapted from Health Education Unit. (1979). A picture of health: A guide to asessing your well-being.* Berkeley, CA: University of California, pp. 72–73.)

In their personal lives nurses model sexual self-care by:

- Making time for sexual nurturing activities.
- Touching others and accepting touch from others.
- Protecting themselves from sexually transmitted disease.
- Making "special times" to spend with their sexual partners.

There are a number of ways in which clients regularly observe the nurse's comfort or discomfort with sexuality. Some of these situations include:

TABLE 15–8 SEXUALITY QUESTIONNAIRE

Discuss the Following with Your Partner:

1. Were there any upsetting experiences that occurred during childhood with regard to sex?
2. What was your first experience with sexual intercourse* like?
3. What emotional conditions are necessary for you to have sexual intercourse?
4. What feelings usually accompany sexual intercourse?
5. Is it difficult to tell your partner what you like sexually? What you don't like sexually? If so, why?
6. What are the more pleasurable physical contacts that are *not* followed by sexual intercourse? Do these activities occur frequently enough?
7. What are the more pleasurable physical contacts that *do precede* intercourse? Do these occur frequently enough?
8. Are there any sexual practices or techniques that you would like to include in your experiences that are not there now? Any that you would like to eliminate?
9. Do you feel comfortable sometimes being the initiator of sexual activity? What is your preference in this area?
10. How do you feel when your partner refuses advances that you make?
11. How would you like your partner to respond if you were not feeling aroused during a sexual encounter? (Not able to get an erection or not lubricating).
12. Are you satisfied with the amount and type of physical affection you have with your partner?
13. What do you think about sexual fantasy? Do you use it and if so, under what circumstances?
14. How do you feel about masturbation? Is it a part of your sexual experience?
15. Do you enjoy reading or watching erotic material? What do you like or dislike about it?
16. How do you see sexual issues affecting other aspects of your relationship?

*Although "Sexual intercourse" refers specifically to heterosexuality, these questions can be revised to accommodate homosexual clients.
(Reprinted with permission from Wells, C. Center for Sexual Communication, 195 Claremont Street, No. 374, Long Beach, CA 90803).

- Asking sexual history questions during routine history taking.
- Male nurses catheterizing female clients or female nurses catheterizing male clients.
- Nurses (male and female) providing intimate, intrusive care to clients during labor and delivery.
- Discovery by a nurse of clients kissing, "petting," masturbating, or having intercourse in the hospital.
- Flirting and seduction that takes place between nurses and certain clients or nurses and other hospital employees.

In clinical interactions nurses model sexual self-care by actions such as:

- Allowing and promoting privacy in the hospital.
- Knocking before entering clients' rooms.
- Allowing sexual partners to share the same room when both are hospitalized on a long-term basis.
- Initiating conversations about clients' sexual concerns, for example: Reactions to mastectomy, prostatectomy, vasectomy, myocardial infarct, cerebral vascular accident, colostomy, hysterectomy
- Influence of medications on sexuality
- Indentifying and accepting cultural variation for touch and sensuality needs.
- Touching clients and accepting touch from clients.
- Providing for touch with elderly clients.

In all of these situations clients observe and learn from behaviors modeled by the nurse. If nurses are able to acknowledge and respect sexuality as a healthy part of life, clients will be more comfortable in talking about their own sexual self-care needs.

On the other hand, if nurses are extremely anxious, defensive, and have no sense of humor, their discomfort with the topic of sexuality is readily conveyed. This type of modeling influences clients. At best clients will avoid these nurses; at worst they will begin to question their own sexual needs and concerns.

CLINICAL APPLICATION

Case Presentation

Leucenda is a 30-year-old journalist who has been divorced for six months. She is employed as a publisher's representative and thoroughly enjoys her work. There were no children from a marriage that lasted four years. She has just had an annual exam with her nurse practitioner. The physical examination revealed no abnormalities and the PAP smear was class I. Her oral contraceptive was refilled.

Although Leucenda had no specific physical complaints, she expressed feeings of insecurity in her new role as a divorced woman. Most of the insecurity is in the area of dating and, in particular, in being sexual with new men. She has avoided going out for this reason.

She has been on birth control pills (O/N ⅟₃₅) for four years and has had no difficulties. At this point she wonders if continuing the pills is "worth it," since she is not optimistic about developing new sexual contacts.

> **Assessment**
>
> • self-care demand
> • assets
> • limitations

Leucenda does not recall how she learned about sex, except that she never discussed it with her parents. She had a pleasant *childhood* with lots of friends, although there was much emphasis on achievement and productivity. Her parents did not fight or disagree in front of her, yet she never saw them acting affectionately or being sexually playful with each other. Her father gave her mother a kiss on the cheek each evening when he returned from work.

Leucenda has a brother two years older and she vaguely remembers some mutual exploration of genitals in the typical "doctor" game when she was a preschooler. After that she remembers very little about sexual experiences until she met her future husband in college. She has never seen her genitals and is not sure if she could locate and name the various parts of her anatomy.

Masturbation has never been a part of Leucenda's experiences. She does not recall *religious training* that forbade masturbation or any particular messages from her parents against it. She does not know why she has never masturbated except to say "I never really thought about it."

Her first *dating experience* (other than group parties) occurred in the tenth grade. She remembers being very much "in love" with a particular boy and dated him exclusively through the eleventh grade. There was some petting, but it was limited to kissing and breast stimulation. Even when she found herself becoming very aroused, she felt uncomfortable with genital exploration. The arousal frightened her, and she would limit the petting to avoid that feeling of "losing control." Possible pregnancy also represented a threat to her career plans. She was an excellent student and wanted to go to college and study journalism.

After breaking up with her boyfriend at the end of her junior year, Leucenda dated several different boys but never any one in particular. In her second year of college she met David, her future husband. She fell very much in love with him, and in her senior year they were engaged. It was after the engagement that Leucenda first experienced mutual genital stimulation. She recalls feeling awkward and unsure. It felt "all right" to be touched but she had "lots of reservations" and she particularly felt "uncomfortable stimulating David's penis."

Her first experience with *sexual intercourse* was with David about six months prior to the wedding. She had gone to the doctor to get birth control pills and was less anxious about pregnancy. The experience was "not that pleasurable," she said; in fact, "it hurt somewhat." David seemed to enjoy himself, and Leucenda felt good about that. Continued intercourse led to less discomfort, but Leucenda seemed to feel that "something was missing." She says she "doesn't feel all that much during intercourse" and rarely had an orgasm.

Leucenda reports that she always had a good *body image* and a healthy *self-concept*. She feels that she is attractive and that this is validated by the way men pay attention to her. She says she is proud of how she has done in her *career* and that she respects and trusts herself. Her additional *assets* include motivation to "discover her sexual self" and the fact that she has friends and a *social life*. She enjoys flirting even though she has been uncomfortable about dating. She recognizes that she has spent very little time nurturing her sexuality. It is an area that makes her anxious and confused, so she tends to avoid it. She rarely spends long periods of time on grooming or any sensual activity, always saying that she is "busy" or "interested in other things." She practices excellent nutrition and exercise *self-care* and is in good physical health.

Leucenda feels "fairly peaceful" about her divorce and is "happy to be out of a bad situation." She demonstrates only minimal ambivalence or sadness about the loss of that relationship. Her major concern is "negative feelings about sex," which come from a deep feeling that "there is nothing in it for me." She completed the assessment tool presented in Figure 15–2. She also completed the sexuality questionnaire (Table 15–8).

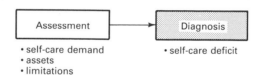

Leucenda expressed an "enlightened feeling" after answering the sexual assessment tools. It became clear to her that she had a self-care deficit in the area of comfort with her body, including her genitals. She said she had "taken her sexuality for granted, thinking it would take care of itself." Leucenda and the nurse arrived at the following self-care deficit:

Discomfort with own body secondary to lack of information and experience

A nursing diagnosis might be:

Body image disturbance or sexual dysfunction

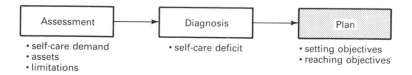

SEXUALITY SELF-ASSESSMENT

Complete the following self-assessment to help you look at the role of sexuality in your life. On the scale below circle the numbers which are most true for you and your life during the last year:

	Almost Never	Seldom	Often	Almost Always
1. Each week I have time just for me.	1	2	③	4
2. Sexual thoughts/feelings occur to me each day.	1	2	③	4
3. Several times each week I take time to explore my body.	①	2	3	4
4. I like the way my body looks.	1	2	③	4
5. I like the way my genitals look. *Don't Know*	1	2	3	4
6. When I am in the mood I take time to be sexual with myself.	①	2	3	4
7. When I am sexual with a partner I feel satisfied.	1	②	3	4
8. I feel comfortable initiating sexual conversations.	1	②	3	4
9. I can be sexual when there is work to be done.	①	2	3	4
10. I have fun being a sexual person.	1	②	3	4

Some suggestions for how you might learn from this self-assessment:

1. Connect all the circles down the length of the page. Look at the pattern that your connected line makes. Turn your page sideways to get an even more clear visual picture of your sexual health. What does it seem to be saying to you?

2. Now add up your total score: _____ *18* _____

   Circle which range it was in:
   (10-19)   20-29   30-40

   If your score was in the 10-19 range you might want to make some changes in your sexual life. Which aspects do you think need the most work? How many "1's" did you mark on this assessment? _3_ These might serve as a clue to help you think about making changes in this area of your life.

3. How would you like this self-assessment to look six months from now? Are you interested in working toward those improvements?

4. Remember to congratulate yourself for the ways in which you are providing for healthy sexuality in your life.

Figure 15–2 Sexuality self-assessment. *(Adapted with permission from Baldi, S., et al. (1980). For your health: A model for self-care. South Laguna, CA: Nurses Model Health)*

Setting Objectives

Leucenda stated that she wanted to change several aspects of her sexuality. She wanted to:

- Become more comfortable with my body, its sensations, and responses to touch.
- Become more comfortable in sexual interactions with men.
- Decrease my fear of 'losing control' in sexual situations.

While these were vague statements, she also identified a number of *specific* self-care objectives:

Within six weeks I will spend at least 30 minutes four times a week on specific activities to nurture my sexuality.

Within six months I will have continued the above process and in addition will have accepted at least four dates with men.

She then completed a self-contract (see Fig 15–3). Initially, the nurse served as the contracting partner, but Leucenda thought that in a few weeks she might be ready to ask a friend at work to be a partner.

Reaching Objectives: Nursing and Client Actions

Leucenda realized that she could become comfortable with her own body only by taking specific small steps in that direction. Table 15–9 presents an example of the specific self-care activities she identified. During this process the nurse served as a consultant and provided basic information about the importance of sexuality to health. Leucenda assumed the major responsibility for identifying and carrying out each self-care activity. Specific nursing and client actions are identified in Table 15–10.

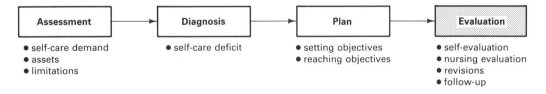

For six weeks Leucenda and her nurse discussed the self-care project every two weeks. Leucenda reported that she could see the value of doing the self-care activities. She felt that she had learned a great deal about her body and feelings about sexuality. She noticed that she frequently had trouble concentrating when studying her genital anatomy or learning about masturbation. The more the nurse talked with her about this, and they discovered that Leucenda had stronger negative feelings about masturbation than she originally thought. Leucenda wanted to overcome these feelings and felt that with continued expe-

SELF-CONTRACT

MY GOALS:

Short-term— by the end of six weeks I will . . . Spend at least 30 min 4x/wk on specific activities to nurture my sexuality.

Long-term— by the end of six months I will . . . Have continued above process and accept at least four dates with men.

ENVIRONMENTAL PLANNING: (all the steps I will take to reach my goal)

1. Arrange for at least 30 minutes extra each day at home in private for nurturing sexuality. Change work schedule if necessary.
2. Take phone off hook and do not answer door during those periods.
3. Buy and keep a diary of my self-care actions each day.
4. Buy the books (or check out from library) recommended by nurse.
5. Buy a special bath lotion and one record for relaxation and fantasy.

THOUGHTS AND ACTIONS

Helpful thoughts:	Helpful actions:
My body really can give me pleasurable sensations. Knowing my body and how it works is great!	Talking with girlfriends about their feelings regarding sexuality.
Non-helpful thoughts:	Non-helpful actions:
Being sexual with yourself is "wrong." Sex is to be experienced only with a partner.	Isolating myself from relationships to avoid sexual experiences.

MY REWARD (if I meet my goal) Short-term: One year membership in the local health club.
Long-term: Trip to Hawaii with friend from work.

THE COST: (if I fail to meet my goal) Bring my lunch to work for one week, no eating out.

REEVALUATION DATE: 8-4 — six weeks evaluation
1-4 — six months evaluation

I agree to help with this project:

Carol
(Support person)

I agree to strive toward this goal:

Lucenda   6-20
(Your signature)   (date)

Figure 15–3 Self-contract. *(Adapted with permission from Baldi, S., et al. (1980). For your health: A model for self-care. South Laguna, CA: Nurses Model Health, p. 47.)*

TABLE 15–9. SAMPLE SELF-CARE ACTIVITY WORKSHEET

Schedule for first six weeks
  Week 1: 10 minutes three times a week   Week 4: 15 minutes four times a week
  Week 2: 10 minutes three times a week   Week 5: 20 minutes four times a week
  Week 3: 15 minutes three times a week   Week 6: 30 minutes four times a week
Activities: During the times listed above, I will choose from one or a combination of
    the following activities to nurture my sexuality:
Sensual skills
    1. Identify the settings and situations in which I feel most sensual
    2. Spend the stated extra time at a specific grooming activity: get a manicure,
       bathing, hair care, use body lotions, perfumes, etc.
    3. Spend the stated extra time completing a relaxation exercise
    4. Get to know my anatomy; study my body in the mirror, complete a genital
       anatomy scale, exercise my levator ani and coccygei muscles
    5. Learn to massage my own body
Communication skills
    1. Read *For Yourself* by Lonnie Barbach; use this to help me clarify my sexual
       values
    2. Complete self-assessment tools and discuss with the nurse
    3. Attend follow-up sessions with nurse
Schedule for remainder of six months
Month 2: Continue 30 minutes four times a week; complete the following activities
    1. Learn how to masturbate and practice for at least part of each weekly time
    2. Develop skills of sexual fantasy through use of reading, imagery, music
Month 3: Continue as above; in addition, accept one date with a man.
Month 4: Repeat above
Month 5: Repeat above
Month 6: Repeat above

Barbach, L. (1987). *For yourself: Fulfillment of female sexuality.* New York: Signet/New American Library.

rience she would be able to relax more and focus on her sensations during self-stimulation.

Leucenda said that she identified strongly with the reports of other women when she read *For Yourself.*[32] She believed that knowing about other women who felt the same way gave her confidence and a more positive body image. In particular, she felt that she had been brought up to believe that "sex is a man's area of expertise," and that since he would take care of it, she really did not need to learn about what felt good to her. She now recognized that getting pleasure from sexual experiences was her responsibility in *cooperation* with her partner. She understood that she must first know and feel comfortable with her own sexual responses.

At the end of six weeks, Leucenda wanted to continue all of the self-care activities and begin learning masturbation exercises. She felt that this would help her with her fear of "losing control."

TABLE 15-10. NURSING CARE PLAN

Reason for Consultation: Routine physical exam; questions about birth control   *Client:* Leucenda

Assessment	Plan	Evaluation	
		Met	*Not met*
Self-care demand	*Setting objectives*		
Need for comfort and integration of sexuality in rest of life	Six weeks:		
	Spend at least 30 minutes four times a week on specific activities to nurture my sexuality.	X	
Assets	Six months:		
Highly motivated to discover sexual self	Continue with above and have accepted four dates with men.	(not yet evaluated; has accepted one date)	
Has social life and friends at work			
Knowledgeable about the self-care process	*Reaching objectives*		
In good physical health	Client actions		
Self-directed	Arrange for 30 minutes a day free to nurture sexuality.	X	
Good relationship with nurse	Take phone off hook, do not answer door.	X	
Limitations	Buy and keep diary of my self-care plan.	X	
Childhood training re: sexuality	Buy and read books recommended by nurse.	(partially done)	
Lack of positive past experiences with sexuality	Buy special bath lotions, perfumes.	X	
Busy work schedule, priority on work	Read *For Yourself*[a] within two weeks.	X	
Lack of knowledge re: own anatomy	Follow plan on activity worksheet (see Table 15.9) and identify which activities are most helpful.	X	
Possible difficulty with resolution re: divorce 6 months ago	See nurse in two weeks.		X

Diagnosis	Nursing actions	
Self-care deficit	Provide education re: normal sexual development.	×
Discomfort with own body secondary to lack of information and experience	Provide consultation re: birth control and preventing risks of sexually transmitted disease.	×
	Offer assistance if client wishes to discuss divorce.	×
	Work on decreased dependence on nurse.	×
	Encourage eventual use of friend as contracting support person.	×
	Model sexual health.	×
		Needed revisions More anxious about masturbation. Take this phase more slowly.
Reevaluation date	Client follow-up	
Every two weeks in office. By phone as needed.	Will return to clinic in six months. Friend is now support person.	

*Barbach, L. (1975) *For yourself: Fulfillment of female sexuality.* New York: Signet/New American Library.

Finally, Leucenda told the nurse that her friend from work had agreed to join the program as a contracting partner. In return, she was going to help her friend in a similar self-care program. After the six-week evaluation period, Leucenda and her nurse ended their formal contact, although Leucenda said she would call if she felt she needed further direction or assistance.

Leucenda said that after only six weeks she already felt more positive about her sexuality. The positive feelings were also giving her new confidence in other areas. She joined a local health club as her sixth-week reward. The exercises there helped her get more in touch with her body, and she also enjoyed meeting the new people. Leucenda had accepted one date, had a pleasant evening, and felt comfortable with the man. She felt that she was ready to repeat this experience with relative ease and continue to take additional risks in order to develop and nurture her sexuality.

SUMMARY

This chapter has presented the significance of sexuality to health. The roles of normal psychosexual development, learning, touch, body image, and culture in sexual health were explored. Specific information about the influence of medications, birth control, and the threat of sexually transmitted disease on overall sexuality was provided. Self-care activities to manage each of these issues were emphasized. Specific self-care activities that nurture sexuality were outlined.

Although this chapter did not address treatment of sexual disturbance, a number of sexual disorders were briefly described. A specific example of how the nursing process can be integrated to help a client learn and maintain sexual self-care was included.

The nurse's own awareness and comfort with sexual issues were described as crucial for effective interventions with clients in this area. Emphasis was placed on development of the nurse's ability to listen without making judgments about sensitive and emotional sexual issues.

STUDY QUESTIONS

Personal Focus

1. How would you rate your level of comfort with your own sexuality? Rate yourself as a model of sexual self-care. What are the ways in which you nurture your own sexuality?
2. What is your definition of sexuality?
3. What is the role of sexuality in you life?
4. Describe the situations and settings in which you feel most sexual.
5. Complete a self-contract regarding one area of your sexual self-care.

Client Focus

1. Discuss the importance of early learning experiences on the development of sexuality. Role-play your explanations of this to a client.
2. With a partner, role-play and practice asking questions regarding a client's sexuality when the client seems hesitant or embarrassed to discuss the issue.
3. Describe the conditions in which you would refer a client for sexual counseling.
4. List the ways in which you can promote sexual health in the clinical setting of your current practice.
5. Practice teaching a client basic self-care activities to prevent sexually transmitted disease.
6. Help a client to complete a self-contract in the area of sexual self-care.

REFERENCES

1. World Health Organization. (1975). *Education and treatment in human sexuality: The training of health professionals* (Report of WHO Meeting, Technical Report Series, No. 572) Geneva: Author, p. 6.
2. Johnson, J. & Klein, L. (1988). *I can cope: Staying healthy with cancer.* Minneapolis, MN: DCI Publishing, pp. 117–118.
3. World Health Organization. *Education and treatment in human sexuality.*
4. Lion, *Human Sexuality*, p. 9.
5. Jourard, M. (1974). *Healthy personality.* New York: Macmillan, pp. 279–281.
6. Wells, C. (1980). Unrealistic aspects of orgasm. *Medical aspects of human sexuality.* 14, 60.
7. Jourard. *Healthy personality*, p. 281.
8. Jourard. Healthy personality, p. 266.
9. Jourard. Healthy personality, p. 11.
10. Sarrel, L., & Sarrell, P. (1984). *Sexual turning points.* New York: MacMillan.
11. Butler, R., & Lewis, M. (1986). *Love and sex after 40: A guide for men and women for their mid and later years.* New York: Harper & Row.
12. Yates, A. (1978). *Sex without shame.* New York: William Morrow, p. 158.
13. Oakes, M. (1975). Blessing way ceremony, puberty rite. *The Co-evolution Quarterly,* 184–185.
14. Yates. *Sex without shame,* p. 74.
15. Spitz, R.A. (1965). *The first year of life.* New York: International Universities Press.
16. Derrogatis, L. (1980). Psychological assessment of psychosexual functioning," In J.K. Meyer (Ed.), *Psychiatric clinics of North America* (Vol. 3, No. 1). Philadelphia: W. B. Saunders, p. 123.
17. Norwood, R. (1988). Letters from women who love too much. NY: Pocket Books.
18. Masters, W., & Johnson, V. (1966). *Human sexual response.* Boston: Little, Brown.
19. Schiavi, R. C. & Schreiner-Engle, P. (1980). Physiologic aspects of sexual function and dysfunction. In J.K. Meyer (Ed.), *Psychiatric clinics of North America* (Vol. 3, No. 1). Philadelphia: W.B. Saunders, p. 82.

20. Jourard. *Healthy personality,* pp. 267–268.
21. Gallo, R. & Montagnier, L. (1988). AIDS in 1988. *Scientific American, 259* (4), 41–48.
22. Heyward, W., & Curran, J. (1988). The epidemiology of AIDS in the U.S. *Scientific American, 259* (4), 72–79.
23. Mann, J., Chin, J., Piot, P., & Quinn, T. (1988). The international epidemiology of AIDS. *Scientific American, 259* (4), 82–89.
24. Surgeon General's report on acquired immune deficiency syndrome. (1988). Washington DC: U.S. Public Health Service.
25. Bancroft, J. (1989). *Human sexuality and its problems.* 2nd ed. NY: Churchill Livingstone.
26. Pearsall, P. (1987). Super marital sex: Loving for life. NY: Doubleday.
27. DeAngelis, B. (1987). How to make love all the time. NY: Rawson Assoc.
28. Masters, W., & Johnson V. (1970). *Human sexual inadequacy.* Boston: Little, Brown.
29. Friday, N. (1973). *My Secret Garden.* New York: Pocket.
30. Friday, N. (1980). *Men in love.* New York: Dell.
31. Barbach, L. (1983). *Shared intimacies.* New York: Bantam.
32. Barbach, L. (1975). *For each other: Sharing sexual intimacies.* New York: Signet New American Library.

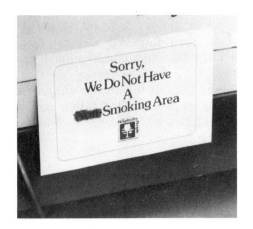

We must go out and re-ally ourselves to Nature
  every day.
We must make root,
Send out some little fibre at least,
Even every winter day.

I am sensible that I am imbibing health
When I open my mouth to the wind

Thoreau

16 Environmental Self-Care

LEARNING OBJECTIVES

Upon completion of this chapter, readers will be able to:

1. Define environmental self-care.
2. List three self-care activities for each of the given environmental self-care areas.
3. Describe the role of the consumer in environmental self-care.
4. List four nursing actions that promote environmental self-care efforts of clients.
5. Assist a client in developing an environmental self-care contract.

DEFINITIONS

Environment   All that surrounds (and therefore influences) a human being, including other human beings, animate and inanimate objects, climate, and so on.

Environmental Self-Care   Actions that are performed to enhance an individual's surroundings. These activities not only prevent illness, they also enhance wellness and promote health maintenance. These may be on a personal, community, or global level.

INTRODUCTION

In recent years, increased attention has been focused on the environment, specifically on areas such as smog, water pollution, nuclear power, and population control. These issues profoundly affect health and daily living.

People relate to their environment in different ways, many of them culturally determined. For example, many native Americans feel an equality with the environment and work in unison with it. Modern science and technology have created environmental problems. Automobile pollution, high noise levels, abuse of natural resources, and waste disposal problems have all tested environmental limits. The threat of nuclear war further tests even the survival of our planet.

To many people, these environmental areas seem too large and too distant to call for much personal time or attention. There are, however, many ways in which people can become aware of and alter environmental conditions within their personal and community spaces. This awareness can lead to the practice of environmental self-care techniques that enhance wellness.

HISTORICAL PERSPECTIVE

Many have long been aware of the environment and its effects on health. Before Pasteur defined the relationship between bacteria and disease, several people identified the relationship between polluted water and disease.[1] Air pollution was first documented in London more than 300 years ago.[2] Remedies for these early pollutions were also documented.[3,4]

Publication of Carson's *Silent Spring* in 1962 promoted a new awareness of the environment.[5] The major focus of her book encouraged people to pause and take stock of the relationship of environmental conditions to their personal wellness.

With attention from the media, a global or worldwide approach to the environment was fostered in the 1970s and continues to grow. This movement centers on factors that affect the quality of life: population growth, finiteness of the earth, utilization of resources, energy, and ecopoisons.[6,7]

Environment and Nursing

Nurses have been involved with environmental concerns since earliest practice in primitive societies. Although clients were not always bathed regularly, nurses had responsibility for laundry, lighting, and other environmental areas.

In the late Middle Ages, much nursing care was done by women in private homes. Often, the sick person's room would be scented with sweet herbs. Red curtains, bedclothes, and other red objects were used in sick rooms before it was believed that red had healing and strengthening powers. Fresh air was not seen as important and the bed curtains were kept drawn.[8]

During the Crimean War, Nightingale focused on environmental conditions at Scutari Hospital. Sanitation in food preparation, dishwashing, and cleansing were some of her first tasks. Her other areas of concentration included ventilation, warmth, noise, and light.[8]

Community health nursing is an area of practice traditionally associated with environmental standards. It was developed in the late nineteenth century as a response to needed care for the sick in their homes. Communicable disease was rampant.[8] Community health nurses brought health care and health teaching directly to the people. With DRGs (diagnostically related groups) and other cost-containment measures, the focus on home care services has become even stronger in the 1990's.

In contemporary practice, the environment is given a significant amount of attention. Specifically in hospitals, environmental planning deals with space, color, lighting, sound, and safety. Mental health nurses have long recognized the importance of environment as part of the therapeutic milieu. The influence of these elements both on clients and health care personnel has become clearly recognized.

Nursing theorists view environment in a variety of ways. Rogers looks at people and environment as coextensive energy fields.[9] Orem talks about environment as elements external to the individual that interact with him or her to affect the self-care system.[10] Parse's theory of "man–living–health" views the person as being in an energy interchange with the environment, participating in a continuously changing process that he or she cocreates.[11] Watson says, "All human caring is related to intersubjective human responses to health–illness conditions; a knowledge of health–illness, environmental–personal interactions; a knowledge of the nurse caring process; self-knowledge, knowledge of one's power and transaction limitations." She also asks, "What are the conditions that facilitate or sustain human care and caring in instances of threatened humanity?"[12]

ENVIRONMENT, HEALTH, AND SELF-CARE

Today, clinical ecology remains an obscure, poorly-defined interest outside the mainstream of acceptable medical practice.[13] There has been much attention to the negative health effects of the environment, however such as the role of air pollution in pulmonary disease. Less attention has been given to the positive health effects of the environment. Environmental self-care focuses on *positive actions* that an individual can take to attain and maintain a healthy personal and community environment.

ENVIRONMENTAL COMPONENTS

There are environmental concerns whether the person is at work, at home, in the hospital, or traveling. Each of the environmental components discussed in this chapter applies to each of these settings.

Many aspects of the environment can influence health. Not all, however, are under the *direct* influence or control of the individual. This chapter focuses on a number of environmental areas that individuals can influence to enhance health. With each topic, relevant self-care activities are included. The environmental areas discussed include air, water, energy, safety, sound, light and color, space, and environmental self-care advocacy.

Air

Air is a universal need. All living things require it. Unclean air has the ability to decrease the quality of life through discomfort and disease. Probably the oldest form of air pollution occurred in prehistory when people lived in caves and experienced smoke contamination from fires that were built for warmth and cooking. Today, because of pollution, many of the cities of the world have unhealthful air much of the time.

Air pollution comes from many sources, both natural and man made. Natural sources of pollution include dust, pollen, and soil particles. Man made sources include by-products of fuel combustion, automobiles, industry, or agricultural burnings.

Many remote lakes in the Northeast are being permanently polluted from fossil-fuel plant emissions, which return to the land in the form of acid rain. These emissions also create a "greenhouse effect," allowing carbon dioxide to build up and preventing heat from escaping back into the atmosphere. As a result, polar ice caps are melting, which will have complex ecological consequences.

In industrial urban areas, smog is exacerbated by temperature inversion, which occurs when a layer of cold air is trapped under a layer of warmer air. This acts as a lid on pollution. When this happens there can be excessive morbidity and mortality in susceptible individuals. Air pollution can cause irritation of nasal and respiratory passages, chest constriction, headache, and emphysema.[14]

Smoking has long been designated as "hazardous to your health." Cancer rates are significantly higher for smokers for all types of cancer, not just lung cancer. Smoking also increases the incidence of other diseases, including cardiovascular disease, chronic obstructive pulmonary disease, ulcers, allergies, and decreases immune response. Pregnant women who smoke are more likely to have smaller, premature babies. Workers who smoke have a higher incidence of absenteeism and therefore cost more to employ.[15] Exposure to passive smoke has also become a known hazard.

Most people think of air pollution as being outside and go indoors to protect themselves from it; however, indoor air pollution is also a significant problem. Americans spend anywhere from 70 to 90 percent of their time indoors. Common sources of indoor pollution include asbestos; molds, bacteria, fungi; radon; cigarette smoke; carbon monoxide from gas appliances, chimneys, and automobiles in garages; and building and furnishing materials that emit vapors such as formaldehyde.[16]

Environmental self-care relative to air requires individual as well as group action and responsibility. Table 16–1 lists self-care activities that promote better air quality.

Water

Water has been used for therapeutic purposes since the time of the early Egyptians. Water was and still is used as a self-care remedy for muscle tension. Consider the rise in the use of hot tubs in the last several years.

Like air, water is a universal need. Without water, no living things could survive. Plants, animals, and human beings all require it. Water pollution continues to occur. The Environmental Protection Agency (EPA) reports more than 700 potentially harmful chemicals have been found in United States drinking water. Even small amounts of groundwater pollution, such as a single gallon of gasoline, can make a town's well water unfit to drink for years.[17]

One particular chemical, polychlorinated biphenyl, accumulates in human

TABLE 16–1. ENVIRONMENTAL SELF-CARE ACTIVITIES: AIR

1. Limit activity according to air pollution level (e.g., do not do strenuous exercise on days with high pollution levels or at high pollution rush hours).
2. Do not smoke or live with smokers. Ask people in the immediate environment to stop smoking.
3. Limit amount of time spent in traffic.
4. Use mass transit or bicycles when possible.
5. Limit use of aerosol sprays.
6. Do not incinerate garbage or trash at home.
7. Keep automobile tuned up, emission-control device serviced.
8. Participate in community and legislative action regarding air concerns.
9. Keep green plants in surroundings.
10. Choose building materials and furnishings that do not emit vapors.
11. Have furnaces, stoves, ovens, and woodstoves checked regularly for safe ventilation.

adipose tissue. Human beings except for lactating women do not usually excrete fat. Polychlorinated biphenyl and the pesticide DDT have been found in human breast milk. These chemicals are now appearing in the human food chain, to be perpetuated for generations.

Historically, polluted water has been associated with disease. Epidemics of typhoid and cholera have been documented since the nineteenth century as being related to contaminated water. The World Health Organization (WHO) states that about 800 million people suffer from one of four water-related diseases. WHO has designated 1981 to 1990 as the "International Drinking Water Supply and Sanitation Decade," with the goal of clean water for all by 1990.[18] As of this date, progress is unclear.

Sources of water pollution include:

1. Untreated sewage, consisting of animal and plant waste in which the oxygen supply in the water is depleted.
2. Treated sludge, containing algae that die and lead to depletion of oxygen in the water.
3. Industrial waste (e.g., toxic chemicals).

Oceans, rivers, lakes, and groundwater supplies are increasingly becoming eutrophicated, meaning that nutrients and sediments in the water increase and the oxygen content of the water decreases. This is a natural aging process for bodies of water. When wastes are discharged in water, however, this markedly accelerates the process and can have a profound effect on both the quality and quantity of our freshwater supply.

Environmental self-care relative to water has a great impact at the legislative level. The Marine Protection Research and Sanctuaries Act of 1972 prohibits ocean dumping of most materials except by permit from the EPA. The Safe Drinking Water Act of 1974 has allowed states to increase resources devoted to the study of waterborne illnesses. Individuals must continue to support protection of water resources and be aware of the hazards of water pollution. Water conservation must also be practiced. Self-care actions for this area are given in Table 16–2. The importance of water relative to diet is presented in Chapter 14.

Energy

Increasing costs of home utilities, solar and wind energy, limitations of natural resources, and dangers of microwaves are all important energy issues. A great amount of literature deals with the controversial advantages and disadvantages of nuclear energy. Safety of nuclear power production is controversial. Recent studies indicate that there may be no safe level of radiation exposure, no dose of radiation so low that the risk of cancer is zero.[19]

The majority of radiation exposure occurs from natural sources, including sources within the earth. Granite, natural gas, and phosphates are examples of these. There is little that can be done to limit human exposure to these sources. Recently, radon has become a national health concern. A colorless, odorless gas

TABLE 16–2. ENVIRONMENTAL SELF-CARE ACTIVITIES: WATER

1. Use biodegradable laundry products.
2. Dispose of chemical wastes so as not to contaminate natural resources.
3. Develop a stored water supply for use in emergency.
4. Determine total fluoride intake: water, toothpaste, dental application, supplements.
5. Participate in community action, lobbying, voting to promote clean water.
6. Determine contaminants in personal water supply, especially if living in a high radon area. Use filtration or bottled water if indicated.
7. Swim only in safe water.
8. Use water conservation devices in the home (flow restricters, shorter showers, minimally full bathtubs, full loads in dishwashers and washing machines).
9. Use drought-tolerant landscaping, resulting in less water usage.
10. Use drip irrigation or water-conserving means of watering landscaping.

produced by the decay of naturally occurring uranium in rock and soil, the gas can travel through cracks or openings in the basement of a home. Studies of uranium miners have shown that exposure to high levels of naturally occurring radon can cause lung cancer. In a survey by the EPA from 1986 to 1988, 10 of 17 states had a significant percentage of homes with levels above the safe range.[20] Homes can be tested and treated for radon. In addition to some background radiation from the sun, other sources of radioactivity are radioactive waste and X-rays.

Often little consideration is given to dental X-rays, X-rays for injuries or illness, or even to parents or nurses who participate in X-ray testing with clients. Microwave ovens and older-model color television sets can also be sources of radiation if not properly serviced and maintained.

Many people purposely expose themselves to the ultraviolet radiation of the sun when they try to tan. The beneficial effects of vitamin D production and a beautiful tan are clearly outweighed by the potential danger to the skin. Skin cancer, damage and thickening of the skin cells, and permanent dilation of superficial blood vessels may appear after years of repeated exposure. Environmental self-care activities relative to energy are found in Table 16–3.

Safety

Environmental safety is an issue that transcends all boundaries. It follows an individual no matter where he or she goes. Many people feel safe at home, and yet more than 240,000 people are killed in their own homes in the United States every year.[21]

In recent years, there has been an increasing concern for the health and safety of those in the workplace. As a result, the Occupational Safety and Health Administration was formed. This federal agency develops safety standards for the workplace and inspects agencies for compliance. The Nuclear Regulatory Commission specifically monitors issues of nuclear safety.

Traveling to and from work can also be hazardous. Automobile accidents

TABLE 16–3. ENVIRONMENTAL SELF-CARE ACTIVITIES: ENERGY

1. Employ X-ray precautions:
   Question necessity and limit use of X-rays, radiation.
   Inform health care provider of pregnancy or possible pregnancy before X-ray procedure.
   Use lead shield for body parts other than those directly involved or if assisting with procedure.
   Wear radiation monitoring badge if exposed at work.
   Keep a record of X-rays, including where filed, to avoid unnecessary repeats.
2. Check microwave oven and color televisions for radiation leaks.
3. Know local evacuation plan for disaster.
4. Provide a temperature-safe environment, neither too hot nor cold.
5. Provide adequate ventilation and fresh air for heat and appliance use.
6. Wear protective clothing, sunscreen, and limit exposure to sun.
7. Participate in community and legislative action regarding energy concerns.
8. Support and participate in anti-nuclear groups.
9. Recycle when possible.
10. Keep auto well-tuned. Use carpools or mass transit.
11. Incorporate solar energy in home and work setting.
12. Test home for the presence of radon and repair as needed.

have been one of the major causes of deaths for the last several years. For every highway fatality, there are nearly 100 injuries.[21] Many states have enacted child and adult restraint laws.

Being aware of safety factors in the home, work setting, and during travel can increase one's quality of life through prevention of accident or injury. Table 16–4 lists self-care activities for environmental self-care relative to safety.

Sound

A causal relationship between noise and hearing loss has been recognized for hundreds of years. Since the Industrial Revolution, society has developed increasing numbers of automobiles, tools, appliances, and machinery that contribute to high levels of noise and thus to increasing amounts of sensorineural hearing losses.[22]

Sound is measured in decibels (dB). The scale runs from 0, which has been designated at the threshold of human hearing, to 140 dB, which is the equivalent of an amplified rock band at close range. Prolonged exposure at 85 dB can induce hearing damage. At 75 dB, the autonomic nervous system becomes aroused, generally without the individual's awareness.[23] Figure 16–1 presents examples of common sound levels.

In addition to hearing loss, four nonauditory effects of loud noise have been identified.

1. Interference with speech communication.
2. Interference with efficiency of performance.

TABLE 16–4. ENVIRONMENTAL SELF-CARE ACTIVITIES: SAFETY

1. Follow safety guidelines at home and work:
   Wet floors marked
   Medicines kept out of reach
   Smoke alarms checked regularly
   Fire extinguisher placed in home
   Fire drills practiced
   Emergency phone numbers posted
   CPR certificate and first aid kept current
   Electrical outlets plugged and unused appliances unplugged
   Plastic bags kept out of reach
   Stairs and floors kept clear, uncluttered
   Children protected from falling out of windows
   Cupboard safety latches used
   Cleaning supplies kept out of reach
   Guidelines for babysitters given
   Swimming pools protected
   Children not left unattended in bathtubs
   Safe toys provided according to age of child
2. Store emergency supplies of food, water, medicine, fuel, paper products, sanitary supplies, baby food, formula, diapers.
3. Use seat belts and car seats; drive within the speed limit.
4. Do not drink and drive or ride with someone who has been drinking.
5. Avoid driving late at night and on holidays when drinking drivers are most common.
6. Drive a car that is "crash-worthy" according to government standards.
7. Keep firearms unloaded and locked away.
8. Teach children safety practices.
9. Actively participate in community to promote safety.
10. Work for safe nuclear power production.
11. Know earthquake, flood, and fire emergency procedures.
12. Practice safety techniques to avoid injury from lightning.

3. Annoyance.
4. Disturbances of physiological function.[24]

Examples of physiological changes include vasoconstriction of small vessels, blood pressure changes, increased corticosteroids in the blood and urine, increased respiratory rates, digestive disturbances, and increased muscle tension.[24]

In one California study, children who attended school near freeways were found to score consistently and significantly lower in reading and math than did children from a socioeconomically matched control group who did not attend schools near freeways.[25]

Sound is everywhere—inside the home, outside, at work. Sometimes people have become so used to sounds in their environments that they do not "hear" them. Fluorescent lights, refrigerators, fans, water heaters, and clocks are common low-level sources of sound. In the hospital, sounds, especially in

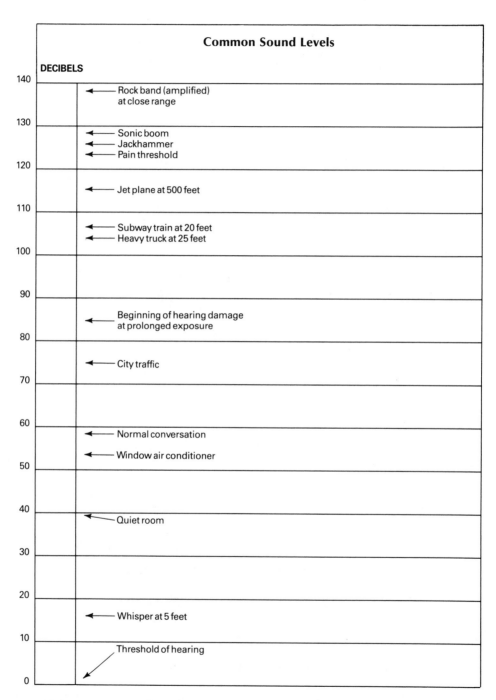

Figure 16–1. Common sound levels.(*Used with permission from Flynn, P.A.R. (1980). Holistic health: The art and science of care. Bowie, MD: R.J. Brady, p. 105.)*

critical-care units, are present 24 hours per day. Although nurses may not "hear" the sounds of the monitors, ventilators, infusion pumps, and suction machines, clients and their families may find these sounds stressful.

Sounds also have positive effects. For example, soft, quiet music can create the opposite physiological effects from those listed above. The Bible relates that David played his harp to provide soothing, relaxing music. Provision of a "quiet time" with a marked decrease in sensory input can also create positive physiological effects. Table 16–5 reviews environmental self-care activities relative to sound (also see Chapter 9 for relaxation and music).

Light and Color

Light and color have a major influence on the immediate environment. Sunlight provides the most complete and natural light source. Its effects are dependent on its full range from ultraviolet to visible colors. Sunlight is essential for human growth. It produces vitamin D within the skin. Vitamin D is essential for absorption of calcium and phosphorus, which leads to mineralization of bone. Sunlight is also central to other important bodily processes, such as immunologic responsiveness, regulation of stress and fatigue, control of viral infections, colds and endocrine function.[26]

Early human beings lived in an environment in which activity was oriented to sunlight. As people moved indoors to protect themselves from the weather, indoor lighting became more important. Some cultures found win-

TABLE 16–5. ENVIRONMENTAL SELF-CARE ACTIVITIES: SOUND

1. Check sound levels of new appliances *before* purchase.
2. Select items that make less noise (e.g., plastic trash cans instead of metal ones).
3. Select sound-absorbent furnishings: thick padded carpets, drapes, upholstered furniture.
4. Use sound "isolators" (e.g., concrete walls, water fountains) that resist passage of sound when possible.
5. Use mufflers on engines.
6. Use earmuffs, earplugs, or other protective devices when exposed to noisy machinery.
7. Play music, TV, radio at safe volumes.
8. Provide for quiet times.
9. Quiet children by singing to them.
10. Provide for music with calming effects.
11. Measure different places in environment with sound-level meter.
12. Tape-record home environment, work environment. Identify sounds that could be decreased or eliminated.
13. Live away from airports, noisy freeways or busy streets if possible.
14. Participate in community/legislative processes to minimize excessive environmental sounds.

dows in dwellings such a luxury that they were taxed.[27,28] Today, many people work and live almost totally indoors. It is important to have artificial light sources that duplicate, as closely as possible, natural light sources.

Providing for complete artificial light can have positive effects. One study found that students who studied for four hours under fluorescent light that simulated sunlight exhibited significantly better visual acuity and less physiological fatigue at the end of the time period than when cool white fluorescent lighting was used.[29] In another report, it was found that an increase in motor and cardiovascular fitness and trends toward lower heart rates and decreased systolic blood pressures followed ultraviolet light treatments.[30] Zamkova and Krivitskaya found that children working in full-spectrum lighting had lower levels of fatigue, improved working capacity, and improved academic performance.[31]

Nursing theorists as early as Nightingale identified the importance of light to health.[32] In hospital settings nurses are often in control of the amount of ambient light. In intensive care units constant 24-hour bright lighting and, conversely, continuous subdued lighting, have both been found to affect clients adversely, inducing disorganized thought, decreased concentration, anxiety, and disorientation.[33]

Light has also been suggested as one modality in the treatment of depression. This phenomenon is particularly significant during the winter months with extremely short daylight hours. The researchers in one study concluded that appropriate artificial light can effect people like natural sunlight.[34]

Color also has psychophysiological effects on people. Blue has been found to be associated with increased relaxation, quiescence, and decreased anxiety. Red elicits increased tension, excitement, and physiological stimulation.[35] Color has a direct impact on the practice of nursing. Hospital planners have long used colors that are soothing in client areas Some mental health facilities have found pink "time-out rooms" the most soothing, calming color for clients.[36]

Color is also important when working with the elderly. Changes in the lens affect the elderly person's ability to discriminate color. The loss is at the blue end of the color spectrum, and the person may be unable to discriminate between blue and green.[37,38]

There are a number of books, such as *Color Me Beautiful*,[39] that discuss the positive mood effects that can be achieved through wearing of color. Other popular books, such as *Dress for Excellence*,[40] describe the impact the colors of clothes have on people in the work environment.

The psychophysiological effects of light and color need to be considered in environmental self-care. Specific self-care activities are found in Table 16–6.

Space

Personal space involves both quantitative and qualitative aspects. Spatial boundaries include immediate personal space as well as personal space within one's home, neighborhood, and community. How this space is used has an

TABLE 16–6. ENVIRONMENTAL SELF-CARE ACTIVITIES: LIGHT AND COLOR

1. Provide for as much use of natural light as possible.
2. Use energy-conserving windows or skylights that admit natural light.
3. Limit use of "tinted" windows that restrict ultraviolet light and other colors from the spectrum.
4. Select soothing environmental colors, especially for the elderly.
5. Select clothing colors that have positive effects on mood.
6. Turn lights off at night when sleeping.
7. Provide for soothing background lighting.
8. Use fluorescent lights with nearly complete color spectrums.
9. Provide for time to be outdoors and exposed to sunlight (see energy and safety precautions). Wear optically correct sunglasses.
10. Provide for a lighting cycle (daytime light, nighttime dark) for people who are in hospitals or confined to home.

impact on health. Friedman states that the stability and comfort of one's home or dwelling may influence self-perception, stress, and health.[41]

Self-care includes providing for personal space that a person considers his or her own within the home. This is particularly important if the home is shared with many others. Having a place for personal belongings and a sense of privacy is important in developing and maintaining self-esteem and a sense of belonging and separateness.[42]

Personal space has been described by Hall as having four distance zones: intimate, personal, social, and public.[43] These zones are generally quite stable; however, they can vary according to culture and situation. In a crowd, the person's intimate zone ends with his or her outer clothing and goes no further. At another time, close personal distance might be 1½ to 2 feet.[43]

The "space issue" can be transmitted beyond the individual to a local, national, and even global level. By the year 2110, the world population will be 10.5 billion. There are conflicting views about the relationship between population and environmental pollution. Ehrlich and Holdren contend there is a relationship between environmental pollution and population levels.[45] Commoner, Carr, and Slanter assert that environmental pollution is more directly related to increased technological levels of productivity.[46]

The helping professions have a particular need to be aware of territoriality when caring for clients. Providing for personal space can serve to orient a client and provide a sense of belonging. In recent years, many hospitals have modified ward settings to semiprivate or private rooms, where the client's territory becomes more clearly defined.

Health care providers frequently enter a client's intimate zone when providing care. Although the touching that happens while caring for a client may be reassuring and comforting, the invasion of space can also increase anxiety. An awareness of the need for personal space is essential is planning for self-care. Specific self-care activities are found in Table 16–7.

TABLE 16–7. ENVIRONMENTAL SELF-CARE ACTIVITIES: SPACE

1. Provide for personal space, time, and privacy for self, family, and friends.
2. Become active in community issues involving space, urban planning, population growth and control.
3. Provide for personal space at work.
4. Provide for outdoor space with plants and sunlight.
5. Ask permission before entering another individual's personal space.
6. Have storage space available for each person's belongings.
7. Make home and work space pleasant (e.g., use plants and decorations to suit personal taste).

Environmental Self-Care Advocacy

People who care for the environment feel more connected to it and more protective of it.[47] Self-care in terms of the environment extends beyond what one can do *not* to contribute to its decline—to what can be *done* to improve existing conditions. What might be done individually and at the community level clearly overlap.

The first step toward addressing the myriad of environmental issues is to improve one's knowledge of the problems. Values enter into this process. How parents and friends have modeled involvement in environmental issues influences future personal action. Specific environmental issues have different significant in particular families. For example, if one comes from a family where allergies and pulmonary disease have been significant problems, participation in community involvement regarding air pollution may have been a highly valued activity. Before any action can take place, the value has to be clear to the individual. What is to be gained from this action? Is there personal benefit? Community benefit? Global benefit?

The second step is to become an active participant. A participating consumer is involved in the decision-making process. The following steps are guidelines for consumer participation in environmental issues:

1. Do a personal and community assessment of environmental needs.
2. Identify problems and attach priorities.
3. Set goals and objectives to resolve the problems.
4. Create consciousness-raising groups or join existing groups.
5. Get influential people to organize.
6. Implement actions by sending newsletters, newspaper articles, advertising, and so on.
7. Evaluate actions and redefine goals and objectives as indicated.

Working and voting for environmentally aware political candidates is another example of environmental self-care advocacy. *There is no more important self-care action than that of preventing nuclear war—which threatens the survival of humanity.* Political activism is one mechanism to accomplish this.

One professional group that actively participates in environmental self-care issues is Nurses' Environmental Health Watch, Inc.* This group's goal is educating nurses and the public about actual and potential threats to human and environmental health. Members are actively involved in networking across the country to accomplish this goal. Many nurses are also active in Physicians for Social Responsibility,† another group which addresses nuclear and other environmental threats to humanity.

NURSES MODEL ENVIRONMENTAL SELF-CARE

Nurses act as models of environmental self-care for family and friends. Figure 16–2 illustrates one environmental assessment tool. Nurses can use it to begin to assess their personal skills in this area. Modeling actions might include:

- Selecting soothing colors for home decorating.
- Providing for quiet time.
- Providing for privacy and personal space.
- Using noisy appliances (vacuum, washer, dryer, dishwasher) when the fewest people are around.
- Using skin protection during exposure to the sun.
- Providing a safe environment.
- Using electronic air filters.
- Avoiding smoke; not allowing smoking in home, work, or car.
- Keeping the telephone bell turned to its lowest volume.
- Having drinking water supply tested for impurities.
- Teaching children about environmental self-care.
- Actively participating in community environmental groups.
- Participating in anti-nuclear groups.

Throughout history, nurses have been involved in caring for the client's environment. Disinfection, linen changes, lighting, and safety precautions are all environmental concerns that have traditionally belonged to nurses.

Today, there are still many ways in which nurses can model environmental self-care for clients. Many of these are continuations or extensions of traditional nursing responsibilities. These might include:

- Playing quiet background music for clients.
- Using vibrating pagers instead of verbal paging or loud beepers.
- Participating in agency committees to select colors, furnishings, lighting, and safety equipment.

---

*Nurses' Environmental Health Watch, Inc., 1808 Aggie Lane, Austin, TX 78757.
†Physicians for Social Responsibility, 639 Massachusetts Ave., Cambridge, MA 02193

- Monitoring sound levels in client areas.
- Maintaining room temperatures for *client* comfort.
- Asking permission *before* entering a client's personal space.
- Wearing uniforms or clothing in quiet, soothing colors.
- Providing for safe disposal of harmful and infectious waste.
- Protecting self and others from unnecessary exposure to radiation.
- Participating in Nurses' Environmental Health Watch or Physicians for Social Responsibility groups.

Each of these self-care actions promotes environmental self-care with clients, family, and friends through modeling by the nurse.

CLINICAL APPLICATION

Case Presentation

Six months ago the Gomez family moved from Mexico to a farming community approximately 50 miles from a large metropolitan city. The family consists of the father, Manuel, age 42; the mother, Juanita, age 35; and the children: Carlota, 7; Jaime, 5; Roberto, 3; and Maria, 8 months. Juanita's mother, Anita, age 70, also lives with the family. The family's house is a cottage in the farm worker's village. It has one large area for living and sleeping, a kitchen, and a bathroom.

Juanita visited the local community health department's family planning center for birth control counseling and a PAP smear. During her health history interview by the nurse practitioner, Juanita expressed frustration with her living conditions. She felt that they had moved to a country where the "living was supposed to be so easy." Although they had not had much money in Mexico, they did have more physical space and privacy and had their own belongings, which had been left behind.

Assessment

- self-care demand
- assets
- limitations

The nurse practitioner completed a *health history* and found that neither Juanita nor any of the family had any physical problems. Anita was also in good physical health.

Developmentally, Juanita was in Erikson's stage of generativity. She was active in providing a home life for her husband and children, preparing meals, and caring for all of the household needs. Juanita's *sociocultural orientation* was Mexican. In her culture, extended families often live together. When she was a child, her grandparents had lived with her family.

Juanita's *current concern* seemed to center around her environment. The physical structure of their cottage was old, the wiring was exposed, and the linoleum was in need of repair. There"might" be a leak in the gas stove. There was one tiny window in the living area in addition to the door. All of these areas required attention.

Juanita completed the environmental self-assessment tool presented in Figure 16–2. All of the assessment tools found in the community health department were available in Spanish.*

A summary of Juanita's assets and limitations revealed these assets:

- Good physical health
- Availability of her mother
- Pleasure working in and around her home
- Concern about environmental safety

Juanita's limitations were:

- New country
- Lack of financial resources
- Spanish-speaking in a primarily English-speaking health system
- Poor condition of her cottage
- Physical overcrowding of her living space
- Lack of knowledge of the "system"
- Lack of awareness of unsafe conditions

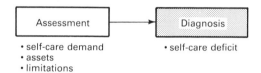

Juanita and the nurse practitioner agreed that Juanita had a self-care deficit. It was expressed as:

Inability to provide for environmental safety without intervention and support

A nursing diagnosis might read:

Potential for injury related to environmental hazard

Although many other issues concerned her, Juanita felt that this was the primary problem area.

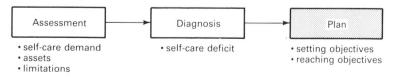

---

*For the purpose of this text, the assessment tool is shown in English.

ENVIRONMENTAL SELF-ASSESSMENT

Complete the following self-assessment to help you look at the role of environment in your life. On the scale below circle the numbers which are most true for you and your life during the last year:

	Almost Never	Seldom	Often	Almost Always
1. I change my immediate surroundings to reflect my favorite colors.	(1)	2	3	4
2. I am aware of the effects of light levels on my health.	(1)	2	3	4
3. I maintain a pleasant environment for myself.	1	(2)	3	4
4. I use non-aerosol sprays.	1	2	(3)	4
5. I know the levels of unsafe elements in my drinking water.	(1)	2	3	4
6. I know which toxic chemicals or other hazards I come in contact with.	(1)	2	3	4
7. I am aware of sources of noise pollution in my environment.	(1)	2	3	4
8. I am aware of sources of radiation in my home.	(1)	2	3	4
9. I avoid smoke-filled rooms.	(1)	2	3	4
10. I participate in environmental decision-making within my local community.	(1)	2	3	4

Some suggestions for how you might learn from this self-assessment:

1. Connect all the circles down the length of the page. Look at the pattern that your connected line makes. Turn your page sideways to get an even more clear visual picture of your environmental health. What does it seem to be saying to you?

2. Now add up your total score: _____ *13* _____

   Circle which range it was in:
   (10-19)   20-29   30-40

   If your score was in the 10-19 range you might want to make some changes in your life. Which aspects do you think need the most work? How many "1's" did you mark on this assessment?
   8 These might serve as a clue to help you think about making changes in this area of your life.

3. How would you like this self-assessment to look six months from now? Are you interested in working toward those improvements?

4. Remember to give yourself a pat on the back for the ways that you practice environmental self-care. Keep up the good work!

Figure 16–2 Environmental self-assessment *Adapted with permission from Baldi, S., et al. (1980). For your health: A model for self-care. South Laguna, CA: Nurses Model Health.)*

Setting Objectives

Juanita and the nurse practitioner together established behavioral objectives that were clear and concise. They discussed their respective roles in attaining objectives. The initial goal was "to call the gas and electric utility companies within 24 hours." Juanita's self-contract is presented in Fugire 16–3.

Reaching Objectives: Nursing and Client Actions. It was agreed that the nurse would provide support and education. Other specific nursing responsibilities were to:

- Provide Juanita with the telephone numbers of the utilities where a Spanish-speaking customer service representative would be located.
- Be available by telephone for support.
- Arrange for interpreter if needed.
- Provide names of additional community service groups that would be able to lend support.

Juanita delineated her responsibilities on her self-contract. They included:

- Telephone the utility companies within 24 hours.
- Return for appointment in one week.
- Call the nurse for support if needed.
- Be at home for the repair person to come.
- Get written documentation of specific needed repairs.
- Telephone progress report to the nurse within 48 hours.

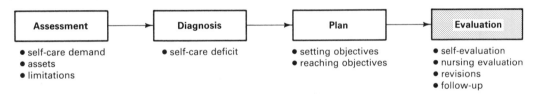

Juanita telephoned the nurse within 48 hours. She had contacted both of the utility companies and both had been to her home. The gas company did find a leak in the stove and repaired it. The repair person also checked each of the gas appliances and connections in the cottage.

The repair person from the electric company found several violations of building codes. While the utility company was unauthorized to make the repairs, a list was itemized for Juanita and the need for immediate attention was emphasized.

The nurse arranged for an interpreter to speak to the landlord with Juanita regarding the repairs. The nurse gave Juanita verbal support for her actions and discussed her alternatives if the landlord was uncooperative. Juanita was given the names of community service groups that would be able to lend support. The nurse confirmed their meeting in five days and reminded Juanita that she was

SELF-CONTRACT

MY GOALS:

Short-term— by the end of six weeks I will . . . *Call the gas and electric company within 24 hrs.*

Long-term— by the end of six months I will . . . *Repaint inside of house.*

ENVIRONMENTAL PLANNING: (all the steps I will take to reach my goal)

1. Get telephone numbers of Spanish-speaking customer service representatives.

2. Go to Bonita's to use telephone.

3. Plan to stay at home when the repairperson will come. Get needed repairs in writing.

THOUGHTS AND ACTIONS

Helpful thoughts:	Helpful actions:
This will make the house safer for the family.	*Making going to Bonita's to call a fun time.*
Non-helpful thoughts:	**Non-helpful actions:**
No one has gotten hurt yet.	*Putting it off until the next time I go to Bonita's.*

MY REWARD (if I meet my goal) *Lunch at McDonald's alone with Bonita.*

THE COST: (if I fail to meet my goal) *Watch Bonita's children for 1 day.*

REEVALUATION DATE: *Call the nurse in 48 hours. Return appointment 1 week (Tues. 3pm).*

I agree to help with this project:

Manuel
_____
(Support person)

I agree to strive toward this goal:

Juanita   *9/5*
_____
(Your signature)   (date)

Figure 16–3. Self-contract. *(Adapted with permission from Baldi, S., et. al. (1980). For your health: A model for self-care. South Laguna, CA: Nurses Model Health, p. 47.)*

to receive her "reward" of lunch with her friend, Bonita, for accomplishing her contract.

During their next meeting, the nurse and Juanita evaluated the contract formally and established another goal. Feelings of both the nurse and Juanita were explored regarding the entire process. Table 16–8 presents a nursing care plan for this clinical situation.

SUMMARY

This chapter emphasized that environmental self-care affects an individual while at home, work, or traveling. The effects on health of air, water, energy, safety, sound, light or color, and space were explored. Although some of the issues related to these topics are out of the *direct* control of the individual, there are many self-care activities that can prevent disease and enhance health. Environmental self-care advocacy was discussed as one vehicle for creating change in the environment.

The role of the nurse as a model of environmental self-care was emphasized. A case presentation, including a self-contract and nursing care plan, was offered as an example of the integration of environmental self-care principles into clinical practice.

STUDY QUESTIONS

Personal Focus

1. Rate yourself as a model of environmental self-care. Give three examples describing the ways you model environmental self-care.
2. Keep a journal for one day. Summarize the effects of air, light, water, energy, and safety on your life that day.
3. How is the physical space arranged for nurses in your clinical setting?
4. Select any one of the environmental components discussed in this chapter. Identify three self-care activities that you might perform within this area to enhance your health. Write a self-contract for that goal.

Client Focus

1. Conduct an interview to assess one hospitalized client's current personal space. With the client, make a list of specific actions that could be taken to enhance his or her environment.
2. List four steps that nurses might take to assist clients in self-care efforts in the area of sound.
3. Describe how clients might be assisted in becoming active advocates of environmental self-care.

TABLE 16–8. NURSING CARE PLAN

Reason for Consultation: Birth control counseling/PAP smear

Client: Juanita Gomez

Assessment	Plan	Evaluation		
		Met	Not met	
Self-care demand	*Setting objectives*			
Increased need for environmental self-care skills	Call the gas and electric company within 24 hours.	X		
Assets	*Reaching objectives*			
Good physical health	Client actions			
Availability of her mother	Make the telephone calls.	X		
Pleasure working in and around her home	Be at home for the repairperson to come.	X		
Concern about environmental safety	Get documentation of specific needed repairs.	X		
Limitations	Call nurse within 48 hours.	X		
Spanish primary language	Nursing actions			
New country, difficult adjustment	Obtain telephone numbers of utilities/Spanish-speaking customer service representatives.	X		
Limited funds				
Crowded living conditions	Be available by telephone.	X		
Doesn't know the "system"	Arrange for interpreter if needed.	X		
Unaware of unsafe conditions	Provide list of community service agencies.	X		
		Needed revisions		
Diagnosis		Add objective about talking with landlord re: needed repairs within 24 hours.		
Self-care deficit				
Inability to provide for environmental safety without intervention and support	**Reevaluation date**	**Client follow-up**		
	Initial: 48 hours.	Check on repair work.		
	Return appointment: one week.	Continue to work on self-care issues in order of priority.		

4. With a client identify one of the environmental problem areas discussed in this chapter. Help the client write a self-contract for that area.

REFERENCES

1. Trieff, N. (Ed.). (1980). *Environment and health.* Ann Arbor, MI: Ann Arbor Science Publishers, pp. 3–4.
2. Evelyn, J. *Fumifugium: or, the inconvenience of the aer, and smoake of London dissipated* 1661. Reprinted by the National Society for Clean Air, Brighton, England.
3. Hodges, L. (1973). *Environmental pollution.* New York: Holt, Rinehart and Winston.
4. Stern, A.C. (1973). *Fundamentals of air pollution.* New York: Academic Press.
5. Carson, R. (1962). *Silent spring.* Greenwich, CT: Fawcett/Crest.
6. Spencer, C. (1989). Help Wanted: A special 16-page activists guide to a better Earth. *Omni, 11,* (12): Special section.
7. Commoner, B. (1971). *The closing circle.* New York: Alfred A. Knopf.
8. Bullough, L., & Bullough, B. (1978). *The care of the sick.* New York: Prodist Press.
9. Rogers, M.E. (1970). *An introduction to the theoretical base of nursing.* Philadelphia: F.A. Davis.
10. Orem, D. (1985) *Nursing: Concepts of practice* (3rd ed.). New York: McGraw-Hill.
11. Parse, R.R. (1981). *Man–Living–Health: A theory of nursing.* New York: John Wiley & Sons, pp. 40–41.
12. Watson, J. (1985). *Nursing: Human science and human care, a theory of nursing.* Norwalk, CT: Appleton-Century-Crofts, p. 29.
13. *National Jewish Center for Immunology and Respiratory Medicine, (1988). Medical and Scientific Update. 7* (4), 1.
14. Leeser, I. (1975). *Community health nursing.* Hyde Park, NY: Medical Examination Publishing, pp. 159–160.
15. Fielding, J.E. (1979). Preventive medicine and the bottom line. *Journal of Occupational Medicine, 21* (2), 79–88.
16. Bellows, K. (ed) (1989). Rooms for improvement. *Special Report on Health.* Knoxville, TN: Whittle Communications.
17. King, J. (1985). Is your water safe to drink? *Medical Self-Care,* Nov/Dec, pp. 44–47.
18. Divine Waters. (1980, August–September). *World Health Organization Magazine,* p. 3.
19. Grawunder, R., & Steinmann, M. (1980). *Life and health.* New York: Random House, p. 458.
20. Graf, T. (1989, January 29). Warnings overstate home radon peril. *The Denver Post,* p. H1.
21. National Safety Council. (1978). *Accident facts.* Chicago: Author.
22. Cooper, R. (1989). Health and fitness excellence. Boston: Houghton Mifflin, p. 393.
23. Flynn, P.A.R. (1980). *Holistic health.* Bowie, MD: Robert J. Brady, pp. 104–105.
24. Trieff. *Environment and health,* p. 353.
25. Savage, D.G. (1983, February 15). Freeway noise linked to poorer school test scores. *Los Angeles Times,* Sec. 1, pp. 1, 15.
26. Wurtman, R.J. (1975). The effects of light on man and other mammals. *Annual Review of Physiology, 37,* 467–483.

27. Collins, J.S. (1961). *The world of light*. New York: Horizon.
28. Hughes, P.C. (1980). The use of light and color in health. In A.C. Hastings (Ed.), *Health for the whole person*. Boulder, CO: Westview Press, p. 287.
29. Maas, J.B., Jayson, J.K., & Kleiber, D.A. (1974). Effects of spectral difference in illumination on fatigue. *Journal of Applied Psychology, 59*, 524–526.
30. Allen, R.M., & Cureton, R.K. (1945). Effect of ultraviolet radiation on physical fitness. *Archives of Physical Medicine and Rehabilitation, 26*, 641–644.
31. Zamkova, M.A., & Krivitskaya, E.I. (1966). Effect of irradiation by ultraviolet erythema lamps on the working ability of school children. *Gigiena i Sanitariia, 31*, 42–44.
32. Chinn, P.L., & Jacobs, M. (1981) *Theory and nursing: A systematic approach*. St. Louis: C.V. Mosby, p. 34.
33. Helvie, C.O. (1981) *Community health nursing: Theory and process*. New York: Harper & Row, pp. 41–42.
34. Hall, E. (1959). *The hidden dimension*. New York: Doubleday.
35. Gerard, R.M. (1958). Differential effects of colored lights on psychophysiological function. Unpublished doctoral dissertation, University of California at Los Angeles.
36. Elias, M. (1980, August 3). Using colors to alter behavior. *Los Angeles Times*, Sec. V, pp. 3, 9, 10.
37. Fozard, J., Wolf, E., Bell, B., McFarland, R. (1977). Visual perception and communication. In J. Birren & K. Schaie (Eds.), *Handbook of the psychology of aging*. New York: Van Nostrand.
38. Corso, J. (1971). Sensory processes and effects in normal adults. *Journal of Gerontology, 26* (1), 90.
39. Jackson, C. (1980). *Color me beautiful*. New York: Ballantine.
40. Malloy, J.T. (1986). *Dress for excellence*. New York: Rawson Assoc.
41. Friedman, M. (1981). *Family nursing: Theory and assessment*. New York: Appleton-Century-Crofts, p. 102.
42. Helvie. *Community health nursing*, p. 67.
43. Hall, E.T. (1959). *The hidden dimension*. New York: Doubleday.
44. Little, K. (1965). Personal space. *Journal of Experimental Psychology, 1*, 238.
45. Ehrlich, P. & Holdren, J. (1975). Impact on population growth. In P.G. Marden & D. Hodgson (Eds.), *Population, environment, and the quality of life*. New York: AMS Press.
46. Commoner, B., Carr, M., & Slanter, P. (1975). The causes of pollution. In P.G. Marden & D. Hodgson (Eds.), *Population, environment, and the quality of life*. New York: AMS Press.
47. Pelletier, K. (1980). In Search of Optimal Health. In T. Ferguson (Ed.), *Medical self-care*. New York: Summit pp. 48–50.

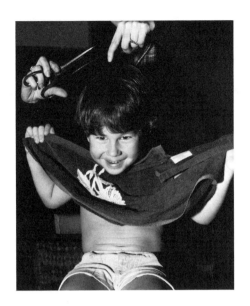

Everyone should be his own physician. We ought to assist, not force nature. What medicine can procure digestion? Exercise. What will recruit strength? Sleep. What will alleviate incurable evils? Patience.

Voltaire

17 Physical Self-Care

LEARNING OBJECTIVES

Upon completion of this chapter, readers will be able to:

1. Identify two physical self-care activities for each of the following age groups: children from birth through kindergarten, school-age children, adolescents, adults, and older adults.
2. Identify three considerations in selecting a health care provider.
3. Discuss two reasons for changing health care providers.
4. Discuss two benefits of maintaining a personal health care record.

DEFINITIONS

Risk A condition that may compromise an individual's health or longevity.
Physical Self-Care Activities performed that care for or protect the body. Physical self-care relates to all areas of self-care and includes health-promoting activities that reduce the risk of disease or disability throughout life.

INTRODUCTION

Physical self-care has gained attention through the efforts of physicians such as Ferguson, Levin, and Sehnert.[1-3] These men encouraged clients to begin to monitor their bodies and symptoms through both observation and the use of basic medical equipment such as otoscopes, stethoscopes, and sphygmomanometers. In 1970, Schnert taught—and largely invented—the first of a modern breed of self-care classes, in which laypeople learned basic medical skills formerly reserved for doctors.[4]

Other chapters of this text have addressed specific self-care areas such as exercise, nutrition, and spirituality. This chapter is designed to identify self-care activities and resources that do not apply directly to any of these single content areas but relate to each of them. These are self-care activities that focus on the physical body, are health promoting, and reduce the risk of disease or disability throughout life.

PHYSICAL SELF-CARE THROUGHOUT THE LIFE SPAN

Many physical self-care skills are age-related. For example, keeping poisons out of reach, having an antidote kit in the house, and having the poison control center telephone number posted by the telephone are all particularly important for parents of young children. Lifeline telephone alert systems for the elderly living alone can provide a sense of security. Table 17–1 reviews physical self-care skills throughout the life span. It is divided into three categories: safety, new health care skills, and substance use or abuse. Table 17–2 suggests materials for a home health care kit.

Health care evaluation of well people has always been of concern to health care providers. The timing of these evaluations and criteria for selection of procedures have been discussed repeatedly. The Council on Scientific Affairs of the American Medical Association (AMA) has reviewed and summarized recommendations by the Canadian Task Force on Periodic Health Examination, The Institute of Medicine, and The American College of Physicians, and various other organizations regarding specific procedures. They conclude:

TABLE 17–1. PHYSICAL SELF-CARE THROUGH THE LIFE SPAN

Developmental Stage	Safety	Substance Use or Abuse	New Health Care Skills
Birth–kindergarten	Parents anticipate safety hazards and intervene *Poison control:* Child safety latches put on cabinets Antidote kit kept in house Poison control number placed by telephone *Automobile safety:* Child put in approved car restraint system Parents fasten own seat belts as models *Electrical safety:* Outlets plugged Plugs in use covered Cords kept out of reach Electrical appliances kept out of reach *Water safety:* Bathtubs, wading pools drained immediately after use Toilet lids kept closed Water safety modeled by parents: not swimming alone, wearing life jackets, not combining alcohol and water sports *Fall prevention:* Stairway kept clear Crib side rails put up Stairways supervised or gated Climbing activity supervised	*Medications:* Clearly labeled with dose and frequency of medication Record of administration posted Kept out of reach and locked Necessary medications stocked (acetaminophen for sudden fevers, etc.) Nursing mothers check with pediatric health care provider *before* taking any medication, alcohol, or "street" drugs Outdated drugs discarded *Alcohol and smoking* Parents model use or abuse Nursing mothers complete alcohol and smoking education programs Physiological effects on small children considered	*Dental:* Initial dental exam provided Instruction given in brushing, flossing Brushing, flossing done by parent before ability developed Fluoride supplements used if required *Decision making:* Child given choices about health care practices Parents model decision-making skills *New health care skills:* Infant sensory stimulation provided Room and motivation provided for crawling and walking Massage provided Sensori-motor skill development encouraged

Emergency care:
 Family members know when and how to seek medical attention
 Emergency numbers placed by all telephones
 Family members and child-care providers know first aid and cardiopulmonary resuscitation (CPR)
 Emergency telephone numbers, parents whereabouts, and emergency medical authorization left with child-care person

School-age

Accident prevention:
 Safety equipment used for bicycling, skateboarding, other sports
 Child put in approved automobile restraint system
 Traffic safety skills developed: street crossing, following traffic signals, bicycle riding
 Safety taught regarding tools, electrical appliances
 Water safety skills developed: swimming, boating, and bathing
Fall prevention:
 Stairways kept clear
 Climbing activities supervised
Emergency care:
 Beginning knowledge of first aid, CPR developed
 Knows own address, telephone number, parents' names, work location

Medications:
 See "Birth–kindergarten"
 Medication safety education provided
 Alternatives explored before medication taken
 Child records own medication
 Drug education programs given regarding "street" drugs
 Parents model use or abuse of prescription, over-the-counter, and "street" drugs
Alcohol and smoking:
 Parents model use or abuse
 Alcohol education programs provided
 Taught dangers of combining alcohol with drugs
 Smoking education programs provided

Dental:
 Responsibility for oral hygiene undertaken
 Accident prevention learned
 Dental examination received every 6–12 months
 Fluoride supplement used if required
 Dental first aid learned
Decision making:
 Some independent decisions made
 Guidance given relative to seeking health care, self-care as an active choice
New health care skills:
 Learn new aspects of human sexual development: puberty, emotions, menstruation, masturbation
 Learn AIDS prevention skills
 Say "No" to Drugs program

Adolescent	Knows how to use telephones and summon emergency assistance Limits taught regarding interpersonal relationships (i.e., abuse, rape, abduction) See "Birth–kindergarten"	*Emergency care:* Knows first aid, CPR Wears Medic-Alert tag, if needed Knows how to summon emergency assistance Limits reviewed regarding interpersonal relationships (i.e., abuse, rape, abduction) *Automobile safety:* Driver education programs taken Seat belts fastened *Sports safety:* Correct equipment used: running shoes, bicycle helmets, motorcycle helmets, skateboarding pads, etc. Sports safety education programs taken	*Medications:* See "School-age" Role of peers as influential models acknowledged *Alcohol and smoking:* Driver education programs taken Education regarding combining alcohol and drugs Alcohol, drug, and smoking education programs taken Knows when, how, where to seek help for substance abuse; for example, Alanon, Alateen, Adult Child of Alcoholics	*Dental:* Annual examination obtained Responsibility taken for oral hygiene See "School-age" *Decision making:* Primarily made independently Minimal guidance given relative to seeking health care, self-care as an active choice *New health care skills:* Breast self-examination done Testicular self-exam done Contraception used PAP smears completed yearly Skin self-exam, skin care undertaken AIDS prevention, safe sex
Adult	*Home safety:* Smoke alarms installed Fire drills held Earthquake drills held Emergency preparedness undertaken (supplies of food, water, fuel, etc.) *Emergency care:* Emergency telephone numbers kept by all telephones	*Medications* See "Birth–kindergarten" During travel, medications kept on person Extra supply of required medicines stocked Alternatives explored *before* medication taken Inform each health care provider of medications taken		*Dental:* Models dental care for children See "Adolescent" *New health care skills:* Contraception used Breast self-exam (male and female) done Testicular self-exam done AIDS prevention, safe sex skills

	Knows current first aid, CPR Has home health kit (see Table 17–2) *Automobile safety:* Models safety for children Seat belts fastened Helmets, safety clothing worn on motorcycles *Sports safety:* Models safety for children Physical exam, cardiac stress test taken aften age 35 Correct sports safety equipment used: running shoes, bicycle helmets, racquetball eye protectors, etc.	Drug reference text kept in home Drug package inserts read Warning labels on drugs heeded Effect of combination of drugs with caffeine known *Alcohol and smoking:* Driver education program taken Knows danger of combining alcohol with medications Alternative of relaxation explored Smoking education programs taken	PAP smears obtained Skin self-exam undertaken Weight kept within normal limits *Preparation for aging:* Calcium, iron intake Maintaining flexibility, strength, endurance
Older adult	*Automobile safety:* Annual evaluation of driving skills completed Seat belts fastened Vision screened annually Car maintained Tires checked *Home safety:* Adequate lighting provided Smoke alarms installed Grab rails in bathrooms, stairways installed Stairways lighted and uncluttered Loose throw rugs eliminated Flashlight kept at bedside	*Medications:* See "Adult" Medications *not* kept at bedside Pharmacist informed of visual deficit; adequate labeling provided Acknowledges that effects of medications may change with age Prescription drugs taken as ordered Outdated drugs discarded Avoiding caffeine Avoiding ETDA for sleep	*Dental:* Dental self-care undertaken Knows cleaning techniques and trouble signs regarding oral appliances Dental exam completed every 6–12 months *New health care skills:* Learns need for new self-care skills with progression of aging process Balance skills learned Retirement planned Dealing with loss learned Breast self-exam (male and female) done

Emergency preparedness
known
Lifeline telephone alert
Emergency care:
Has emergency friend or family
member to call upon
Emergency numbers kept by
each telephone
Knows current first aid, CPR
Learns how to recognize elder
abuse and seek assistance
Sports safety:
Regular assessment of physical
condition completed
Correct sports safety equip-
ment used: running or walk-
ing shoes, bicycle helmets,
etc.

Alcohol and smoking:
See "Adult"
Knows effects of alcohol may
change with age, new medica-
tion
Long-term effects of tobacco
use realized
Does not smoke in bed

Testicular self-exam done
Skin self-exam undertaken
PAP smear completed
AIDS prevention, safe sex
skills
Sunscreen
Cholesterol levels

399

TABLE 17–2. HOME HEALTH CARE KIT

These tools will enable individuals to do their own screening. If a call to the health care provider becomes necessary, more accurate information will be available.
Thermometer   Antipyretics, e.g., acetaminophen   Stethoscope/sphygmomanometer   Cool mist vaporizer   Tongue blades   Tweezers   Watch with second hand   Flashlight   Otoscope   Vaginal speculum   Measuring tape   Dental kits[a]   Emergency stock of regular medication such as antihypertensives   In-home pregnancy kits as needed   Hot water bottle/heating pad

[a]Dental emergency kits are available from Dental Aide Products, Rahway, NJ. They are small kits that provide tools and instructions necessary for temporary relief of pain or discomfort.

1. Periodic evaluation of healthy people is important for early detection of disease and for recognition and correction of certain risk factors that may precede disease.
2. The *optimal frequency* of the periodic evaluation and the procedures to be performed *vary with the client's age, socioeconomic status, heredity, and other individual factors.*
3. The testing of any individual or group should be pursued only when adequate treatment or intervention can be arranged for the abnormal condition that is identified.[5-11]

Tables 17–3 to 17–6 present normal health screening intervals and the content of each particular screening. These figures, only intended as *guidelines* for the well client, include history and physical examination, procedures, immunizations, and counseling issues of particular importance. If an individual has a strong family history for a particular disease or other health risk factors, these must be considered.

Screening for older adults has particular ethical interest. As health care costs continue to escalate, it is not uncommon to see routine screening measures dropped for older adults with the unspoken message, "What would I do anyway?" The research, however, regarding screening in the elderly is in-

TABLE 17–3. HEALTH SCREENING FOR THE NORMAL INFANT

Services	Birth Visit	Second Visit[a]	Subsequent Visits[b]
History and physical examination			
Length and weight	*		*
Head circumference	*		
Urine stream	*		
Check for congenital abnormalities	*		*
Development assessment			*
Procedures			
PKU screening test		*	
Thyroxin T4		*	
Vitamin K		*	
Silver nitrate prophylaxis	*		
Immunizations			
Diphtheria			*
Pertussis			*
Tetanus			*
Measles			*
Mumps			*
Rubella			*
Poliomyelitis			*
Parental counseling, with referrals as necessary and desired			
Infant nutrition and feeding practices (especially breast feeding)		*	*
Parenting		*	*
Infant hygiene		*	*
Accident prevention (including use of automobile restraints)		*	*
Family planning and referral for services		*	*
Child care arrangements		*	*
Medical care arrangements		*	*
Parental smoking, use of alcohol and drugs		*	*
Parental nutrition, physical activity, and exercise		*	*
In response to parental concerns		*	*

[a]Second visit should occur within 10 days or before leaving the hospital.
[b]Four visits during the rest of the first year, or enough to provide immunizations on schedule. (Reprinted with the permission of the Institute of Medicine, Ad Hoc Advisory Group on Preventive Services, Washington, DC, April 13, 1978.)

TABLE 17–4. HEALTH SCREENING FOR THE WELL POPULATION

Services	Preschool[a]	School Child[b]	Adolescent[c]	Adult Entry[d]	Young Adult Years[e]	Middle Adult Years[f]	Older Adults[g]
History and physical examination and referrals when necessary							
Height and weight	•	•	•	•	•	•	•
Development assessment	•	•	•				
Blood pressure	•	•	•	•	•	•	•
Vision / Glaucoma	•	•	•		•	•	•
Hearing	•	•	•			•	•
Speech	•	•	•				
Screening for scoliosis (9–10 years or at first visit)		•	•				
Skin			•	•	•	•	•
Breast examination in women				•	•	•	•
Rectal examination						•	•
Mammography						•	•
Electrocardiogram (one baseline value at 40 or 45)							•
Laboratory examinations							
Serum cholesterol (once during age periods specified)			•	•	•	•	
VDRL, if not otherwise required or obtained recently				•			
Papanicolaou smear (women)			•	•	•	•	•
Gonococcal culture (women)				•			
Rubella titer (women)							
Blood glucose							•
Hematocrit						•	•
Urine analysis for sugar and protein						•	•
Stool guaiac						•	•
Immunizations							
Completion of immunization schedule	•						
Tetanus		•				•	•
Diphtheria		•				•	•

Pneumovax (high risk only until old age)

Hepatitis B (high risk only)

Influenza, when and as required (especially over age 65)

Counseling with referrals as necessary and desired

Nutrition

Hygiene/Dental health

Accident prevention

Physical activity and exercise

Alcohol, other drug use

Cigarette smoking

Family relations, social problems, sexual development and adjustment

Family planning (contraception if appropriate)

Sleep

Obesity

Antecedents of adult disease

Teaching breast, testicular, skin self-examination

Retirement

Living arrangements

In response to parental or individual concerns

[a]Two health visits, one at 2 to 3 years and one at school entry.
[b]Two health visits, one at 6 to 7 and one at 9 to 10 years of age.
[c]Two health visits, the first preferably about age 13.
[d]One health visit. Screen for susceptibility to measles, rubella.
[e]Three health visits, about age 25, 30, and 35.
[f]Four health visits, about age 40, 45, 50, and 55.
[g]Health visit at age 60, and every 2 years thereafter.
[h]To be performed once during the interim between examinations.
[i]Counseling about effects of parental use on children.

References: Institute of Medicine, Ad Hoc Advisory Group on Prevention Services, Washington, DC, April 13, 1978; Williams, W., Hickson, M., et al. (1988). Immunization policies and vaccine coverage among adults. *Annals of Internal Medicine.* 108:616–625; U.S. Preventive Services Task Force. (1989). *Guide to Clinical Preventive Services.* Washington, D.C.: Department of Health and Human Services.

TABLE 17–5 HEALTH SCREENING FOR THE PREGNANT WOMAN AND FETUS

Services	Initial Visit[a]	Subsequent Visits[b]
History		
General medical	*	
Family and genetic	*	
Previous pregnancies	*	
Current pregnancy	*	*
Physical examination		
General	*	
Blood pressure	*	*
Height and weight	*	
Fetal development		*
Laboratory examinations		
VDRL	*	
Papanicolaou smear	*	
Hemoglobin/hematocrit	*	
Urinalysis for sugar and protein	*	*
RH determination	*	
Blood group determination	*	
Rubella HAI titer	*	
Amniocentesis (for women over 35)[c]	*	
Counseling with referrals as necessary and desired		
Plans for pregnancy continuation	*	*
Nutrition during pregnancy	*	*
Nutrition of infant, including breast feeding	*	*
Cigarette smoking	*	*
Use of alcohol, other drugs during pregnancy	*	*
Sexual intercourse during pregnancy	*	*
Signs of abnormal pregnancy	*	*
Labor and delivery (including where mother plans to deliver)	*	*
Physical activity and exercise	*	*
Provisions for care of infant	*	*
In response to parental concerns	*	*

Labor and delivery[d]

Postpartum visit[d] (including family planning counseling and referral, if desired)

[a]Initial visit should occur early in the first trimester.

[b]Subsequent visits should occur once a month through the 28th week of pregnancy; twice a month from the 29th through the 36th week, once a week thereafter.

[c]If desired, amniocentesis should be performed at about the 13th or 14th week for women who are over 35 or who have specific genetic indications.

[d]Although not a "preventive" service, labor and delivery should be included in a package of pregnancy-related services.

(Reprinted with permission of the Institute of Medicine, Ad Hoc Advisory Group on Preventive Services, Washington, DC, April 13, 1978.)

complete.[12] The recommended screening techniques in Table 17–6 are designed to provide cost-effective health screening for the elderly.

SELECTING A HEALTH CARE PROVIDER OR OTHER SELF-CARE RESOURCE

Most people generally think of physicians when they think of health care services. Many other health care providers and self-care resources are available, however, and these can be used in conjunction with traditional medical care.

How does an individual select a health care provider or self-care resource? Often little thought is given to this process. Many people continue with their parents' physician just because it is less complicated than switching. Another common source of referral is through friends. Sometimes people have little apparent choice. They are assigned the person on-call in the emergency department.

Many people begin the search by obtaining names from the telephone book's *Yellow Pages*. Most professional associations maintain an information and referral service of their members. For example, if someone needs a physician in the area, he or she might call the AMA and obtain a list of referrals. This process might give the individual three to five names. Another common referral source is the local hospital, which will probably give a list of referrals from the staff roster. These referrals (AMA or local hospital) have undergone some screening by the referral organization, but excellence is by no means assured. Calling the head of a clinical department (e.g., medicine or obstetrics) at a local medical school may lead to referrals to highly qualified physicians. Specialty board certification (often unknown by laypersons) can be considered another excellent screening guide.

Other professional associations also maintain referral sources. The American Nurses' Association (ANA) supplies lists of nurses in advanced practice by clinical specialty.

Before an actual appointment is made for health care, an interview appointment may be arranged with *each* of the health care providers under consideration. Many providers do not charge for this service; however, that question needs to be asked *before* the appointment is made. This applies whether the health care provider is in private practice, a community health agency, or a health maintenance organization.

The prospective client should be encouraged to take a *written* list of questions to the session. Some examples of typical questions to consider are found in Table 17–7. After the interviews with each of the prospective health care providers, a selection is made. Hopefully, this relationship will become a collaborative one, focused on wellness, with the health care provider encouraging and fostering self-care skills.

There are many self-help groups and self-care resources located in almost

Table 17–6. HEALTH SCREENING FOR THE ELDERLY

	1st visit	f/u	2nd yr.	3rd yr.	4th yr.	5th yr.	6th yr.	7th yr.	8th yr.	9th yr.	10th yr.
Enter date											
Enter age											
Enter date of first visit under that title and fill in schedule											
Enter appropriate value or finding in open boxes under each exam date.											
Diphtheria/tetanus			X	X	X	X	X	X	X	X	X
Influenza											
Pneumococcal	X		X	X	X	X	X	X	X	X	X
Exercise amount		f/u if nec									
Calcium[a]		X	X	X	X		X	X	X	X	
Fiber[a]		X	X	X	X		X	X	X	X	
Fluid[a]		X	X	X	X		X	X	X	X	
Caffeine[a]		X	X	X	X		X	X	X	X	
Smoking		X	if nec								
Alcohol use		X	if nec								
Accident risk[a]		f/u if nec	X	X	X		X	X	X	X	
Social support[a]		X	X	X	X		X	X	X	X	

Procedure								
Blood pressure-value								
Pulse-value								
Height/weight[a]	X	X	X	X	X	X	X	
Annual cancer exam[c]	X							
Pap smear[b]	X	X	X	X	X	X	X	X
Hearing screen[a]	X	X	X	X	X	X	X	
Vision screen[a]	X	X	X	X	X	X	X	
Urinary incontinence[a]	f/u if nec	X	X	X	X	X	X	
Complete physical[a]	X	X	X	X	X	X	X	
Medication review[a]	X	X	X	X	X	X	X	
Depression[a]	f/u if nec	X	X	X	X	X	X	
T4 + TSH-value[a]	X	X	X	X	X	X	X	
Stool for occult blood	X							
Mammography	X							

[a]After 74, all procedures tied to Complete Health Review done biannually.

[b]If no previous Pap, need two, one-year apart. Otherwise, no further testing recommended after age 65.

[c]Includes skin, oral, breast, thyroid, lymph, prostate and pelvic.

(Reprinted with persmission from Albert, M. (1987). Health screening to promote health for the elderly. *The Nurse Practitioner, 12* (5), 55.

TABLE 17–7. QUESTIONS FOR PROSPECTIVE HEALTH CARE PROVIDERS

Professional qualifications

1. What are his or her credentials (license, board certification, degrees, other certification)?
2. Where did he or she go to school?
3. Does he or she belong to professional organizations?
4. Is he or she affiliated with a hospital? How many? Which ones?
5. Is he or she affiliated with a clinic?
6. Is he or she a member of an HMO or PPO?
7. Does he or she have a medical school or nursing school teaching appointment?
8. Is he or she involved in any research? What? Are clients or their records part of any research?
9. Are his or her personal qualities pleasing?

Office organization

1. Is the office close to home? Work?
2. Are laboratory and X-ray services available in the office or building?
3. Is he or she part of a group practice?
4. Is practice covered 24 hours a day, seven days a week? Appointment hours? Evenings? Weekends? Are home visits made?
5. Who takes "call"?
6. Is there telephone availability? Charge?
7. What is the process for health education within the practice? Does another health care provider perform that service? Fees?
8. How does he or she feel about second opinions?
9. What are the typical indications for referral? What is the process?
10. What is the length of an appointment?
11. How long is the wait for initial appointments? Emergency appointments?
12. Is there an opportunity to ask questions during office visits?
13. What other health care workers are employed in the office? What are their qualifications?
14. Does he or she keep medical records? Available to clients? Copies given? Charges?
15. Are students of any kind in the practice (medical, nursing, medical assistants, lab technicians, X-ray technicians, and so on)?

Financial

1. What are the fees for service?
2. What are the arrangements for insurance? Payment required at each office visit? Charge for completing forms? Payment for cancelled visits?
3. How is payment handled? Complete payment at visit? Partial payment? Monthly billing available?
4. What is the charge for the initial visit? What is included?

Value placed on self-care

1. What are the health care provider's feelings about self-care?
2. Does the health care provider smoke? Permit smoking in the office? Appear to be in good physical and emotional health? Overweight or underweight?
3. Does he or she use alternative treatment methods? Nutrition? Biofeedback? Exercise? Acupressure?
4. What is his or her philosophy about nutrition, exercise, relaxation, and so on?
5. Does the health history include life-style information such as smoking, drinking, occupation, stress, life changes, exercise, and nutrition?

every community. Big Brother, Make Today Count, and the American Cancer Society are examples. Guidelines to assist people in locating self-care resources are found in Table 17–8. These guidelines may be used by both clients and nurses.

Health care is an a state of transition. Physicians in particular are suffering bruised relationships with their clients as the result of highly technological advances, consumerism, and threats of liability.[13] People need to feel free to be assertive in regard to their health needs. Consumerism applies to one's own health care. Clients who are uncomfortable with their relationships with health care providers should feel open about discussing it. Conflicts regarding any of the areas listed in Table 17–7 can occur. For example, if working parents with an ill child find that their pediatrician does not have evening telephone availability or has no Saturday office hours, they should have a frank discussion with the doctor. If the problem is not able to be satisfactorily resolved, the parents should feel confident about seeking the services of another provider or resource. The problems that prompted them to look for another provider or resource need to be addressed with future prospective candidates.

TABLE 17–8. LOCATING SELF-CARE RESOURCES

There are many self-care resources in most communities. Many are simple to find and easy to use. These are *general guidelines* to assist in locating these resources.

1. Use the telephone book. Many agencies are cross-referenced in both the general listing and the classified section.

2. Clinics and hospitals in the community have many services and programs that are not advertised. Call and ask for a health educator. These people are excellent resources for referrals within the community.

3. University or community college student health centers may offer community outreach programs or provide referrals.

4. Professional organizations such as the American Medical Association, American Nurses' Association, and the American Dietetics Association generally have local offices. Even if you do not require their specific services, the organization can be helpful in locating other health care services.

5. Local newspapers frequently have articles highlighting available local services.

6. Official health care agencies such as county health departments generally have compilations of local service agencies.

7. There are a variety of written resources. Many books are published with addresses and telephone numbers of the national offices of self-care organizations. Local addresses and numbers may be obtained from the organizations. An example of these publications is: Art Ulene and Sandy Feldman, *Help Yourself to Health: A Health Information and Services Directory* (New York: Putnam, 1980).

8. Go to the resource yourself *before* referring a client. This can help avoid surprise and embarrassment. Be sure to telephone before going. Many of these organizations change locations, cost for services and operating procedures frequently.

MAINTAINING PERSONAL HEALTH RECORDS

Keeping personal health records can yield many benefits. A cumulative record can give a health care provider valuable insight into the client's family history and potential risk of developing diseases with familial tendencies. Records can give consulting specialists a clearer picture of past health history and life-style. Descriptions of X-rays, laboratory tests, dates, location, and results may avoid unnecessary duplication.

In addition to health record forms, Figures 17–1 and 17–2 illustrate examples of forms used in emergency situations. Emergency telephone numbers should be posted near each telephone in the home. A visitor in the home (for example, a babysitter or overnight guest) would then find them readily accessible.

The emergency consent form is for minors who require parental consent for health care when a parent is not available. If an emergency occurs a presigned consent can save needed time.

NURSES MODEL PHYSICAL SELF-CARE

Historically, nurses have been involved in promoting physical self-care for clients. Immunization clinics, hearing exams, and blood pressure checks all have had strong nursing support. Physical self-care, however, is an area easily "forgotten" by many nurses. Since large numbers of nurses deal with life and death crises daily, these preventive tasks and skills are easily put off until later.

There are many ways in which nurses can model physical self-care in their personal lives. Modeling behaviors could include activities such as:

- Providing for their own
    Pap smears
    Breast self-exams (BSE) and testicular self-exams (TSE)
    Physical examinations
    Dental examinations
    Renewal of CPR certification
- Wearing seat belts.
- Maintaining current immunizations.
- Posting emergency telephone numbers.
- Reporting to employee health center for physical examinations when requested.

Teaching these skills is often not part of nursing care. Yet opportunities frequently arise in which teaching can be integrated, such as:

- Teaching BSE and TSE during baths.
- Instructing about medication safety and poison control center telephone numbers in conjunction with medications sent home.

Emergency Telephone Numbers

_____

name of family member   date of birth   patient file number

_____

name of family member   date of birth   patient file number

_____

address (include directions for finding house if it's not easy to find, so emergency vehicles can arrive promptly)

Fire _____

Police _____

Rescue squad _____

Emergency room at hospital _____

Poison control center_____

Family doctors _____

                name   family member(s) seen   office phone   home phone

                name   family member(s) seen   office phone   home phone

Dentist _____

       name   office phone   home phone

Pharmacy_____

        name   phone

24-hour pharmacy_____

          name   phone

Father's work phone_____ Mother's work phone_____

Person to contact
in emergency_____

           name   address   phone

Taxi_____

Gas company_____

Electric company_____

Oil company _____

Water company_____

Other numbers_____

_____

Figure 17–1. Emergency telephone numbers form. *Used with permission from Sehnert, K. (1981). The family doctor's health tips. Deephaven, MN: Meadowbrook Press, p. 93.)*

Emergency Consent Form

If your minor-aged child needs emergency medical care and you aren't available to give your formal consent, the care may be delayed — with serious, even fatal, consequences. Leave an up-to-date Emergency Consent Form with your Emergency Telephone Numbers list each time you leave a child with a babysitter, and call the sitter's attention to it. The sitter will need to bring it to the hospital if emergency care is necessary. The form below is satisfactory.

To whom it may concern: In the event of any medical emergency I/we hereby give my/our consent to Dr. _____
or whoever he/she designates to care for our child/children _____

_____ .
name(s)

_____
signature

_____
relationship   date

Address and directions to emergency room:

_____

_____

_____

_____

_____

_____

Figure 17–2. Emergency consent form. *Used with permission from Sehnert, K. (1981). The family doctor's health tips. Deephaven, MN: Meadowbrook Press, p. 94.*

- Giving local emergency telephone number stickers as part of hospital admission kits and during discharge teaching.
- Providing seat belt and child-restraint instruction when preparing for discharge.

Clients will be more likely to learn and practice these skills at home if they have seen that they are a valued, intergral part of the health care provider's approach.

CLINICAL APPLICATION

Case Presentation

Don is a 21-year-old college student. He has come to the student health center for his annual pre-sports physical examination. Don comes from a middle-class, suburban family and is the oldest of three children. He is studying microbiology with the career goal of becoming a medical technologist.

As part of Don's pre-physical examination questionnaire, the nurse practitioner gave him a self-assessment tool for physical self-care. He verbalized a strong interest in further information at the beginning of their appointment.

```
┌─────────────────────┐
│     Assessment      │
└─────────────────────┘
```
• self-care demand
• assets
• limitations

The sample of Don's physical self-assessment questionnaire is found in Figure 17–3. He exhibited knowledgeable and responsible behavior in many of the areas, including:

- Wearing seat belts.
- Keeping his immunizations current.
- Having regular physical examinations.
- Visiting the dentist regularly.

One of the areas identified as limited was testicular self-examination (TSE). When questioned by the nurse practitioner, Don revealed that he "had never heard about doing that before." He stated that he did not think "young, healthy, athletic males needed to be concerned about cancer." The nurse told him that the majority of testicular tumors, particularly malignant ones, were found in males aged 20 to 40. In asking additional assessment questions, the nurse practitioner wanted to know Don's:

- Family history of testicular cancer and genitourinary problems.
- Personal medical history with particular attention to genitourinary (G-U) injuries, surgeries, urinary tract infections, orchitis, epididymitis, sexually transmitted diseases, vasectomy, undescended testes, circumcision, indirect hernias, phimosis, prostate disease, hydrocele, and hypospadias.
- Level of comfort or discomfort with touching his penis and scrotum.
- Comfort or discomfort with discussing and working in this area with a female nurse.
- Knowledge of anatomy and physiology.
- Knowledge of abnormal G-U signs and symptoms, such as lesions, alterations in size, shape, consistency, pain, swelling.

After this exploration, the nurse practitioner and Don made summaries of his assets and limitations. His assets included:

- Knowledge of basic anatomy and physiology.
- Comfort with touching his penis and scrotum.
- Comfort with working with a female nurse.

PHYSICAL SELF-ASSESSMENT

Complete the following self-assessment to help you look at the status of your physical health. On the scale below circle the numbers which are most true for you and your life during the last year:

	Almost Never	Seldom	Often	Almost Always
1. I get regular physical examinations.	1	2	3	(4)
2. I do a monthly breast self-exam or testicular self-exam.	(1)	2	3	4
3. I keep a personal health history.	1	(2)	3	4
4. I make sure my immunizations are current.	1	2	3	(4)
5. I wear a seat belt.	1	2	3	(4)
6. I have emergency numbers by the telephone.	1	2	(3)	4
7. I keep my CPR certificate current.	1	2	(3)	4
8. I visit the dentist yearly.	1	2	3	(4)
9. I know the credentials of my health care professionals.	(1)	2	3	4
10. I know my family medical history and take preventive action to decrease my risk.	(1)	2	3	4

Some suggestions for how you might learn from this self-assessment:

1. Connect all the circles down the length of the page. Look at the pattern that your connected line makes. Turn your page sideways to get an even more clear visual picture of your physical health. What does it seem to be saying to you?

2. Now add up your total score: _____ ɔ7 _____

   Circle which range it was in:
   10-19   (20-29)   30-40

   If your score was in the 10-19 range you might want to make some changes in your life. Which aspects do you think need the most work? How many "1's" did you mark on this assessment?
   ̄3̄ These might serve as a clue to help you think about making changes in this area of your life.

3. How would you like this self-assessment to look six months from now? Are you interested in working toward those improvements?

4. Remember to give yourself a pat on the back for the ways that you are physically healthy. Keep up the good work!

Figure 17–3. Physical self-assessment. *(Adapted with permission from Baldi, S., et al. (1980). For your health: A model for self-care. South Laguna, CA: Nurses Model Health.)*

- No personal or family history of pathology.
- Practice of other self-care skills (exercise, sleep, and so on).

His limitations included:

- No knowledge about how to do TSE.
- Need for current review of male anatomy and physiology of the G-U system.
- No knowledge of specific G-U disease signs and symptoms.

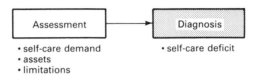

After completing the assessment phase, Don and the nurse collaborated on a diagnosis. They identified his self-care deficit at:

Inability to perform TSE due to lack of knowledge and skill

A nursing diagnosis might read:

Knowledge deficit related to the inability to perform TSE.

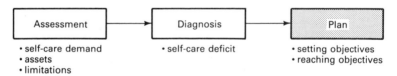

Setting Objectives

Don completed a self-contract. Don and his nurse considered several factors in establishing his goal:

- Sufficient time to learn the skill.
- Time intervals for TSE.
- Dates to perform TSE.

They arrived at a six-month goal:

Will perform TSE on the first of every month.

The goal was developed with consideration of the following:

- TSE should be performed monthly.
- Don felt that he could accomplish the goal.
- The date was easily remembered because he paid all his bills on the first of the month.

Figure 17–4 presents Don's self-contract.

SELF-CONTRACT

MY GOALS:

Short-term— by the end of six weeks I will . . . _n/a_

Long-term— by the end of six months I will . . . _perform TSE on the first of every month._

ENVIRONMENTAL PLANNING: (all the steps I will take to reach my goal)

1. Attend TSE class.
2. Ask Rob for support/rewards.
3. Do TSE in the shower — hang instructions there.
4. Mark the calendar when exam done.
5. Make 6-mo follow-up appt. with Nurse Practitioner

THOUGHTS AND ACTIONS

Helpful thoughts:	Helpful actions:
Doing this will help me take better care of my body.	Posting the instructions in the shower.
Non-helpful thoughts:	Non-helpful actions:
I'm too young to get cancer.	Putting it off until tomorrow.

MY REWARD (if I meet my goal) _Monthly – A new tape._
6 month – Cheap Trick Concert Dec. 7

THE COST: (if I fail to meet my goal) _Type Rob's papers for ½ semester_

REEVALUATION DATE: _June 1_

I agree to help with this project:

Rob May
(Support person)

I agree to strive toward this goal:

Don _5-1_
(Your signature) (date)

Figure 17–4. Self-contract. *(Adapted with permission from Baldi, S., et al. (1980). For your health: A model for self-care. South Laguna, CA: Nurses Model Health, p. 47.)*

Reaching Objectives: Nursing and Client Actions

Skills that are practiced only monthly are particularly difficult to reinforce. There are long intervals between practice times and it is easy for clients to forget. In addition, the level of the skill will not change. That is, after the client has learned TSE, he will not do it any better or any more often, as happens with exercise or relaxation. The reinforcement process thus had to be handled carefully. Don felt, at least initially, that a support person would be helpful in reminding him to do his TSE and to give him his rewards. He chose his roommate, Rob, who agreed to post a reminder note on their bathroom mirror on the last day of every month.

Rob also did not know about TSE. As a result, he attended a group class at the student health center on campus. After the class, he posted the photographic brochure about how to do TSE in their bathroom on the shower wall. He covered the paper with plastic contact paper to protect it from the water. This served as an additional reminder to do TSE properly.

Don's environmental planning to reach his goal included:

- Receiving instruction in TSE at the student health center.
- Gaining the support of his roommate, Rob, who agreed to remind him and give him his rewards.
- Planning to do TSE in the shower. His hands and body are warm, he is undressed, and the examination is smoother and easier to perform with water and soap.
- Marking the calendar on the refrigerator when he had done TSE. This would let Rob know that he had completed his exam.
- Making a follow-up appointment for six months with the nurse practitioner.

The nurse practitioner agreed to assist Don in the following ways:

- Give him instructions in TSE, including when and where to do TSE; characteristics of normal testicles, epididymis, and spermatic cords; when to call the nurse practitioner; abnormal signs and symptoms.
- Have Don perform TSE for her as a return demonstration to validate his technique.
- Provide him with written and pictorial information to take home.
- Send him postcard reminders for the first three months.

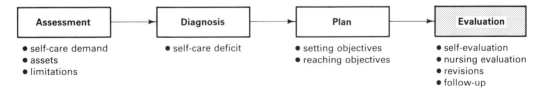

The self-contract goal was for six months. The return appointment was made at the time of the original appointment. During the evaluation session,

TABLE 17–9. NURSING CARE PLAN

Reason for Consultation: Pre-sports physical exam

Client: Don

Assessment	Plan	Evaluation	
		Met	*Not met*

Self-care demand
  Increased need for physical self-care skill: TSE
	Setting objectives
	  Six months:
	  "I will perform TSE on the first of every month."
		X (was late twice)	

Assets
  Comfort with touching his penis and scrotum
	Reaching objectives
	  Client actions
	    Receive instruction in TSE at student health center.
		X	

Comfort in working with a female nurse	Ask Rob for support/rewards.	X	
No personal or family history of pathology	Hang TSE instructions in shower.	X	
Practicing other self-care skills	Record completed TSE on calendar on refrigerator.	X	
Some knowledge of anatomy and physiology	Make follow-up appointment for six months.	X	

Limitations
  No knowledge of TSE
	Nursing actions
	    Give TSE instruction.
		X	

Need for male anatomy and physiology review	Return demonstration on model.	X	
No knowledge of G–U signs and symptoms	Give written/pictorial information.	X	
	Send postcard reminder in three months.	X	
Diagnosis	Reevaluation date	*Needed revision:* None	
Self-care deficit Inability to perform TSE due to lack of knowledge and skill	December 1	Client follow-up Monthly postcards for three months. Inform about other self-care programs available at student health center.	

Don felt that he had achieved his objective. He had done TSE monthly for the first six months. Twice, he was one or two days late.

Don found it particularly helpful having the TSE procedure posted in the shower. Rob had made sure he had given a new tape to Don every month and had taken him to the concert for his six-month reward.

At the follow-up appointment, the nurse practitioner asked Don what his next goal would be. He expressed an interest in learning more about self-care. The nurse practitioner reviewed the schedule of self-care classes available in the student health center. Don selected relaxation as a skill that he thought might help him with the stress of collegiate examinations and competitive sports. Table 17–9 presents a nursing care plan for this clinical situation.

SUMMARY

This chapter discussed self-care activities that contribute to physical self-care. Activities that influence a person's overall health were reviewed, including physical and dental examinations, hearing and vision screening, immunizations, laboratory tests, and breast and testicular self-examinations.

Self-care educational activities were also included in this chapter. Those presented were safety, new health care skills, substance use/abuse and normal health care screening. The processes of selecting a health care provider and maintaining personal health care records were discussed.

The role of the nurse as a model of physical self-care was explored. A case presentation described the way in which the nursing process and the self-care process can be used simultaneously to promote health. Self-contracting provided a primary method for behavior change in this presentation.

STUDY QUESTIONS

Personal Focus

1. Rate yourself as a model of physical self-care.
2. Discuss one physical self-care activity applicable to your developmental level. What would you need to do in order to integrate this into your life-style?
3. What are the criteria you use in selecting your personal health care providers?
4. How do you maintain your personal health care records?

Client Focus

1. Discuss two physical self-care activities that might be integrated into the care you are now giving one client?

2. What information is important to give clients when they are contemplating a change in health care providers?
3. How would you help a client to select a new health care provider?
4. Practice teaching a client how to keep a personal health care record.
5. Help one client complete a self-contract in the area of physical self-care.

REFERENCES

1. Ferguson, T. (Ed.). (1980). *Medical self-care.* New York: Summit.
2. Levin, L. with Katz, A.H., & Holst, E. (1976). *Self-care: Lay initiatives in health.* New York: Prodist Press.
3. Sehnert, K. (1972). The patient as a paramedical. *Virginia Medical Monthly,* 409–413.
4. Ferguson. *Medical self-care,* p. 21.
5. Spitzer, W.O., Bayne, R.D., Charron, K.C., et al. (1984). Task force report: The periodic health examination. *Canadian Medical Association Journal, 130:* 1270–1284.
6. U.S. Preventive Services Task Force (1989). *Guide to clinical preventive services.* Washington, D.C.: Department of Health and Human Services.
7. Medical Practice Committee, American College of Physicians. (1981). Periodic health examination: A guide for designing individualized preventive health care in the asymptomatic patient. *Annals of Internal Medicine, 95,* 729–732.
8. American Cancer Society. (1980). ACS report on the cancer-related checkup. *CA 30,* 194–232.
9. Council on Scientific Affairs. (1983). Medical evaluations of healthy persons. *Journal of the American Medical Association, 249* (12), 1633.
10. Albert, M. (1987). Health screening to promote health for the elderly. *The Nurse Practitioner, 12* (5), 42–58.
11. Lindberg, S.C. (1987). Adult preventive health screening: 1987 update. *The Nurse Practitioner, 12* (5), 19–41.
12. Albert. Health screening to promote health, p. 42.
13. Gibbs, N. (1989, July 31). Sick and tired. *Time. 134,* (5), 48–53.

Appendix A. The Social Readjustment Rating Scale

THE SOCIAL READJUSTMENT RATING SCALE

Life Event	Mean Value
1. Death of a spouse	100
2. Divorce	73
3. Marital separation from mate	65
4. Detention in jail or other institution	63
5. Death of a close family member	63
6. Major personal injury or illness	53
7. Marriage	50
8. Being fired at work	47
9. Marital reconciliation with mate	45
10. Retirement from work	45
11. Major change in the health or behavior of a family member	44
12. Pregnancy	40
13. Sexual difficulties	39
14. Gaining a new family member (e.g., through birth, adoption, oldster moving in, etc.)	39
15. Major business readjustment (e.g., merger, reorganization, bankruptcy, etc.)	39
16. Major change in financial state (e.g., a lot worse off or a lot better off than usual)	38
17. Death of a close friend	37
18. Changing to a different line of work	36
19. Major change in the number of arguments with spouse (e.g., either a lot more or a lot less than usual regarding childrearing, personal habits, etc.)	35
20. Taking out a mortgage or loan for a major purchase (e.g., for a home, business, etc.)	31
21. Foreclosure on a mortgage or loan.	30
22. Major change in responsibilities at work (e.g., promotion, demotion, lateral transfer)	29
23. Son or daughter leaving home (e.g., marriage, attending college, etc.)	29
24. Trouble with in-laws	29

25.	Outstanding personal achievement	28
26.	Wife beginning or ceasing work outside the home	26
27.	Beginning or ceasing formal schooling	26
28.	Major change in living conditions (e.g, building a new home, remodel-ing, deterioration of home or neighborhood)	25
29.	Revision of personal habits (dress, manners, association, etc.)	24
30.	Troubles with the boss	23
31.	Major change in working hours or conditions	20
32.	Change in residence	20
33.	Changing to a new school	20
34.	Major change in usual type and/or amount of recreation	19
35.	Major change in church activities (e.g., a lot more or a lot less than usual)	19
36.	Major change in social activities (e.g, clubs, dancing, movies, visiting, etc.)	18
37.	Taking out a mortgage or loan for a lesser purchase (e.g., for a car, TV, freezer, etc.)	17
38.	Major change in sleeping habits (a lot more or a lot less sleep, or change in part of day when sleep)	16
39.	Major change in number of family get-togethers (e.g., a lot more or a lot less than usual)	15
40.	Major change in eating habits (a lot more or a lot less food intake, or very different meal hours or surroundings)	15
41.	Vacation	13
42.	Christmas	12
43.	Minor violations of the law (e.g., traffic tickets, jaywalking, disturbing the peace, etc.)	11

USING THE SOCIAL READJUSTMENT RATING SCALE: PREVENTIVE MEASURES

The following suggestions are for using the Social Readjustment Rating Scale for the maintenance of your health and prevention of illness:

1. Become familiar with the life events and the amount of change they require.
2. Put the scale where you and the family can see it easily several times a day.
3. With practice you can recognize when a life event happens.
4. Think about the meaning of the event for you and try to identify some of the feelings you experience.
5. Think about the different ways you might best adjust to the event.
6. Take your time in arriving at decisions.
7. If possible, anticipate life changes and plan for them well in advance.
8. Pace yourself. It can be done even if you are in a hurry.
9. Look at the accomplishment of a task as a part of daily living and avoid looking at such an achievement as a "stopping point" or a time for "letting down."

10. *Remember,* the more change you have, the more likely you are to get sick. Of those people with over 300 Life Change Units for the past year, almost 80% get sick in the near future; with 150 to 299 Life Change Units, about 50% get sick in the near future; and with fewer than 150 Life Change Units, only about 30% get sick in the near future.

So, the higher your Life Change Score, the harder you should work to stay well.

(Reprinted with permission from: Holmes, T.H. & Rahe, R.H. (1967). The social readjustment rating scale. *Journal of Psychosomatic Research,* .11, 213–218.)

Appendix B. Self-Contracting for Health

DIRECTIONS

This appendix has been designed to encourage you to work on the process of self-contracting. Completing each of the following steps will enable you to:

1. Set a realistic goal to improve one area of your life.
2. Identify three possible rewards for yourself.
3. Complete one self-contract.

STEP 1: SET YOUR GOAL!

Can you think of something to work on to make yourself more healthy? Success at setting a goal that you can reach is based on many factors. You must:

Choose the right time to start	+	Set one goal at a time	+	Allow enough time

Use the 50% rule	+	Get a good baseline	+	Remember free days	+	Take the risk

Choose the Right Time to Start

Look at your life right now. Are you experiencing or expecting any unusual stress in your life? _____ If you are under some particular stress right now you may not want to add another stress of changing a specific behavior. _____ If this is not a good time for you to start, when do you think might be better?

Set One Goal at a Time

Pick only *one* goal! Write down what you would like to have accomplished by six weeks and by six months. Don't plan to lose 50 pounds, run a marathon, and find a new job all in the next month. *Start slowly.*

By six weeks I will: _____

By six months I will: _____

Allow Enough Time to Work on Your Goal

Are you being realistic? Most behavior change requires a time commitment. How much daily time does your goal require?

Circle appropriate box: To reach my goal I will have to spend:

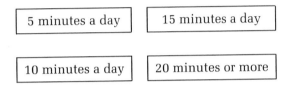

| 5 minutes a day | 15 minutes a day |

| 10 minutes a day | 20 minutes or more |

Do you have that much time to work on your goal each day?

Yes _____   No _____

If you checked *no*, go back and plan for a goal that would take less time. Review all of your commitments.

Take a Look at Your Daily Schedule

Complete this form for a *typical weekday* in your life during the last month. Include things like showering, driving, laundry time.

Time		What I am doing	Comments/How I feel about this activity
6:00	A.M.		
7:00	A.M.		
8:00	A.M.		
9:00	A.M.		
10:00	A.M.		
11:00	A.M.		
12:00	noon		
1:00	P.M.		
2:00	P.M.		
3:00	P.M.		
4:00	P.M.		
5:00	P.M.		
6:00	P.M.		

7:00	P.M.
8:00	P.M.
9:00	P.M.
10:00	P.M.
11:00	P.M.
12:00	mid.
1:00	A.M.
2:00	A.M.
3:00	A.M.
4:00	A.M.
5:00	A.M.

Is the time available for you to work on your goal?

Yes _____   No _____

If not, what could you change to make the time available in your daily schedule?

Remember to be realistic but also flexible. Some people plan extensive changes for themselves only to find that they have no time to complete the "absolute essentials" each day. Look at how well you organize and plan your time. Decide what to leave out for a while and what must take a higher priority.

50 Percent Rule

Simply cut your goal *in half!* Take whatever goal you set for yourself and reduce it by half. (For example, if your goal was to run 6 miles, change it to 3 miles; or to lose 20 pounds, change it to 10 pounds.)

Write your *new goal* here:

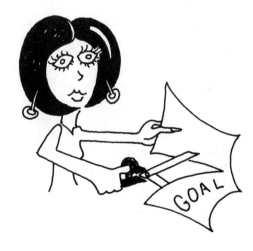

This 50 percent rule is *very important*. When starting to make self-contracts most people make the mistake of expecting too much of themselves rather than too little. When you do this, you set yourself up for failure and disappointment. It becomes much harder to help yourself stay healthy.

Get a Good Baseline

Before starting on your goal, be sure that you have the right information about how you are doing right now—so that you will know exactly what you need to change. For example, many people make a guess that they walk 3 to 4 miles in their normal daily activities. When they wear pedometers and measure it, they might actually only be walking ½ mile—or 6 to 7 miles without even knowing it! Getting a measure of how much you eat, what food, and when, for example, provides a baseline for measuring improvement.

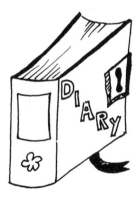

Before you begin your program, spend a week or so keeping a diary of details about how you are doing right now with the problem you want to resolve.

Remember Free Days

This rule is very important. Be realistic and build on your program at least *two free days per week*. On these days you do not have to be perfect. Do not necessarily decide ahead of time which days they will be. It is a major advantage if you wake up particularly tired one day to just be able to rest—and to know that you are not breaking your contract.

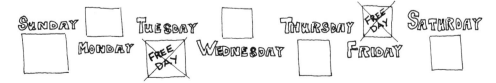

Take A Risk

Are you willing to *risk*? Did you pick something to work on that is so simple you can be sure you will not fail—but it is not a challenge for you at all? Risks are required to get healthier and to feel better about yourself. Do you feel ready to do that?

Yes _____   No _____

What else is going on in your life right now? Be sure that you have the time and energy to invest in your actual program. Take a small risk where you have a chance to succeed.

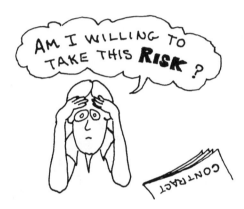

STEP 2: SET THE SCENE

Make a detailed list of all of the activities you will do to help yourself meet your goal—both to get started and to keep going.

For example: Do you need to buy new walking shoes? Plan to do grocery shopping only when you have just eaten? Arrange for help with the kids one extra hour per day?

Sketch out each weekly step to achieve in order to reach your larger six-week goal and six-month goal. For example, if your six-month goal is to run 2 miles, decide how far you want to run at your three-month point, your one-month point, and so on. Maybe your first step will be to be able to walk ¼ mile. These small steps are very important to achieve your goals.

STEP 3: RECORDS AND REMINDERS

Keep some sort of record of your success. Choose whichever method works best for you. Many people like to keep a calendar in a noticeable place at home and write on it each day. Others prefer to keep something private in their purses, or desks.

You need to know how you are doing as you go along—and your memory just can't do it alone! You might want to use little stars to mark your success days.

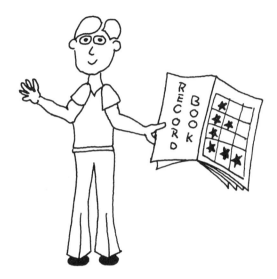

Plan a way to have lots of reminders of your goal around. Make little cards with notes to yourself about what you want to achieve in the next six weeks. Paste them around in special places in your home, work, and car settings. Each time you see them you will be reminded of your goal. You have probably heard of people who paste pictures of thin models on their refrigerators when they are trying to lose weight. This is the same idea. Put your hints and reminders in your special places, like maybe in the bathroom or on the steering wheel? Do you need a friend to help you decide these places?

The best places for my reminders are:

1.
2.
3.
4.

STEP 4: THOUGHT PATTERNS AND ACTION PATTERNS

Think about all of the things that you "think about" and "do" that *either* help you get more healthy (and meet your goals) or do the opposite and cause problems for you.

Do you have some examples? Put them here:

Did you have trouble thinking of things? Perhaps these will help:

Some typical *helpful* thought and actions

Thoughts	Actions
I'm going to feel so much better in six weeks.	I've just finished dinner so I'll go to the store now.
My friends and family like my change and have complimented me on it.	I'll do my relaxation exercise now. That drink isn't necessary.

Some typical *nonhelpful* thought and actions

Thoughts	Actions
My friends haven't noticed the change anyway—why keep trying?	I'm starving! This is a good time to go grocery shopping!
I'll start my diet tomorrow.	I'll just buy one more pack of cigarettes.
If smoking was that bad, so many people wouldn't be doing it.	I need this drink to help me relax.

Think about specific thoughts and actions you take that sabotage your efforts to get healthier. Write them down. Think of a positive thought and action to counteract each sabotaging one. Write them down and look at them frequently.

STEP 5: CHOOSE A REWARD

It is a good idea for you to pick three levels of rewards. The small ones can be for when you meet the six-week goal; the larger ones can be saved for when you reach your six-month or even one-year goal.

What do you give yourself or do for yourself that is a special treat? For example: a dinner out? a weekend trip? a new book? Many people find it *extremely hard* to think of ways to praise/reward themselves.

Fill in this worksheet:

Level 1 Rewards (small gifts to myself)

1.
2.
3.

Level 2 Rewards (medium gifts to myself)

1.
2.
3.

Level 3 Rewards (the sky is the limit!: for example, a trip to Europe!)

1.
2.
3.

If you would probably buy yourself a new record whether or not you reach your goal, do not pick that as your reward. Pick something *very special* that you would normally not do for yourself. Make sure that you only give yourself that present or reward when you have actually done what you said you would—the reward is for meeting the goal. No cheating!

At first your rewards should be small items that can be given every day. This is the best way to get started. You might need help from your friends or family, but remember that you make the final decision. Pick rewards for both your short-term and long-term goals that you will really want to work for! Eventually, you might not need these special rewards when your new activities themselves become rewarding. For example, in a while you will experience feeling better when you eat more nutritious foods, relax, play, and so on, and that will naturally help you want to stay healthy.

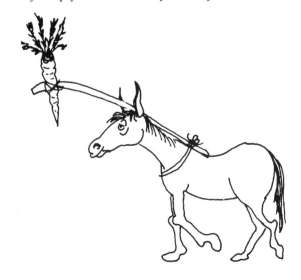

One big mistake that many people make is forgetting or deciding not to give themselves the rewards once they have reached their goals. Think about this and plan ahead to prevent this problem. For this project to work, *you must give yourself every reward that you have earned.*

STEP 6: A COST IF I DON'T SUCCEED?

There are many pros and cons as to whether or not you should build this into your program. If you decide to have a "punishment" attached to your program, be sure to pick something that really would "hurt" you. Have your friends help you decide what these costs for nonsuccess might be. One example might be for you to give your friend a check made out to a political organization that you violently oppose. If you do not meet your goal, the check goes to the organization. If you do succeed, the check gets torn up.

Be sure to put a positive fun reward into your program whether or not you decide also to use a "cost". What are some possible "costs" you might want to include in your program? Write them here:

1.
2.
3.

STEP 7: PLAN EVALUATION TIMES

Decide when you want to evaluate your success. It can be at one week, six weeks, or whenever you feel would be *best for you.* Do not wait too long, though—as you will need to look at your program regularly and keep praising yourself.

At your evaluation time you will:

- Praise yourself—for trying and/or for succeeding.
- Decide if you need to change your program. *That's O.K.!* You can make it easier or harder.
- Be sure that you are getting some *pleasure* out of your project. It will not work if your plans are so difficult that you dread each day of the program.
- At those points ask yourself:

 Am I feeling better? Yes _____ No _____
 Do I like myself better? Yes _____ No _____

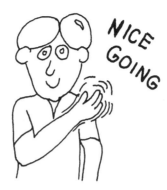

STEP 8: DO I WORK ALONE OR WITH A PARTNER?

Some people like to work alone and have great success with privacy. Other people prefer to have one partner or even a small group of people to help them with their projects. This decision depends on your personality, how well you know yourself, and how you think you could best succeed. There are some advantages to having a partner "cheer you on," help you remember your goal, and provide emergency help when you feel like giving up. For others the privacy of a "secret" program is fine. Which type are you? Think about this and make a decision before you start your program.

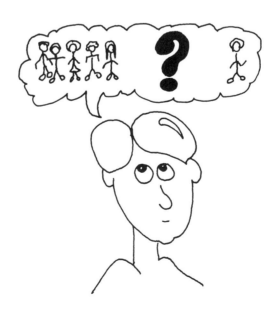

STEP 9: SIGN THE ACTUAL CONTRACT

Chapters 7 through 17 each have sample completed contracts. Identify one self-care area that you would like to improve and complete the blank self-contract that follows.

The activity of completing and signing the contract is *vital*. Even if you have decided not to use a partner to help you, be sure that you write out your contract and post it in a special and visible place. This method keeps giving you hints and reminders to continue your program.

FINAL HELPFUL HINTS

Here are some thoughts for you about building your self-care program. You can look back at them frequently. You may want to copy them down and paste them on your mirror.

1. Begin with small steps.
2. Find your own style—what works for you will be different from what works for your best friend.
3. Give yourself permission to change your mind—your life is not cast in stone.
4. Accept your failures or disappointments—these are part of life's adventures.
5. Give yourself permission to begin *again* and *again* and *again*—trying is better than giving up.
6. Remember that how well you do will largely depend on your own beliefs and values—if you value your health and believe that you can influence your health, you will be more successful!

(Reprinted with permission from Baldi, S. et al. (1984, 2nd ed.) *For your health: A model for self-care.* Laguna, CA: Nurses Model Health: p. 33–39. Rick Walti, graphic artist.)

SELF-CONTRACT

MY GOALS:

Short-term — by the end of six weeks I will . . . _____

Long-term — by the end of six months I will . . . _____

ENVIRONMENTAL PLANNING: | (all the steps I will take to reach my goal)

THOUGHTS AND ACTIONS

Helpful thoughts:	Helpful actions:
Non-helpful thoughts:	Non-helpful actions:

MY REWARD | (if I meet my goal)

THE COST: | (if I fail to meet my goal)

REEVALUATION DATE:

I agree to help with this project: I agree to strive toward this goal:

_____   _____
(Support person)   (Your signature)   (date)

Appendix C. Contract Samples

Two-Week Self-Contract:
Plan to Increase Amount of Walking

I will increase my average daily pedometer reading by an extra quarter mile per day, from my present two miles to an average of two and one-quarter miles per day during the two weeks of this self-contract. I will enlist the help of _____ .

My responsibilities:

1. To focus on increasing my walking while at work, especially during my lunch hour.
2. To reward myself on each day that I reach two and one-quarter miles on my pedometer with 30 minutes (or more) of reading for my own enjoyment. I will forego this reward if I don't reach my walking goal.
3. To record my data in my journal at 10:00 each night.

My helper's responsibilities:

1. To walk with me, when possible, during my lunch hour and to generally support my effort to exercise more.
2. To help me review the results of this action plan in two weeks.

Date: _____   Signed: _____
Review Date: _____   Helper: _____

(Reprinted with permission from Farquhar, J.W. (1978). *The American way of life need not be hazardous to your health.* New York: W.W. Norton, p. 51. Copyright © by John W. Farquhar.)

I, _Dorothy Edwards_, will _cough and deep breathe 5 times each hour after surgery tomorrow_ in return for _Nancy Meyers reading me the Bible, one minute for each time I cough and take a deep breath._

Signed _Dorothy Edwards_

Signed _Nancy Meyers, RN_

Date _2-25-81_

Bonus clause: Nancy will give Mrs. Edwards a one-minute back rub for each time over five that Mrs. Edwards coughs and takes a deep breath.

(Reprinted with permission from Steckel, S. (1982). *Patient contracting.* Norwalk, CT: Appleton-Century-Croft, p. 87.)

Sample Health Contract

Goal: to attain & maintain BP 150/90 or < by April 2

Evaluation
February 2 see flow sheet for BP, continue goal, reassess March 2

Client Responsibilities:

1. Monitor & record BP at home twice a week
2. Take prescribed drug as ordered
3. Record any side effects
4. Practice relaxation 15 min. day

5. . . . .

1. February 2 unsuccessful, wife to learn, reassess March 2
2. February 2 self reports success
3. February 2 useful, continue
4. March 2 unsuccessful, will try again, reassess April 2

5. . . . .

Nurse Provider Responsibilities

1. Collect data, formulate diagnoses & plans, set priorities & collaborate
2. Monitor response
3. Prescribe medical therapy with MD consultation p.r.n.
4. Provide information re: hypertension
5. Assess understanding & reinforce teaching
6. Teach technique for taking BP
7. Provide relaxation counseling

8. . . . .

1. See H&P, problem list, progress & flow sheets, lab reports
2. See flow sheet
3. See progress & flow sheets

4. January 2 overview, booklets, group class February 2
5. Booklets reviewed February 2 March 2
6. January 2, wife February 2
7. February 2, March 2 refer to client using technique well (name & phone)

8. . . . .

Signed by client with date, revised date & initials, revised date & initials
Signed by provider with date, revised date & initials, revised date & initials

(Reprinted with permission from Brykczynski, K. (1982). Health contracting. *Nurse Practitioner*, 28.)

SELF-CONTRACT

Date _September 18,_

Self: _Mary Baxter_

Other: _Jane Paulson_

Goal: _to reduce my smoking_

Agreement

Self: _I agree to smoke only during the first 15 minutes of any hour (1:00 to 1:15, 2:00 to 2:15, etc.). If I do not want a cigarette during an interval, I will wait for the next hour interval before I smoke._

Others: _Jane Paulson (my roommate) agrees to praise me whenever she sees me not smoking and to refuse to talk to me while I am smoking._

Consequences

Provided by Self:
(if contract is kept) _If I stick to the above agreement, at the end of each week (ending Sat. at 6:00 PM) I will reward myself with a movie._

(if contract is broken) _If I do not keep the above agreement during a particular week, I will do my roommate's laundry that Saturday evening (no movie)._

Provided by Other:
(if contract is kept) _Jane will (1) praise me for not smoking, (2) ignore me when I am smoking, and (3) do my laundry each week that I keep the contract._

(if contract is broken) _For each week that I fail to keep the contract, Jane is authorized to (1) insist that I do her laundry and (2) limit my access to her stereo albums._

Signed _Mary Baxter_

October 18,
Review Date

Jane Paulson
Witness

(Reprinted with permission from Mahoney, M.J., & Thoreson, C.E. (1974). *Self-control: Power to the person.* Monterey, CA: Brooks/Cole, p. 53.)

STATEMENT OF AGREEMENT
REGARDING SHARING OF HEALTH CARE

We, _____ Jane D. _____ (client)

and _____ Doris S. _____ (facilitator)

agree on the following health care goals for _____ Jane D. _____
   1. Have vaginal infection clear up
   2. Learn more about my body and how it works
   3. Learn what to do to stop having so many sore throats
   4. Go to the "Stress Management" class

I, _____ Jane D. _____ (client) understand
my part in achieving the goals of health care and agree to participate in the following ways:
   1. Follow the medication instructions for 3 weeks
   2. Don't wear tight jeans
   3. Stop scratching
   4. Refrain from intercourse until the pain and itching stop
   5. Attend the "Stress Management" class
   6. Check Our Bodies, Ourselves out of the Center Library
   7. Return to Center if problem is not clearing in one week, or if unable to keep agreement

I, _____ Doris S. _____ (facilitator) agree to
participate in achieving the goals of health care in the following ways:
   1. Initiate the mutual record of health care today and encourage Jane D. to write her comments.
   2. Be available for questions and discussion by phone. Give Jane D. the specific hours that I'm at WHM.
   3. Give Jane D. enrollment card for class on "Stress Management"
   4. Inform Jane D. about new class being formed on "Women's Health and Human Wholeness."

I understand that this health care agreement is not legally binding and that my keeping this agreement is my own responsibility, and that if this agreement is not kept, the goals as stated above may not be achieved. If the health care plan is not satisfactory, it is my responsibility to return to the WHM and work out another plan.

_____ (client)

_____ (facilitator)

1 copy to client
1 copy to client's record

(Reprinted with permission from Bermosk, L.S., & Porter, S.E. (1979). *Women's health and human wholeness.* New York: Appleton-Century-Crofts, p. 138.)

Nurse–Client Contract and Agreement

Statement of Health Goal: _____ *Decreased feelings of stress and tension* _____

I _____ *Jim Johnson* _____ promise to _____ *use progressive relaxation* _____
        (client)

_____ *techniques (four-muscle groups) upon arriving home from work each day* _____
        (Client Responsibility)

for a period of _____ *one week* _____ , whereupon,

_____ *Kathy Turner* _____ will provide _____ *a copy of* _____
        (nurse)

_____ *Herbert Benson's book, Relaxation Response* _____
        (Nurse Responsibility)

on _____ *Saturday, March 7th* _____ to me.
        (date)

If I do not fulfill the terms of this contract in total, I understand that the designated reward will be withheld.

Signed: _____
        (client)

         _____
        (date)

         _____
        (nurse)

         _____
        (date)

(Reprinted with permission from Pender, N. (1987). *Health promotion in nursing practice* (2nd ed.). Norwalk, CT: Appleton & Lange, p. 231.)

Index

Page numbers in italics indicate figures or tables

Page numbers in italics indicate figures or tables

Page numbers in italics indicate figures or tables

Page numbers in italics indicate figures or tables